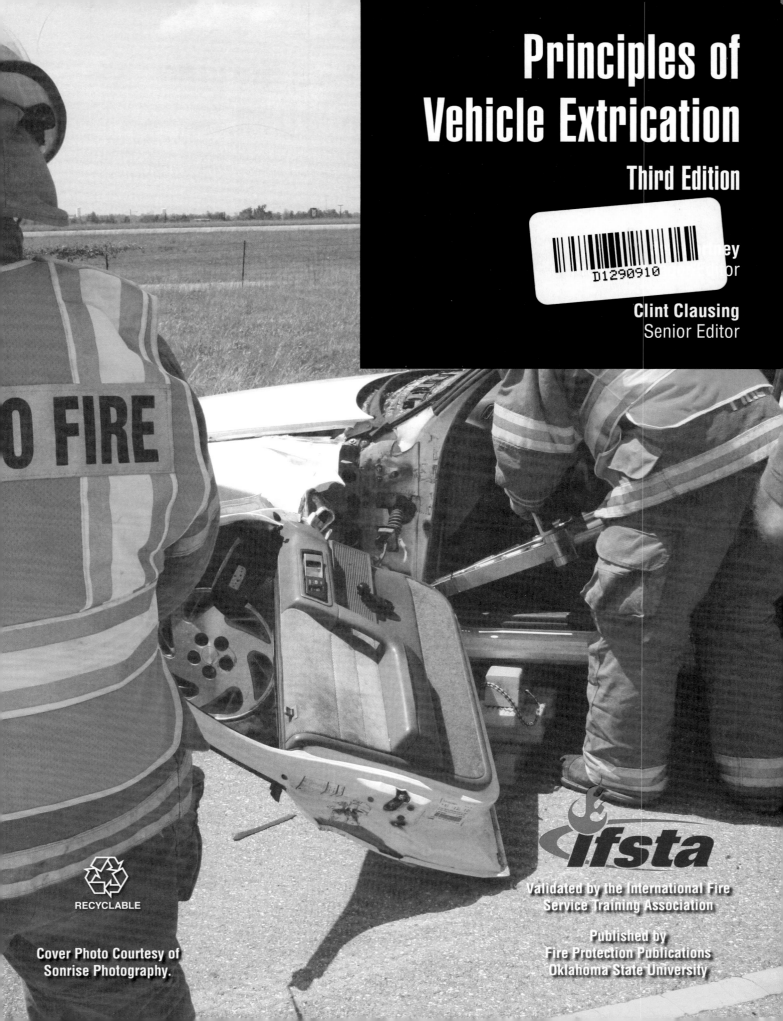

Principles of Vehicle Extrication

Third Edition

D1290910

[...]ley
[...]or

Clint Clausing
Senior Editor

ifsta

Validated by the International Fire
Service Training Association

Published by
Fire Protection Publications
Oklahoma State University

RECYCLABLE

Cover Photo Courtesy of
Sonrise Photography.

The International Fire Service Training Association

The International Fire Service Training Association (IFSTA) was established in 1934 as a *nonprofit educational association of fire fighting personnel who are dedicated to upgrading fire fighting techniques and safety through training.* To carry out the mission of IFSTA, Fire Protection Publications was established as an entity of Oklahoma State University. Fire Protection Publications' primary function is to publish and disseminate training texts as proposed and validated by IFSTA. As a secondary function, Fire Protection Publications researches, acquires, produces, and markets high-quality learning and teaching aids as consistent with IFSTA's mission.

The IFSTA Validation Conference is held the second full week in July. Committees of technical experts meet and work at the conference addressing the current standards of the National Fire Protection Association® and other standard-making groups as applicable. The Validation Conference brings together individuals from several related and allied fields, such as:

- Key fire department executives and training officers
- Educators from colleges and universities
- Representatives from governmental agencies
- Delegates of firefighter associations and industrial organizations

Committee members are not paid nor are they reimbursed for their expenses by IFSTA or Fire Protection Publications. They participate because of commitment to the fire service and its future through training. Being on a committee is prestigious in the fire service community, and committee members are acknowledged leaders in their fields. This unique feature provides a close relationship between the International Fire Service Training Association and fire protection agencies, which helps to correlate the efforts of all concerned.

IFSTA manuals are now the official teaching texts of most of the states and provinces of North America. Additionally, numerous U.S. and Canadian government agencies as well as other English-speaking countries have officially accepted the IFSTA manuals.

ISBN 978-0-87939-380-9   Library of Congress Control Number: 2009939284

Third Edition, First Printing, November 2009   *Printed in the United States of America*

10   9   8   7   6   5   4   3

If you need additional information concerning the International Fire Service Training Association (IFSTA) or Fire Protection Publications, contact:

Customer Service, Fire Protection Publications, Oklahoma State University
930 North Willis, Stillwater, OK 74078-8045
800-654-4055   Fax: 405-744-8204

For assistance with training materials, to recommend material for inclusion in an IFSTA manual, or to ask questions or comment on manual content, contact:

Editorial Department, Fire Protection Publications, Oklahoma State University
930 North Willis, Stillwater, OK 74078-8045
405-744-4111   Fax: 405-744-4112   E-mail: editors@osufpp.org

Chapter Summary

Table of Contents

List of Tables

Preface

This third edition of **Principles of Vehicle Extrication** was written to update the information contained in the second edition. Since the second edition was published, there have been many changes in the design of land-based vehicles, and in the technology built into them. There have also been many improvements in the tools and techniques used to extricate victims from entrapment in crashed vehicles. This edition addresses those differences.

Acknowledgement and special thanks are extended to the members of the material review committee who contributed their time, wisdom, and knowledge to this manual:

IFSTA Principles of Vehicle Extrication
Third Edition Validation Committee

Chair
Jerome Harvey
Georgia Forestry Commission
Macon, GA

Committee Members

Alan Braun
University of Missouri Fire and Rescue
Institute
Cole County Fire Protection District

Shane Campbell
Midwest City Fire Department
Midwest City, OK

Ralph Catlett
Valdosta Fire Department
Valdosta, GA

Kevin Ferrara
USAFE Fire Academy
Ramstein AB, Germany

George Hollingsworth
Fairfax County Fire & Rescue Department
Burke, Virginia

Jeffrey Kelly
Orlando Fire Department
Winter Garden, FL

Paul Pestel
City of Russellville Fire Department
Russellville, AR

Eddie Pyle
Louisiana State University
Fire & Emergency Training Institute
Baton Rouge, LA

Mark Rabdau
Eagle Fire & Rescue
Eagle, ID

Timothy Robinson
Concord Fire Department
Concord, NH

Alan Sanders
Midwest City Fire Department
Midwest City, OK

Peter Schecter
Keystone Municipal Services
Philadelphia, PA

Committee Members (Concluded)

Chris Scott
Rockford Fire Department
Rockford, IL

Ian Yocum
Tualatin Valley Fire & Rescue
Aloha, OR

Steven Taylor
Rescue Engineering Institute
Fort Wayne, IN

It would not be possible to develop a book of this scope without the assistance of many individuals and organizations. We thank all of the following for contributing photos, information, and/or their facilities and equipment.

AAAA Wrecker, Oklahoma City, OK
 Justin W. Hurley
Barnes Wrecker Service, Midwest City, OK
Buda Fire Department, Buda, TX
 Chief Clay Huckaby
Camperland of Oklahoma, Tulsa, OK
 Gary Burger, Jr.
Capital Region Ambulance
 Kim Kline
Cole County Sheriffs Department, Jefferson City, MO
 Shawn Gerstner
Collin County Community College
 Pat McAuliff
Dallas-Fort Worth International Airport Department
of Public Safety, TX
 Sgt Brian Canady
Del City Fire Department, Del City, OK
 Darren Appleby
 Steve Davis
 Nathan Newman
 Ryan Weaver
Fenton Motors, Stillwater, OK
 Scott Foster
Frontier City Amusement Park, Oklahoma City, OK
 Jeni Scott
 Andrea Pennock
 Jillian Howell
 Jerrad Aubritton
 Brittany Duffin
 Roy Gilbert
 Andrew Hinkle
 Paul Levy
 Richard Willcox
G & M Body Shop, Stillwater, OK
 Derek McCubbin

Jefferson City Fire Department, MO
 Dave Ruetz
 Michael Vaught
Jefferson City Police Department, MO
 Celeste Suchanek
John Deere and Company
 Pamela Barry
LaBoit, Inc. Specialty Vehicle Manufacturer
 Jeff Blais
Lake Ozark Fire District, Lake Ozark, MO
 Mark Amsinger, Fire Chief
 Scott L. Apprill
 Caleb Freese
 Tanner Garber
 Chris L. Mare
 Jason B. Nelson
McKinney Fire Department, McKinney, TX
 Mark Wallace, Fire Chief
 Ronald Moore, Training Battalion Chief
 Nancy Eastham
MerCruiser, Stillwater, OK
 Bart Foster
 Tim Wilson
 Matt Stanek
Midwest City Fire Department
 Alan Sanders
 Jeffery Ingram
 Jerimy Meek
 Michael Todd
Midwest EMS, Midwest City, OK
 Michael A. Carter
 Brandi Whitney

Nicoma Park Fire Department, Nicoma Park, OK
Eric Beaty
Josh Fields
Bryant Gantter
Justin Hill
Night & Day Limousine, Stillwater, OK
Paul McCully
Oklahoma State University Transportation Services, Stillwater, OK
Chris Hoffman
Osage Fire Protection District, MO
Allyssa Gipe
Barry Gipe
Kevin Wieberg
Justin Braun
Owasso Fire Department, Owasso, OK
Bradd Clark, Fire Chief
Mark Stuckey, Assistant Fire Chief
Kris Anderson
Shane Atwell
John Bishop
Mike Blevins
Eric Gomez
David Hurst
Barry Ingram
Kip Jennings
Loyd Mosier
Steven Nelson
Rick Parris
Lucas Shearer
Matt Trout
Robert Williams
Joe Wakely
Jeff Yeats
P & K Equipment / John Deere, Stillwater, OK
Alan Nietenhoefer
Brett Fruits
Ron Shirley Pontiac / Buick / GMC, Stillwater, OK
Ron Shirley II
RSC, Stillwater, OK
Chad Clark
Sonrise Photography
Jennifer Ayers
Camron Ayers

Stillwater Fire Department, Stillwater, OK
Rex Mott
Jay Willis
Todd Jones
Stan Kent
Rick Lozier
Tom Oosting
Puddin Payne
Stet Sodowsky
Tyler Sparks
Mike Wilda
Jerad Warlick
Stillwater Public Schools Transportation Services, Stillwater, OK
Matt Parcell
Vicki Jamison
SVI Trucks
Jake Sorensen
Thomas Ford, Stillwater, OK
David Thomas
U.S. Department of Transportation
Tina Foley
Wilson Chevrolet / Jeep, Stillwater, OK
Scott Heddleston
Wittwer Construction, Stillwater, OK
William Acord
Alan Braun
Marty Burch
Ed Chapman
Randy Curry
Grady Davis
Kevin Ferrara
Jerel Flora
Sean, Hannah, and Mara Lily Fortney
Ron Jeffers
Larry Jenkins, Fairfax County Fire Department
Phil Linder, Thomson Metals & Disposal
Rich Mahaney
John Perry, Albuquerque, N.M.
Robert J. Tremberth
Brian Wozniak, Newtown Fire Association

xvi

Special thanks to Leslie Miller, Senior Editor, for working with the validation committee during its initial meetings and editing the first few chapters.

Thanks are also extended to the faculty and staff of the Oklahoma Fire Service Training for their timely and efficient assistance on this manual.

Last, but certainly not least, gratitude is also extended to the members of the Fire Protection Publications Principles of Vehicle Extrication, 3rd Edition, Project Team whose contributions made the final publication of this manual possible.

Principles of Vehicle Extrication, 3rd Edition, Project Team

Project Manager/Writer
Jeff Fortney, Senior Editor

Copy Editor
Clint Clausing, Senior Editor

Editorial Reviewer
Clint Clausing, Senior Editor

Technical Reviewer
Chris E. Wagers
Topeka Fire Department
Topeka, KS

Production Manager
Ann Moffat, Coordinator, Publications Production

Illustrators and Layout Designers
Errick Bragg, Senior Graphic Designer
Ben Brock, Senior Graphic Designer
Missy Hannan, Senior Graphic Designer
Ruth Mudroch, Senior Graphic Designer
Clint Parker, Senior Graphic Designer

Curriculum Development
Melissa Noakes, Curriculum Developer
Justin House, Curriculum Developer

Photography
Brett Noakes, Photographer

Editorial Assistant
Tara Gladden

Library Researchers
Susan F. Walker, FPP Librarian

Research Technicians
Elkie Burnside
Gabriel Ramirez
Mike Sturzenbecker
Joseph Raymond

Introduction

Chapter Contents

Introduction

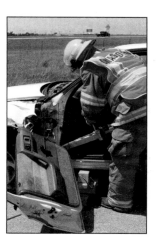

Vehicle extrication incidents can occur everywhere that land-based vehicles operate — on streets and highways, on improved and unimproved rural roads, on railroads and light rail tracks, on farms and ranches, on industrial facilities and construction sites, and in remote wilderness areas. Often, victims are entrapped or entangled in the involved vehicles requiring rescue personnel to perform vehicle extrication in order to free them. Response to vehicle extrication incidents is inherently dangerous and results in many injuries and deaths to response personnel because exposure to vehicular traffic and other hazardous conditions.

The majority of vehicle extrication incidents are handled by firefighters, either career or volunteer. Others are handled by members of dedicated rescue squads or rescue companies, either public or private. Some are handled by law enforcement personnel. The concepts and techniques described in this manual can be applied by any or all of these groups provided that they are properly trained and equipped. Within the pages of this manual, performing vehicle extrication safely and efficiently are recurring themes.

The term "extrication" means different things to different people, and in some jurisdictions it includes more or less than in others. According to NFPA® 1670, *Standard on Operations and Training for Technical Rescue Incidents* (2009), extrication is defined as "the removal of trapped victims from a vehicle or machinery." While the **IFSTA Aircraft Rescue and Fire Fighting** manual addresses extrication from aircraft, this IFSTA manual focuses on extricating victims of entrapment in land-based vehicles and also addresses freeing victims from entrapment in machinery. Some land-based-vehicle extrication incidents — those occurring on elevated or underground sections of light rail or subway systems, and roadways — are considered to be technical rescue situations and are therefore beyond the scope of this manual.

Purpose

This training manual is written for personnel who respond to vehicle extrication incidents. These responders include the following individuals:

- Firefighters
- Law enforcement officers/personnel
- Emergency medical services personnel
- Industrial and transportation emergency response members

- Public works employees
- Utility workers
- Members of private industry
- Military responders
- Other emergency response professionals

This edition of **Principles of Vehicle Extrication** is designed to provide these rescue personnel with an understanding of the current challenges, techniques, skills, and equipment available for the safe and effective extrication of victims trapped in land-based vehicles of all types. The information in this manual deals only with the mechanics of freeing victims from entrapment in vehicles and related machinery. While the manual includes a chapter on emergency medical service considerations, it *does not* include specific emergency medical treatment protocols.

NOTICE

No one should expect to become proficient at vehicle extrication simply by reading this or any other book on the subject. The information contained in this manual must be combined with hands-on training delivered by qualified instructors with experience on extrication incidents.

The tools, equipment, and techniques described in this manual represent the current state of the art as practiced by rescuers throughout the world, but they are not the only ways that extrication can be performed safely and efficiently. No single tool nor any single technique will be safe and effective in every situation. Readers are encouraged to master a variety of extrication tools and techniques.

Scope

This manual addresses Sections 6.4.1 and 6.4.2 of NFPA® 1001 (2008); Chapter 4, Chapter 5 (Sections 5.1 through 5.5), and Chapter 10 of NFPA® 1006 (2008); and Chapters 4, 8, and 12 of NFPA® 1670 (2009) published by the National Fire Protection Association. The scope of this manual covers the information necessary to meet Awareness-level, Operations-level, and Technician-level vehicle extrication training.

The text begins with an introduction to vehicle extrication, scene management, and incident command. It continues with a review of extrication-related equipment and techniques. Extrication of victims trapped in passenger vehicles, buses, medium and heavy trucks, trains, and industrial and agricultural vehicles are also discussed. Finally, special situations and topics in vehicle extrication are discussed.

Manual Organization

The 3rd edition of **Principles of Vehicle Extrication** gathers the knowledge, skills, and abilities listed above into 12 chapters. The chapters include:

Chapter 1- Introduction to Vehicle Extrication

Chapter 2 - Extrication Incident Management

Chapter 3 - Vehicle Science and Anatomy

Chapter 4 - Extrication Equipment

Chapter 5 - Extrication Techniques

Chapter 6 - Passenger Vehicle Extrication

Chapter 7 - Bus Extrication

Chapter 8 - Medium and Heavy Truck Extrication

Chapter 9 - Railcars Extrication

Chapter 10 – Industrial/Agricultural Vehicle and Machinery Extrication

Chapter 11 - Special Extrication Situations (Special Operations)

Chapter 12 - EMS Rescue Considerations

Learning objectives, located at the beginning of each chapter, will assist the reader in focusing on the appropriate topic and knowledge. The numbers of the JPRs are also listed at the beginning of chapters where they are referenced. **Appendix A** contains a guide that coordinates the JPRs to the specific page of the chapter that relates to the requirements.

Study questions are located at the end of each chapter to ensure that the reader has a good comprehension of the material in the chapter. The questions are based on the learning objectives. Please note that these questions should not be used for certification or course examinations. **Appendix B** provides a list of websites of online and downloadable emergency response guides for hybrid vehicles. The information in **Appendix B** was current at the time this manual went to print. The manual also contains a glossary of essential terms that will be of interest to the reader.

Terminology

IFSTA has traditionally provided training materials that are used throughout the U.S. and Canada. In recent years, the sales of IFSTA materials have expanded into a truly international market and resulted in the translation of materials into German, French, Spanish, Japanese, Hebrew, Turkish, and Italian. Writing the manuals, therefore, requires the use of *Global English* that consists of words and terms that can be easily translated into multiple languages and cultures.

This manual is written with the global market as well as the North American market in mind. Traditional fire service terminology, referred to as *jargon*, must give way to more precise descriptions and definitions. Where jargon is appropriate, it will be used along with its definition. The glossary at the end of the manual will also assist the reader in understanding words that may not have their roots in the fire and emergency services. The sources for the definitions of fire-and-emergency-services-related terms will be the *NFPA® Dictionary of Terms* and the IFSTA **Fire Service Orientation and Terminology** manual.

NFPA® Copyright Permission

One of the basic purposes of IFSTA manuals is to allow fire service personnel and their departments to meet the requirements set forth by NFPA® codes and standards. These NFPA® documents may be referred to throughout this manual. References to information from NFPA® codes and standards are used with permission from National Fire Protection Association®, Quincy, MA 02169. This referenced material is not the complete and official position of the National Fire Protection Association on the referenced subject which is represented only by the standard in its entirety.

Key Information

Various types of information in this book are given in shaded boxes marked by symbols or icons (sidebars, information, key information, and case histories). Smart Operations tips and What Does This Mean To You notices are given in boxes indicated by a safety-alert icon. See the following examples:

Sidebar

Atmospheric pressure is greatest at low altitudes; consequently, its pressure at sea level is used as a standard. At sea level, the atmosphere exerts a pressure of 14.7 psi (101 kPa) {1.01 bar}. A common method of measuring atmospheric pressure is to compare the weight of the atmosphere with the weight of a column of mercury: the greater the atmospheric pressure, the taller the column of mercury.

Information

Some experts make this differentiation: Acids are *corrosive*, while bases are *caustic*. In the world of emergency response; however, both acids and bases are called *corrosives*. The U.S. Department of Transportation (DOT) and Transport Canada (TC), for example, do not differentiate between the two. Any materials that destroy metal or skin tissue are considered corrosives by these agencies.

Key Information

Volatility refers to a substance's ability to become a vapor at a relatively low temperature. Essentially, volatile chemical agents have low boiling points at ordinary pressures and/or high vapor pressures at ordinary temperatures. The volatility of a chemical agent often determines how it is used.

Three key signal words are found in the book: **WARNING, CAUTION,** and **NOTE.** Definitions and examples of each are as follows:

- **WARNING** indicates information that could result in death or serious injury to industrial fire brigade members. See the following example:

WARNING!

Any clothing saturated with a cryogenic material must be removed immediately, particularly if the vapors are flammable or oxidizing. The industrial fire brigade member could not escape flames from clothing-trapped vapors if the vapors were to ignite.

- **CAUTION** indicates important information or data that industrial fire brigade members need to be aware of in order to perform their duties safely. See the following example:

CAUTION

All personnel working at hazardous materials incidents must use appropriate personal protective equipment, including appropriate respiratory protection equipment.

- **NOTE** indicates important operational information that helps explain why a particular recommendation is given or describes optional methods for certain procedures. See the following example:

NOTE: *Vapor* is a gaseous form of a substance that is normally in a solid or liquid state at room temperature and pressure. It is formed by evaporation from a liquid or sublimation from a solid.

Notice on Use of State and Province

In order to keep sentences uncluttered and easy to read, the word "state" will be used to represent both state and provincial level governments. This usage is applied to this manual for the purposes of brevity and is not intended to address or show preference for only one nation's method of identifying regional governments within its borders.

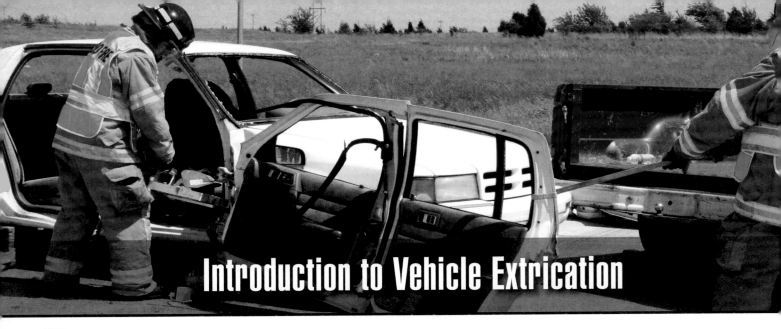

Introduction to Vehicle Extrication

Chapter Contents

Key Terms

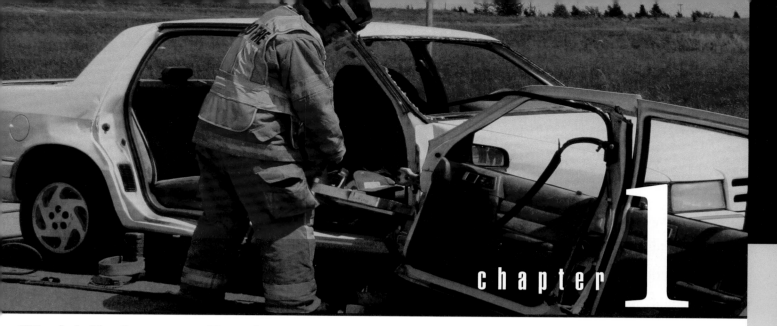

Job Performance Requirements

This chapter provides information that addresses the following job performance requirements (JPRs) of NFPA® 1001, *Standard for Fire Fighter Professional Qualifications* (2008), NFPA® 1006, *Standard for Technical Rescuer Professional Qualifications* (2008), NFPA® 1670, *Standard on Operations and Training for Technical Search and Rescue Incidents* (2009).

NFPA® 1001 JPRs

6.4.1

6.4.2

NFPA® 1006 JPRs

4.1.1	4.3.2	5.2.4	10.1.1	10.1.6	10.2.2
4.1.2	5.1	5.2.5	10.1.2	10.1.7	10.2.3
4.2	5.2.1	5.2.7	10.1.3	10.1.10	10.2.4
4.3	5.2.2	5.3.3	10.1.4	10.2	
4.3.1	5.2.3	10.1	10.1.5	10.2.1	

NFPA® 1670 JPRs

4.1	4.1.10.1.1	4.2.2	4.4.1.3	4.5.1.4	8.2.1	12.3.1
4.1.1	4.1.10.1.2	4.2.3	4.4.2.1	4.5.1.5	8.2.2	12.3.2
4.1.2	4.1.10.2	4.2.4	4.4.2.2	4.5.2.1	8.2.3	12.3.3
4.1.3	4.1.10.3	4.2.5	4.4.2.3	4.5.2.2	8.3.1	12.3.4
4.1.3.1	4.1.10.4	4.2.6	4.4.2.4	4.5.3.1	8.3.2	12.4.1
4.1.3.2	4.1.10.5.1	4.2.7	4.4.2.4.1	4.5.3.2	8.3.3	12.4.2
4.1.4	4.1.10.5.2	4.2.8	4.4.2.4.2	4.5.3.3	8.3.4	
4.1.5	4.1.11	4.3.1	4.4.2.4.3	4.5.3.4	8.4.1	
4.1.6	4.1.11.1	4.3.2	4.4.2.4.4	4.5.3.5	8.4.2	
4.1.7	4.1.11.2	4.3.3	4.5.1	4.5.4	12.1	
4.1.8	4.1.11.3	4.3.4	4.5.1.1	4.5.5.1	12.2.1	
4.1.9	4.1.11.4	4.4.1.1	4.5.1.2	4.5.5.2	12.2.2	
4.1.10.1	4.2.1	4.4.1.2	4.5.1.3	8.1	12.2.3	

Introduction to Vehicle Extrication

Learning Objectives

1. Define extrication, disentanglement, and rescue.

2. Identify organizations relevant to extrication operations.

3. Describe the roles performed by organizations relevant to extrication operations.

4. Identify the responsibilities of the rescue organization.

5. Define authority having jurisdiction (AHJ) and standard operating procedures (SOPs).

6. Identify basic facts about hazard and risk assessment surveys.

7. Identify basic facts about operation capability and training requirements.

8. Identify basic facts about extrication equipment and personal protective equipment.

9. Identify basic facts about After Action Reviews (AAR).

10. List success factors related to extrication operations.

11. Describe the roles and responsibilities of personnel responding to an extrication incident.

Chapter 1
Introduction to Vehicle Extrication

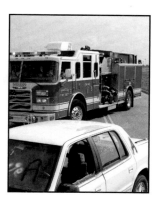

Case History

Emergency personnel responded to a report of a two vehicle head-on collision with several patients trapped inside the vehicles. Visibility was extremely limited due to the late hour and an intense fog lingering in the area. An incident command post was quickly established and scene size-up was conducted.

The two vehicles were positioned across the roadway and adjacent to each other. A total of four patients were found at the scene. Vehicle #1 contained one female patient. The male driver was found lying on the road next to the vehicle. Both driver and passenger were conscious and breathing. Vehicle #2's driver, a male, was pinned between the steering wheel and the seat. The driver's side door and left front tire further pinned the driver. The driver was conscious and able to communicate with rescuers. The female passenger of Vehicle #2 was found unconscious in the back seat and in critical condition.

The incident commander requested additional ambulances. Responders set up portable scene lighting and assisted ambulance personnel in packaging the patients of Vehicle #1. Rescue personnel used spreaders to gain access to the driver of Vehicle #2 and remove those vehicle components trapping the driver. The rescue personnel were able to extricate the three patients within the vehicles and package all four patients for transport in less than half an hour. The patients were then transported to local medical facilities for treatment.

Fire and emergency services organizations play an integral part in performing vehicle extrication and machinery rescue **(Figure 1.1, p.12)**. The ever-increasing number of automobiles, trucks, buses, and trains around the world has correlated with an increasing number of vehicle collisions and vehicle extrication incidents. These incidents range from a baby or pet locked inside a parked automobile to a worker caught in industrial machinery to severely injured passengers trapped in a wrecked automobile, truck, bus, or train. Some agencies respond to this type of incident on a regular basis, others less frequently. Regardless of the frequency with which the personnel in these organizations respond to such incidents, to do their jobs well they need to understand the challenges they face and have the training and equipment necessary to safely perform in these situations.

In order to limit confusion about key terms used in this manual, the following definitions apply:

- Extrication — Removal and treatment of patients who are trapped by some type of man-made machinery or equipment **(Figure 1.2, p. 12)**.

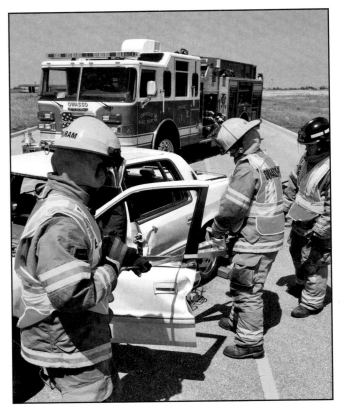

Figure 1.1 Fire and emergency services personnel practicing vehicle extrication techniques. *Courtesy of Sonrise Photography.*

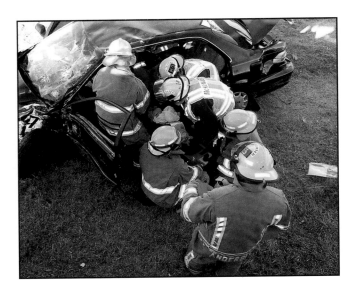

Figure 1.2 Rescuers extricating a patient from a wrecked vehicle. *Courtesy of McKinney Fire Department (TX).*

- Disentanglement — That part of vehicle extrication that relates to the removal and/or manipulation of vehicle components to allow a properly packaged patient to be removed from the vehicle. Sometimes referred to as removing the vehicle from the patient **(Figure 1.3)**.

- Rescue — Removing a patient from an untenable or unhealthy situation or atmosphere **(Figure 1.4)**.

This chapter provides an overview of vehicle extrication, and it forms a foundation for the rest of the manual. Key vehicle extrication terms are defined, regional and national standards that relate to the rescue technician are discussed, and organizations relevant to vehicle extrication in North America are identified. In addition, the respective roles and responsibilities of rescue personnel engaged in extrication duties are discussed. The responsibilities of the rescue organization are described and the critical knowledge, skills, and abilities necessary to safely and effectively perform vehicle extrication are identified. The factors involved in a successful extrication are discussed, along with the principles of vehicle extrication and vehicle anatomy. The roles and responsibilities of all participants involved in an extrication incident are also discussed.

Relevant Organizations

In North America, there are a number of governmental agencies and nongovernmental organizations that have some responsibility and authority relevant to vehicle extrication. Some have the authority to legislate and regulate, others do not. In some cases, these organizations investigate transportation crashes and issue findings upon which new laws and regulations are based. In other cases, they may have authority to dictate design criteria to promote vehicle safety or broad authority to regulate how the highways are used, by whom, and under what conditions. These organizations are:

- United States Department of Transportation (US-DOT)

- National Highway Traffic Safety Administration (NHTSA)

- Insurance Institute of Highway Safety (IIHS)

- American National Standards Institute (ANSI)

- National Fire Protection Association® (NFPA®)

- Transport Canada

- Transportation Emergency Rescue Committee

- National Transportation Safety Board (NTSB)

United States Department of Transportation (USDOT)

The U.S. Department of Transportation was created through an act of the U.S. Congress on October 15, 1966. Its mission is to develop and coordinate policies that will provide an efficient, economical national transportation system which meets our national needs and defense while protecting the environment. The USDOT is responsible for creating and administering policies and programs that are designed to protect and improve the safety, adequacy, and efficiency of the U.S. transportation system and services. Information about the USDOT, its policies, and its programs can be found at *www.dot.gov*.

National Highway Traffic Safety Administration (NHTSA)

Established by the Highway Safety Act of 1970, the NHTSA is a part of the U.S. Department of Transportation. The NHTSA is responsible for reducing deaths, injuries, and economic losses resulting from motor vehicle crashes. The NHTSA does this by setting and enforcing safety performance standards for motor vehicle equipment and by funding state and local highway safety programs. Among its many services, the NHTSA investigates safety defects in motor vehicles and helps states and local communities reduce the threat posed by impaired drivers. The NHTSA also promotes the use of safety belts, child safety seats, and air bags. Highway safety information may be obtained from NHTSA on its web site at *www.nhtsa.dot.gov*.

Insurance Institute for Highway Safety (IIHS)

The IIHS is an independent research organization funded by a host of well-known insurance companies. The institute focuses on both crash avoidance and the crashworthiness of vehicles. At its state-of-the-art test facility, the institute conducts scientifically controlled crash tests on a variety of vehicles to test their safety performance. The institute also evaluates physical and environmental factors that may contribute to vehicle crashes. Evaluations are conducted on red-light cameras (automated cameras that identify vehicles that fail to stop for red traffic lights), traffic law enforcement technologies, and the elimination of roadside hazards. Information about IIHS programs can be obtained from its web site at *www.iihs.org*.

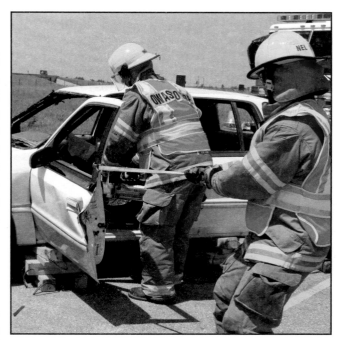

Figure 1.3 Rescue personnel conducting disentanglement procedures.

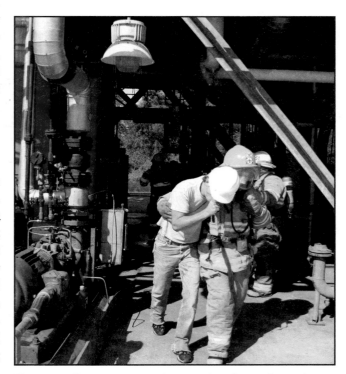

Figure 1.4 Rescuers removing a patient from a hazardous location.

American National Standards Institute (ANSI)

Founded in 1918 by a small group of engineering societies and governmental agencies, ANSI is a private, nonprofit membership organization that manages the voluntary standardization and conformity assessment system within the United States. The organization works to improve the quality of life within the U.S. and the global competitiveness of U.S. businesses by seeking to bring about coordinated, cohesive standards. While ANSI does not develop standards, it facilitates that process and has approved more than 13,000 national and international standards to date. Information about ANSI and its activities can be found on its web site at *www.ansi.org*.

National Fire Protection Association® (NFPA®)

The NFPA® is an organization concerned with fire safety standards development, technical advisory services, education, research, and other related services. Its members come from the educational and scientific sectors of the fire protection field, both private and public. The NFPA's® primary service to the fire protection field is the development of technical consensus standards. The NFPA®, which was organized in 1896, also develops fire training and public fire education materials. Information about NFPA® and its activities can be found on its web site at *www.nfpa.org*.

Transport Canada

Similar to the USDOT, Transport Canada, which is a part of the Canadian federal government, is the primary regulatory agency relevant to vehicle and highway safety in Canada. It is the agency responsible for most of the transportation policies, programs, and goals set by the Government of Canada to make sure that the national transportation system is safe, efficient, and accessible to all its users. The surface transportation section of Transport Canada works with other levels of government, the automotive industry, safety councils, consumer groups, and others to provide information pertinent to vehicle safety such as the risks and benefits of seat belts, air bags, child safety seats, and daytime running lights. Information about Transport Canada and its activities can be found on its web site at *www.tc.gc.ca*.

Transportation Emergency Rescue Committee (TERC)

TERC was formed in 1986 and sanctioned by the International Association of Fire Chiefs. Its original mission was to serve as a competent source of guidance and information on transportation emergencies for those involved in providing emergency services. The organization has an international membership base. The members of these organizations share their vehicle extrication expertise by conducting schools, seminars, and competitive exercises. Their goals are as follows:

- Develop a three-level system for vehicle extrication training
- Develop guidelines to be met by vehicle extrication instructors
- Develop safety guidelines for training
- Disseminate information about vehicle extrication through a newsletter or other source
- Develop a registration system for extrication judges

Information about TERC-USA and TERC-Canada and their activities can be found at *www.tercus.org* and *www.terccanada.ca*.

National Transportation Safety Board (NTSB)

The National Transportation Safety Board is an agency of the U.S. Department of Transportation. The NTSB is tasked with determining the probable cause of transportation accidents involving the release of hazardous materials and those transportation accidents of a recurring nature. Additional information regarding the NTSB can be found at its web site at *www.ntsb.gov*.

Responsibilities of the Rescue Organization

To perform vehicle and machinery rescue operations safely and effectively, rescue organizations should meet a number of responsibilities. First and foremost, they should comply with all laws (local, state/provincial, and federal) and regulations that apply to their jurisdiction. Members of the organization should be trained to implement appropriate components of local, state/provincial, or federal/national response plans. In the United States, for example, these plans would include the National Search and Rescue Plan, the Federal Response Plan, and the National Incident Management System (NIMS).

Rescue organizations should also conform to national standards of performance such as those created by the National Fire Protection Association. NFPA® Standard 1006, *Standard for Rescue Technician Professional Qualifications*, and NFPA® 1670, *Standard on Operations and Training for Technical Search and Rescue Incidents*, both identify a number of responsibilities the rescue organization or authority having jurisdiction (AHJ) should meet in order to conduct rescue operations. These requirements include many of the following elements:

- Conducting hazard/risk assessment surveys
- Developing written response plans and standard operating procedures (SOPs)
- Setting minimum entrance requirements
- Determining operational capabilities
- Conducting training **(Figure 1.5, p. 16)**
- Identifying and providing appropriate equipment and personal protective equipment
- Establishing a safety program

These requirements should be met before conducting any operations at a vehicle or machinery rescue incident.

Hazard and Risk Assessment Surveys

Prior to conducting rescue operations, the organization should conduct a hazard/risk assessment survey of the response area to identify potential hazards, assess the level of risk within the locale, and determine possible rescue situations that may occur. The organization should then examine the cultural, social, physical, and environmental factors that can influence the frequency, scope, or magnitude of possible incidents and compare them to the impact they may have upon the organization's ability to respond safely to an incident. This assessment should be documented, undergo periodic review and survey, and be updated on a regular basis (or as needs arise) to determine if additional types of rescue situations may occur within the local area that require a higher level of response.

Authority Having Jurisdiction (AHJ) — Term used in codes and standards to identify the legal entity, such as a building or fire official, that has the statutory authority to enforce a code and to approve or require equipment. In the insurance industry it may refer to an insurance rating bureau or an insurance company inspection department.

Standard Operating Procedures (SOPs) — Standard methods or rules in which an organization or a fire department operates to carry out a routine function. Usually these procedures are written in a policies and procedures handbook and all firefighters should be well versed in their content. A SOP may specify the functional limitations of fire brigade members in performing emergency operations.

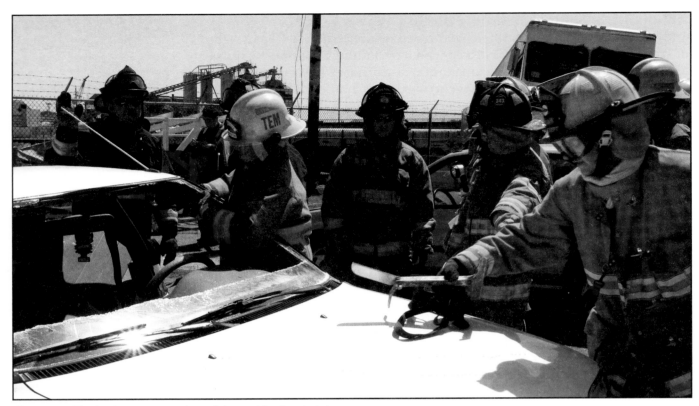

Figure 1.5 Extrication personnel receiving extrication training.

Hazard and Risk Assessment — Formal review of the hazards and risk that may be encountered while performing the functions of a firefighter or emergency responder; used to determine the appropriate level and type of personal and respiratory protection that must be worn.

Weapons of Mass Destruction (WMD) — Any weapon or device that is intended or has the capability to cause death or serious bodily injury to a significant number of people through the release, dissemination, or impact of one of the following means: toxic or poisonous chemicals (or their precursors), a disease organism, or radiation or radioactivity.

The AHJ must assess the potential of an incident response involving nuclear and/or biological weapons, chemical agents, or weapons of mass destruction (WMDs). This assessment must include the potential of secondary devices at the incident scene. If the AHJ determines such risks exist, appropriate training and equipment must be provided to emergency response personnel.

Written Response Plans and Standard Operating Procedures

In addition to conducting the hazard/risk assessment survey, each rescue organization should develop a formal, written incident response plan that details the operational procedures for vehicle and machinery extrication responses. This plan should identify all organizations that are associated with the plan including automatic and mutual aid agencies, particularly those that could provide external resources during an incident. To be effective, this plan should be formally reviewed and adopted by all participants in the plan, updated as necessary, and provide a method for implementing all changes and revisions within each of the organizations involved.

The written response plan should reference the AHJ's standard operating procedures (SOPs). SOPs are created by the AHJ to address a broad range of topics related to vehicle and industrial machinery rescue to ensure these operations are conducted in the safest possible manner for patients and rescuers alike. These SOPs should be in a written format, and all personnel should become familiar with their content. These procedures or guidelines should be reviewed on a recurring basis and updated as needed to meet the organization's needs.

Because of the inherent dangers posed by vehicle and machine rescue situations, it is important to ensure rescuers are psychologically, physically, and medically able to perform their duties. In the SOPs, the AHJ should outline the minimum entrance and fitness requirements for personnel to perform their duties during training exercises and actual emergencies. The minimum requirements for rescue personnel may include the following items:

- Minimum age
- Medical condition(s)
- Physical and psychological fitness
- Level of emergency medical care training
- Educational level
- Hazardous materials incident and contact control training

SOPs should describe the organization's safety program. A key component of any rescue organization is a safety program that ensures all personnel are trained to recognize and control the hazards/risks associated with vehicle and machinery rescue operations in order to minimize danger posed to patients and rescuers. Rescuers performing tasks at vehicle and machinery rescue incidents should be trained to meet the safety requirements for emergency operations, special operations, and protective clothing and protective equipment sections of NFPA® 1500, *Standard on Fire Department Occupational Safety and Health Program*. Rescue personnel should not be armed except when authorized to carry weapons by their organization.

The AHJ's SOPs should address the role of an incident safety officer to be assigned by the incident commander at each incident and during training exercises. This individual should meet the appropriate requirements of NFPA® 1521, *Standard for Fire Department Safety Officer*, and should be able to identify, evaluate, and mitigate, if possible, any hazardous situations or conditions, and unsafe procedures found at an incident. Additional information on the roles and responsibilities of the safety officer can be found in **IFSTA's Fire Department Safety Officer** manual.

Emergency medical care should also be addressed in the organization's policies and procedures. Basic life support (BLS) should be considered the minimum level of emergency medical care to be provided during technical search and rescue operations. BLS personnel should be standing by whenever training exercises or rescue operations are underway in which there is a high potential for injury **(Figure 1.6, p. 18)**. Chapter 12 contains additional information regarding this topic. Some organizations may choose to provide advanced life support (ALS).

In developing its SOPs, the organization should bear in mind that the methods and procedures used during vehicle and machinery extrication may also be used during training, body recovery, and evidence identification and gathering operations with a level of urgency equal to the organization's risk/benefit analysis. For example, if the hazard identification and risk assessment identifies the potential for emergency responses and vehicle/machine extrication operations involving nuclear, biological, or chemical materials, the organization should establish policies to govern these responses and provide adequate training and equipment for rescuers to use in such emergencies.

Secondary Device — Bomb placed at the scene of an ongoing emergency response that is intended to cause casualties among responders; secondary explosive devices are designed to explode after a primary explosion or other major emergency response event has attracted large numbers of responders to the scene.

Automatic Aid — Written agreement between two or more agencies to automatically dispatch predetermined resources to any fire or other emergency reported in the geographic area covered by the agreement. These areas are generally where the boundaries between jurisdictions meet or where jurisdictional "islands" exist.

Mutual Aid — Reciprocal assistance from one fire and emergency services agency to another during an emergency based upon a prearrangement between agencies involved and generally made upon the request of the receiving agency.

Basic Life Support (BLS) — Maintenance of airway, breathing, and circulation, as well as basic bandaging and splinting, without the use of adjunctive equipment.

Advanced Life Support — Advanced medical skills performed by trained medical personnel, such as the administration of medications, or airway management procedures to save a victim's life.

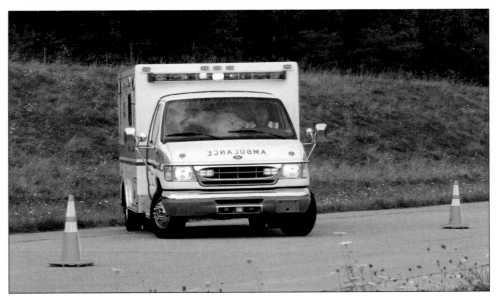

Figure 1.6 Basic life support personnel and ambulance on standby during an extrication training exercise.

The AHJ should establish a policy for the adoption and implementation of an incident management system and a personnel accountability system as outlined in NFPA® 1561, *Standard on Emergency Services Incident Management System.* This policy will provide for training all rescue personnel in the activation and implementation of both systems at each incident. The policy should also address the incident commander's responsibility in briefing rescuers on the appropriate safety considerations at each incident and for establishing a personnel rotation that will reduce rescuer fatigue and stress. In the United States, the policy should conform to the National Incident Management System - Incident Command System (NIMS-ICS).

The AHJ should also establish procedures or guidelines that address rescue team evacuation and accountability measures to be followed in imminent danger situations. These SOPs should also address the methods used to notify rescue personnel of an evacuation (for example: radio, visual, audible warning signals and devices).

The organization should develop SOPs in accordance with the operational capability level of the organization (as described in the next section). No operations or procedures should be allowed that exceed the level of capability set by the organization. The AHJ should provide adequate supervisory personnel who are proficient to operate at the organization's chosen level of capability.

National Incident Management System - Incident Command System (NIMS-ICS) — The U.S. mandated system that defines the roles, responsibilities, and standard operating procedures used to manage emergency operations. Also be referred to as NIMS- ICS.

Operational Capability and Training Requirements

The AHJ should establish the level of capability at which the organization will perform technical search and rescue operations. This level should be selected based on the types of hazards identified during the hazard/risk assessment survey conducted by the organization, the level of personnel training, and the resources (internal and external) available to the organization. Rescue organizations should conduct sufficient training of all personnel to meet the organization's level of operational capability. The awareness level is the minimum level to which the organization may train. Organizations at the operations level should train to and respond at the operations level and so on. The organization should also provide for the continuing education necessary to maintain the organization's level of operational capability. Plans should also be developed for incidents that require a higher level of capability than the local jurisdiction provides.

- *Awareness Level* – Personnel at the awareness level should be able to meet the NFPA® 1670 operational requirements for the Awareness Level. Some of these duties and tasks may include the following:
  — Conducting incident size up
  — Recognizing the need for vehicle/machinery rescue
  — Identifying general hazards at an incident
  — Identifying the resources required to mitigate the incident
  — Initiating a response to an incident
  — Initiating site and traffic control and scene management procedures.

- *Operations Level* – Personnel at the operations level should be able to meet the NFPA® 1670 operational requirements for the Operations Level. Some of these duties and tasks may include the following:
  — Conducting incident size up
  — Recognizing and controlling incident hazards
  — Controlling traffic at the incident scene
  — Locating patients and determining their survivability
  — Making the incident scene safe
  — Mitigating fluid releases
  — Determining the condition of patients
  — Protecting patients during extrication operations
  — Preparing patients for extrication and transport
  — Acquiring and tracking extrication resources
  — Operating extrication hand tools and equipment safely

- *Technician Level* – Personnel at the technician level should be able to meet the NFPA® 1670 operational requirements for the Technician Level. Some of these duties and tasks may include the following:
  — Conducting incident size up
  — Recognizing and controlling incident hazards
  — Controlling traffic at the incident scene
  — Locating patients and determining their survivability
  — Making the incident scene safe
  — Mitigating fluid releases
  — Applying advanced stabilization techniques **(Figure 1.7, p. 20)**
  — Determining the condition of patients
  — Protecting patients during extrication operations
  — Treating patients and preparing them for extrication and transport
  — Acquiring and tracking extrication resources
  — Operating specialized extrication equipment safely

Additionally, each member of the emergency response organization must be trained on the appropriate requirements of NFPA® 472, *Standard for Com-*

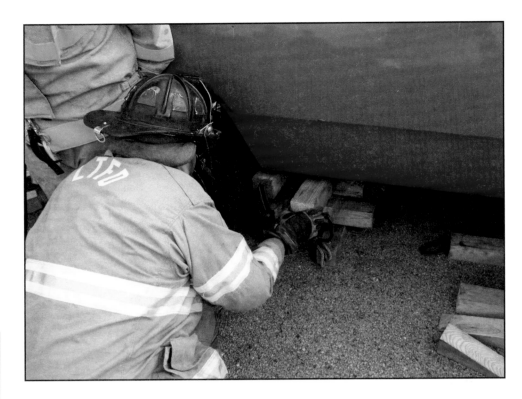

Figure 1.7 Extrication personnel using cribbing to stabilize a pickup truck.

Personal Protective Equipment (PPE) — General term for the equipment worn by firefighters and rescuers; includes helmets, coats, pants, boots, eye protection, gloves, protective hoods, self-contained breathing apparatus, and personal alert safety systems (PASS devices). Also called Bunker Clothes, Protective Clothing, Turnout Clothing, or Turnout Gear.

petence of Responders to Hazardous Materials/Weapons of Mass Destruction Incidents, that correspond to the level of the organization's rescue capability. It is important for the organization to review its training program and its performance regularly. Procedures should be established for conducting an annual review of the organization's training program to ensure personnel are adequately trained to function in a variety of hazardous conditions and environments. Procedures should also be established for conducting an annual review of the organization's performance in relation to the appropriate standards.

All training should be documented, and the organization should have a system for managing and maintaining this documentation. All training documentation should be available for review and inspection by rescue teams members and personnel they authorize to view it.

Extrication Equipment and Personal Protective Equipment

The rescue organization should identify the equipment and resources available (both internally and externally) and acquire equipment that is applicable to the organization's level of capability. The types, quantities, and locations of this equipment should be listed in the organization's SOPs or inventory control system. The SOPs should describe the procedures for accessing the equipment during emergency situations. This inventory list should be updated on an annual basis or as new equipment is added or removed from service. The organization should maintain each piece of equipment in accordance with the manufacturer's recommendations. All rescue personnel should be properly trained in the use of each piece of equipment.

To safely perform vehicle and machinery extrication, rescuers should have adequate personal protective clothing and equipment suited to the hazards the rescuers will face **(Figure 1.8)**. The organization should identify and acquire the appropriate type or types of personal protective clothing and equipment needed to provide this protection. All personnel should be trained in the capa-

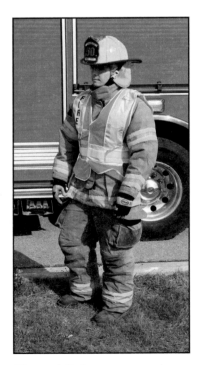

Figure 1.8 A rescuer wearing personal protective equipment.

bilities and limitations of each piece of protective clothing or equipment. They should also be trained to perform proper inspection, care and maintenance, and use of the personal protective clothing and equipment issued to them or made available for their use. To be effective, personal protective clothing and equipment should be worn properly when conducting emergency operations or training exercises.

When needed, NFPA® 1981 compliant self contained breathing apparatus (SCBA), supplied air respirators (SAR), or other appropriate, approved respiratory protection should be available for use and worn by rescue team members during rescue incidents. At a minimum, the air for these systems should meet ANSI/CGA G7.1, *Commodity Specification for Air*, for Grade D air. SAR equipment must be equipped an emergency supply of self-contained breathing air to be used during egress should the primary air supply fail.

After Action Reviews (AAR)

After Action Reviews (also known as post incident analysis or PIAs) are learning tools used to evaluate a project or incident to identify and encourage organizational and operational strengths and to identify and correct weaknesses. Many civilian and military organizations have successfully used the AAR process to improve their organizational operations and processes. Regularly scheduled AARs have become a standard practice within the interagency wildland fire community resulting in the capture and dissemination of crucial knowledge throughout the organizations involved. The AAR process and its importance to rescue organizations will be discussed in greater detail later in this chapter.

Knowledge, Skills, and Abilities for Safe Extrication Operations

One of the most important skills for rescue personnel on vehicle extrication incidents is the ability to recognize existing and potential dangers to themselves and others. Rescue personnel are trained and equipped to help those who cannot help themselves, and they are willing to accept the risks involved in rescue operations. However, all on-scene rescue personnel should resist the urge to rush into the scene before it is safe to do so — and thereby add more patients to the incident. It is essential that all rescuers remember that they did not cause the problem; they are not responsible for the patients being in that situation, and they are not obligated to sacrifice themselves in a heroic attempt to save a patient — especially not in an attempt to recover a body. During any emergency incident, the safety and survival priorities for emergency response personnel are — *self, fellow rescuers, bystanders, and patients.*

IFSTA Principles of Risk Management

1. Activities that present a significant risk to the safety of members shall be limited to situations where there is a potential to save en dangered lives.

2. Activities that are routinely employed to protect property shall be recognized as inherent risks to the safety of members, and actions shall be taken to reduce or avoid these risks.

3. No risk to the safety of members shall be acceptable when there is no possibility to save lives or property.

Self-Contained Breathing Apparatus (SCBA) — Respirator worn by the user that supplies a breathable atmosphere that is either carried in or generated by the apparatus and is independent of the ambient atmosphere. Respiratory protection is worn in all atmospheres that are considered to be Immediately Dangerous to Life and Health (IDLH). Also called Air Mask or Air Pack.

Supplied Air Respirator — Atmosphere-supplying respirator for which the source of breathing air is not designed to be carried by the user; not certified for fire fighting operations. Also known as an Airline Respirator.

To safely and successfully extricate a patient trapped in a vehicle, rescuers should be able to all of the following:

- Assess the situation (perform size-up)

- Make informed decisions about how to stabilize the situation (stop it from getting worse)

- Devise and implement a plan of action that protects the rescuers and patient(s) from further injury and results in all patients being freed from entrapment

To fulfill these general requirements, rescuers should have a significant amount of specific knowledge and a variety of skills and abilities. Although not listed in any order of importance or priority, rescuers should have an understanding of the following:

- *Available resource capabilities and limitations* — Local emergency response personnel should know the capabilities and limitations of all resources that would be immediately available and those that would be available with some delay. One of the best ways of learning these capabilities and limitations – and of increasing the capabilities and reducing the limitations – is through realistic joint training exercises held on a regular basis.

- *How to activate the local emergency response system* — An important part of using the available resources to their fullest extent is knowing how to access those resources quickly when needed. Regardless of whether additional resources are available from within the primary agency, mutual aid units, or private providers, rescuers should be aware of how to activate the emergency response system.

- *Vehicle construction* — Knowledge of how vehicles are constructed is critical to the safety of rescuers, trapped occupants, and bystanders. Knowing the operational characteristics and locations of supplemental restraint systems (including air bags, seat belt pretensioners, and other safety devices) can protect both rescuers and trapped occupants. Knowledge of vehicle construction is also an important element in freeing trapped vehicle occupants as quickly and safely as possible.

- *Vehicle crash dynamics* — Knowing what happens to vehicles and their occupants when they collide with stationary objects or other vehicles is important to understanding the nature of the extrication problems involved. For example, knowing how vehicles designed with crumple zones react to impact compared to those without such features is important to assessing how occupants may be trapped in the wreckage. Different types of collisions may also indicate the types of injuries that occupants may have suffered.

- *How and why patients become entrapped in vehicles* — Rescuers should combine their knowledge of vehicle construction with the dynamics of vehicle crashes to understand how and why vehicle occupants are entrapped in the wreckage of their vehicles. This knowledge can be obtained through years of experience or, more efficiently, by studying data and video footage of controlled crash tests conducted by research organizations.

- *Mechanisms of injury* — Understanding how the inertial forces produced during vehicle crashes cause injuries to vehicle occupants helps rescuers determine the proper packaging and handling techniques in a given situation.

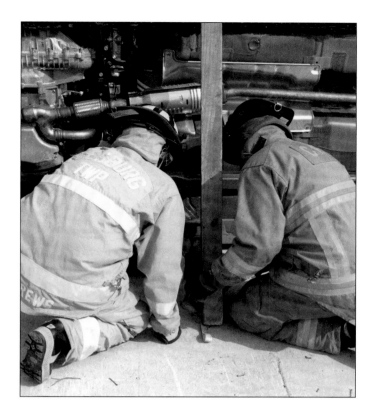

Figure 1.9 Extrication personnel using a wooden shore post to stabilize an overturned vehicle.

Matching the packaging and handling techniques to the patient's potential injuries minimizes patient trauma and maximizes a patient's chance for survival.

- *Vehicle stabilization* — Stabilizing wrecked vehicles is an important safety and patient care consideration. There are a variety of techniques and equipment commonly used to stabilize crashed vehicles, and rescuers should be well trained in their application **(Figure 1.9)**.

- *Scene control and protection* — Controlling the perimeter of a crash scene is also of critical importance to the safety of rescuers, trapped patients, and bystanders. If the wrecked vehicles are still on the roadway, the scene should be protected from oncoming traffic. There may be other hazards, such as spilled fuel, hazardous materials, or downed power lines that threaten those at the scene. When vehicles plunge into creeks, rivers, or other bodies of water, rescuers must also contend with hypothermia and drowning as additional hazards. All potential safety hazards should be identified and addressed if the extrication operation is to be conducted safely.

- *Procedures to protect rescuers* — Procedures should be implemented for mitigating general and specific hazards at the scene and for maintaining traffic control. As mentioned earlier, these measures are necessary to protect everyone at the scene, including the rescuers. It is critically important that rescuers be protected so that they can perform their duties.

- *How to use available tools and equipment safely and effectively* —Rescuers should be able to select and use the most appropriate tools and equipment according to the manufacturer's recommendations. Using tools and equipment safely requires hands-on training by qualified instructors and first-hand experience under the supervision of qualified supervisors.

- *How to access trapped patients* — Rescuers should know the procedures for accessing patients trapped in a vehicle and be able to follow them in a way that results in the patients being freed from entrapment. This may involve the use of a variety of tools and equipment to manipulate and/or remove major vehicle components.

- *Patient assessment* — Before trapped patients can be transported to a medical facility, they should be medically assessed to determine the nature and extent of any injuries they may have suffered during the crash. From the standpoint of patient survival, this can be one of the most critical steps in the entire extrication operation. If an injury is overlooked during this assessment, it can possibly develop into a life-threatening problem because of the movement and manipulation of the patient during extrication.

- *How to provide on-scene medical care* — Rescuers should have adequate training to provide on-scene medical care to injured or ill patients including providing on-scene treatment of the injured to prepare them for transport.

- *How to protect and package trapped patients* — Rescuers should be able to properly protect and package patients in accordance with the findings of their medical assessment and within their medical training and capability. Packaging can include everything from simple bandaging to applying a Cervical-collar with full spinal immobilization and traction devices to immobilize and prepare a patient for transport to further medical care.

- *How to transfer injured patients to EMS personnel for transportation* — Rescuers should be able to transfer injured patients to EMS personnel for transportation to an appropriate medical facility. This includes properly preparing the patient for transfer as well as following local protocols and passing on critical information about the patient's condition.

- *How to ensure that the area and vehicles are left in a safe condition when the incident is terminated* — The rescue organization should ensure that a vehicle extrication scene is left in a safe and environmentally stable condition. Wrecked vehicles should be removed from the scene and any other hazards mitigated before the scene is abandoned. Any hazards that cannot be immediately mitigated should be isolated to prevent members of the public from inadvertently entering a hazardous area.

Obtaining all this knowledge and developing all these skills and abilities takes time, training, and experience. No one should expect to become proficient in vehicle extrication merely by reading this or any other text on the subject. In addition to instructional materials such as this manual, hands-on training delivered by competent qualified instructors and first-hand experience under the supervision of knowledgeable and conscientious company officers are absolutely necessary.

Success Factors

To be successful, vehicle and machinery extrication operations involve four incident priorities:

- *Personnel protection/life safety* — Protecting both the patients involved in the incident, bystanders in the immediate area, and the emergency response personnel operating on the scene. Meeting this priority involves a safe response by emergency personnel, implementing the incident command system, providing scene safety by controlling and protecting the scene from oncoming traffic or interference from curious bystanders, determining the condition of patients and how their condition may impact the types of tools and procedures used, conducting the operation in a safe manner, and protecting trapped patients during the operation.

- *Incident stabilization* — Taking the steps necessary to prevent the situation from getting any worse than it was when emergency response personnel arrived; some of these steps are as follows:
  - Maintaining scene control and protection while the operation is being conducted
  - Stabilizing the vehicles
  - Stabilizing and removing trapped patients
  - Eliminating sources of ignition
  - Providing fire protection and hazardous materials control as needed

- *Property and environmental conservation* — Preventing *unnecessary* damage to property during and immediately after the operation. Meeting this priority involves the following activities:
  - Developing and adopting procedures that result in as little property damage as possible and are consistent with achieving incident objectives
  - Using nondestructive techniques that accomplish the objective as fast or faster than other more destructive techniques
  - Providing security for unprotected property at the conclusion of the operation
  - Protecting the environment by preventing gasoline, hydraulic fluids, battery acids, coolants, or other contaminants from running into sewer drains or streams

- *After Action Review (AAR)* — Continuous operational improvement can occur when an organization implements an AAR process. Immediately following an incident, the personnel should conduct an AAR with the incident leader serving as the facilitator. Participants should be encouraged to focus on:
  - What was preplanned?
  - What really occurred?
  - What caused that to happen?
  - What worked and what didn't work?
  - What should be done next time?

Roles and Responsibilities of Personnel Responding to an Extrication Incident

Vehicle extrication incidents involve a number of separate and distinct functions that should often be performed simultaneously. These functions can be and sometimes are performed by members of a single response agency. However, to perform these functions most efficiently, groups of personnel from more than one agency are usually required **(Figure 1.10, p. 26)**. The following sections describe the roles and responsibilities of these various groups.

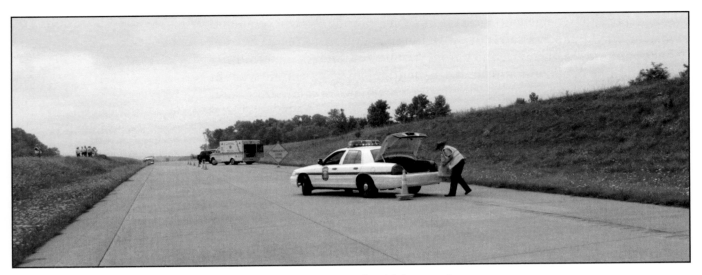
Figure 1.10 Motor vehicle accidents often require the response of multiple agencies.

- *Rescue Personnel* — Group which is directly responsible for stabilizing crashed vehicles, accessing patients, stabilizing patients, disentangling patients, packaging patients for removal from wrecked vehicles, and transferring crash patients to EMS personnel.

- *Law Enforcement* — Group which is responsible for directing traffic around vehicle crash scenes, crowd control at these scenes, and investigating these incidents if they occurred on public streets or highways.

- *Emergency Medical Service (EMS)* — Group which is responsible for evaluating, treating, and transporting (if necessary) vehicle crash patients to appropriate medical facilities once patients are removed from wrecked vehicles. If local protocols permit, the EMS group may begin its work prior to the patients being extricated from the vehicles.

- *Fire Service* — Group which is responsible for providing fire protection (engine or fire companies) to protect extrication teams, patients, EMS personnel, and any others working in and around crashed vehicles.

- *Other Response Agencies* — Other response agencies can be of assistance during extrication incidents by providing support to the extrication organization. Some of these agencies include, but are not limited to:

  — Utility companies

  — State and Provincial Department of Transport

  — Private industrial response teams

  — Towing and recovery companies

Summary

Vehicle and machinery extrication is a broad and diverse field and one in which most emergency response organizations are involved. The importance of following regional and national standards was discussed. A number of national as well as state/provincial and local organizations relate in some way to the field. Rescue organizations have numerous responsibilities that should be addressed in order for those organizations to function safely. To be successful, those involved in vehicle extrication operations should possess a variety of skills, knowledge, and abilities. They should have a thorough knowledge of vehicle anatomy, extrication principles, and the roles and responsibilities of those involved in extrication operations. Potential rescuers should be carefully selected for their physical and emotional strength and for their willingness and ability to learn the many aspects of safe and effective vehicle extrication operations.

Review Questions

1. Which organization develops fire safety standards, fire training, and public fire education materials?

2. Which standards identify the responsibilities the rescue organization or authority having jurisdiction (AHJ) should meet in order to conduct rescue operations?

3. What formal document details the operational procedures for vehicle and machinery extrication responses and should reference the AHJ's SOPs?

4. What are the responsibilities of each of the three levels of vehicle and machinery extrication personnel?

5. What is the purpose of conducting After Action Reviews (AAR)?

6. What are the four incident priorities that lead to successful vehicle and machinery extrication operations?

7. What are the roles and responsibilities of rescue personnel during vehicle and machinery extrication operations?

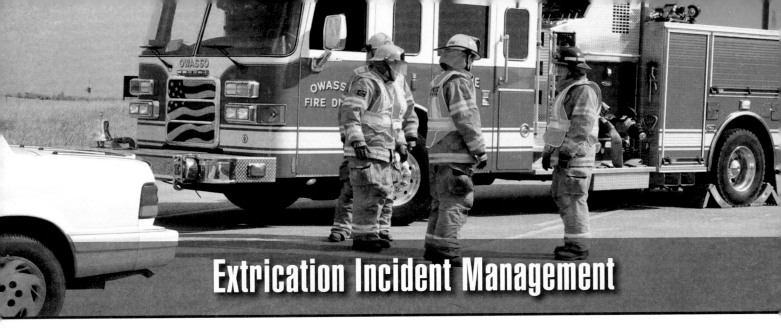

Extrication Incident Management

Chapter Contents

Key Terms

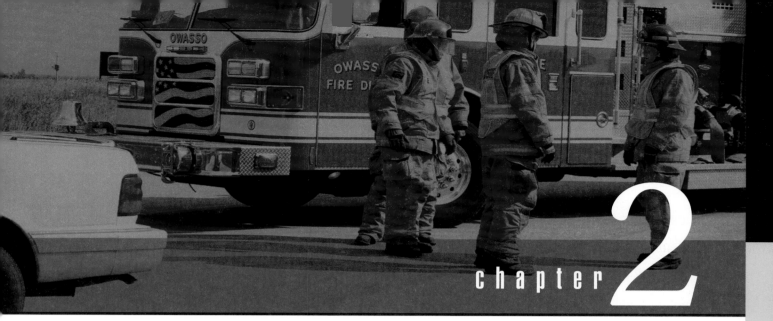

Job Performance Requirements

This chapter provides information that addresses the following job performance requirements (JPRs) of NFPA® 1001, *Standard for Fire Fighter Professional Qualifications* (2008), NFPA® 1006, *Standard for Technical Rescuer Professional Qualifications* (2008), NFPA® 1670, *Standard on Operations and Training for Technical Search and Rescue Incidents* (2009).

NFPA® 1001 JPRs

6.4.2

NFPA® 1006 JPRs

4.1.1	5.2.3	5.3.1	10.1.1	10.1.9	10.2.4
4.1.2	5.2.4	5.3.3	10.1.2	10.1.10	
4.3.2	5.2.5	5.4	10.1.3	10.2	
5.2.1	5.2.6	5.4.1	10.1.6	10.2.1	
5.2.2	5.2.7	5.4.2	10.1.7	10.2.2	
5.2.1	5.3	10.1	10.1.8	10.2.3	

NFPA® 1670 JPRs

4.1.1	4.5.3.3	12.3.4
4.1.3.1	8.2.3	12.4.2
4.1.6	8.3.3	
4.1.9	8.3.4	
4.5.1.4	8.4.2	
4.5.2.1	12.2.3	
4.5.3.1	12.3.3	

Learning Objectives

1. Identify standards that related to managing an extrication incident.

2. Identify basic facts about safety requirements for extrication incidents.

3. Describe the importance of training to extrication incident safety.

4. Identify facts about the early stages of an emergency extrication response.

5. Describe the duties performed by outside agencies during an extrication operation.

6. Describe Incident Command/Management as it relates to extrication operations.

7. Identify key components of an extrication operation.

8. Describe the duties performed by extrication personnel at an extrication operation.

Chapter 2
Extrication Incident Management

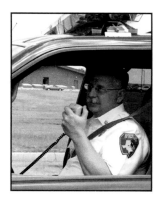

Case History

An initial, two unit response consisting of an engine and a brush/mini-pumper was dispatched to a single vehicle accident with an unknown number of patients involved. The first officer on the scene assumed command, established a command post, and assigned an extrication officer. The incident commander requested a truck company response. Because of the position of the incident vehicle, the extrication officer determined it was necessary to dig a trench to access and remove the passenger doors. Hydraulic tools were deployed from the brush/mini-pumper to begin door removal operations. When the truck company arrived, it deployed its light tower, air bags, and hydraulic tools to assist the extrication operation. A higher ranking department officer arrived and assumed command of the operation. With the passenger doors removed, rescuers were able to access the patients, stabilize their conditions, and package them for removal on back boards. The patients were then transferred to ambulance personnel for transport to medical treatment.

The safe and effective handling of extrication incidents demands a well-organized extrication operation. This includes providing an appropriate response and using a clearly defined incident command/management system to manage the scene and the available resources. The keys to effective response, organization, and management are planning and training. Pre-incident planning and realistic training enable emergency crews to become familiar with the district, standard operating procedures, other agencies, and the incident command/management system. Well-trained rescuers know what can and cannot be done with the resources available. Knowledge of the capabilities and limitations of equipment and personnel improves the decision-making of those in charge.

This chapter examines some of the basic safety principles involved in extrication operations. Also addressed is emergency response. Finally, implementing an incident command/management system and managing a rescue scene are discussed.

Standards

As described in Chapter 1, if a survey of the jurisdiction reveals a sufficient number of potential situations where an extrication capability may be needed, the AHJ must then determine the operational level that may be required. Having done that, the AHJ must then decide how best to provide that level of extrication capability to the citizens of the jurisdiction.

In addition to NFPA® 1670 on which this manual is based, the management of extrication operations is governed by NFPA® 1561, *Standard on Emergency Services Incident Management System*, and NFPA® 1500, *Standard on Fire Department Occupational Safety and Health Program*. In the United States, Homeland Security Presidential Directive/HSPD-5 directs that all state and local governments and tribal entities adopt NIMS-ICS. Local emergency organizations should make sure that their command structure will interface with "outside" organizations in an emergency.

Each of these standards requires that an incident command/management system be adopted by the agency. In addition, they require that agency personnel be trained in the implementation and use of the system. Finally, these standards require that the adopted incident command/management system be used on all emergency incidents.

Extrication Incident Safety

Success in an extrication operation is defined by how effectively it was conducted and how safely it was conducted. These two criteria cannot be separated when assessing the outcome of an extrication incident. However, since the subsequent chapters of this manual deal specifically with the knowledge, skills, and abilities needed to conduct extrication operations effectively, the discussion in this section focuses exclusively on conducting extrication operations safely.

Conducting extrication operations safely involves a number of different but interrelated components. Each of the following components is important to incident safety during extrication operations:

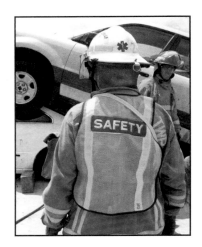

Figure 2.1 Incident safety officers monitor vehicle extrication scenes for potential hazards.

- Training
- Operational assignments
- Medical branch/group
- Rehabilitation (Rehab) station
- Mitigation of potential hazards at the extrication scene
- Appointment of Incident Safety Officer **(Figure 2.1)**
- Effective personnel accountability system

Training

Training firefighters and other rescuers to function safely during extrication operations involves a number of different considerations. First, each individual must be trained to use the most appropriate rescue tools and techniques for the task at hand so that his or her assignments are carried out safely. Next, each individual must be trained to function as a member of a rescue team. *Freelancing* – acting individually without supervision and without coordination with other members of the team – is counterproductive and may be quite dangerous. Finally, each individual must be made aware of standard operating procedures (SOPs) and any other operational plans developed during pre-incident planning, and with his or her role within those plans. These plans and SOPs should be practiced during training until they are second nature.

Operational Assignments

Before an extrication team leader makes an operational assignment during an extrication incident, the officer making the assignment should consider the situational requirements and match each to a rescuer in the officer's crew who is most qualified to safely carry out the assignment. When making this assessment, the supervisor must attempt to answer the following questions:

- Who has the necessary knowledge?
- Who has the necessary experience?
- Who has the necessary competence?
- Who has the necessary skill?
- Who has the necessary ability?
- Who has the necessary physical strength and stamina?
- Who has the necessary emotional strength and stability?

If the organization has a valid system of certifying professional competencies, the likelihood of choosing the right subordinate for an assignment is greatly increased. If the officer and the members of his or her crew have trained together and worked together on other incidents, this assessment can often be done in an instant. It is equally important to train with and assess the capabilities and limitations of mutual aid resources that may be needed on extrication incidents. However, if the assessment is not done, or is done too casually, the results could be disastrous. The likelihood of failure is increased by assigning a potentially hazardous task to someone who may be technically or physically incapable of completing the assignment safely.

Subordinates also have a personal responsibility regarding operational assignments. Every rescuer has not only the right but the obligation to refuse to accept an assignment if the rescuer is not qualified or lacks the necessary resources to safely complete the task. This right to refuse is especially true of those who are responsible for the safety of others, such as a rescue team leader. Before refusing an assignment, the rescuer or team leader must discuss the safety concerns with whoever is making the assignment and attempt to reach an agreement on how the assignment can be altered to reduce the level of risk and still meet the objective. If the discussion fails to satisfy the individual's safety concerns, the individual must decide whether to accept or refuse the assignment within the parameters of departmental policy. Every refusal of an assignment should be documented and investigated after the incident is terminated.

When an individual refuses an assignment, the individual can still be used in some other capacity during the incident. Those lacking the necessary training or experience to perform the actual rescue may be given assignments that support those who are performing the rescue.

Medical Component

Because extrication is an inherently dangerous endeavor, rescuers do sometimes suffer injuries. Rescuers are often required to place themselves at risk in order to rescue someone in distress. In most cases, the rescuers' training and experience, the reliability of their equipment, and the safety margin built into their procedures allows them to complete their sometimes risky assignments safely. However, despite the best efforts of rescuers to protect themselves and supervisors to protect those for whom they are responsible, the unforeseen sometimes happens and rescuers get hurt.

Because of this potential for injury, at least one ambulance should be on standby for the rescuers at every emergency incident. The ambulance or ambulances designated for the rescuers should be at least basic life support (BLS), and advanced life support (ALS) if available. Whatever their levels of capability, these ambulances are in addition to any other ambulances that may be standing by to transport the patient or patients being rescued.

In addition to these transportation capabilities, large and/or complex mass-casualty extrication incidents will require one or more medical triage stations. Ideally, a triage station should be dedicated to the rescuers on scene, separate from the one set up for those being extricated.

Rehabilitation (Rehab) Station

In every prolonged extrication operation, and especially those that are conducted in less than ideal weather conditions, there is a need to establish a rehab station for the rescue personnel. Even in relatively hospitable conditions, rescuers often have to perform heavy physical labor such as operating heavy power tools, struggling with heavy debris, or installing cribbing and shoring. All such physically demanding activities can dehydrate and fatigue rescuers. Even under ideal circumstances, these rescuers need to be relieved from time to time for rest and rehydration. The frequency with which crews will need to be rotated during an extrication operation will vary with the conditions in the restricted (hot) zone, the type of PPE being worn by the rescuers, and the types of activities in which they are engaged. For more information on this topic, refer to the BRADY/IFSTA **Emergency Incident Rehabilitation** manual.

Mitigating Potential Hazards

Some of the most common hazards that rescuers may encounter during extrication operations are as follows:

- Vehicular traffic **(Figure 2.2)**
- Downed electrical power lines
- Leaking vehicle fluids
- Leaking flammable gas lines
- Broken water mains or sanitary sewer lines
- Uncontrolled release of toxic and corrosive hazardous materials

These and countless other hazards can make extrication operations more difficult and can put rescuers at serious risk. Therefore, the actual extrication operation might have to be delayed until the hazards at the scene have been mitigated. These hazards must first be recognized, identified, and isolated and then a mitigation plan developed and implemented. In this phase of an extrication operation, rescuers must exercise discipline and resist the temptation to enter the hot zone prematurely in an attempt to conduct an extrication operation. Depending upon the nature of the hazard and its severity, what started as an extrication operation may already have turned into a body recovery operation. It is certainly unjustified to put rescuers in serious jeopardy to recover the remains of someone who is already dead.

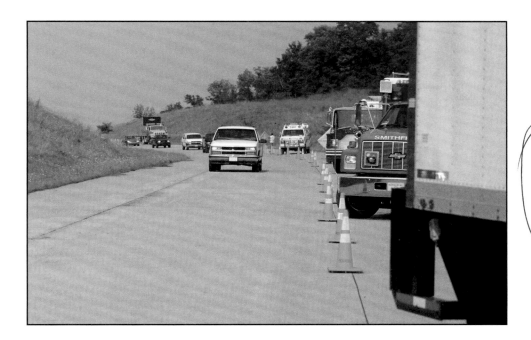

Figure 2.2 Vehicle traffic can pose a hazard to rescuers and patients during vehicle extrication operations.

Appointment of Incident Safety Officer

Every extrication operation requires an incident safety officer. On very small extrication incidents that do not require a large organization, the IC may be able to function as the incident safety officer. This practice should be discouraged and an incident safety officer should be assigned. On larger incidents, the IC should delegate the authority to a safety officer whose only responsibility during the incident is to observe the operation and make sure that it is conducted in the safest possible manner. Rank is not always a reliable indicator of an individual's qualifications to be the safety officer on a technical extrication incident. To be effective, the safety officer must have sufficient knowledge and understanding of the hazards involved as well as the tools and techniques of the specific rescue discipline. For more information on this topic, refer to the IFSTA **Fire Department Safety Officer** manual.

Effective Personnel Accountability

There are a number of different personnel accountability systems in use by agencies across North America. Depending upon the organization of a particular extrication incident, personnel accountability may or may not be a responsibility of the incident safety officer.

If using an accountability system is to become a part of the organizational culture, extrication organizations must train their personnel in the operation of the system that fits their particular organization, include the system in their SOPs, and require its use on every incident. In any operation that requires rescuers or rescue crews to enter a hazard zone – especially a zone in which the rescuers are not visible from the incident command post – an effective personnel accountability system is needed. To prepare for these incidents, extrication organizations should stress the use of teamwork during training. In addition, they should establish a rapid intervention team (RIT) on every incident requiring rescuers to enter an IDLH atmosphere.

Rapid Intervention Team (RIT) — Two or more fully equipped and immediately available firefighters designated to stand by outside the hazard zone to enter and effect rescue of firefighters inside, if necessary; also known as Rapid Intervention Crew (RIC).

Emergency Extrication Response

This section deals with many of the basic issues involved in responding to and dealing with emergency extrication incidents. Receiving information and dispatching calls are discussed, along with implementing the response plan. The operational considerations that must be addressed at the rescue scene are also discussed.

Receiving Information and Dispatching Calls

An important part of an effective rescue response is making sure that the responding resources arrive at the correct location as quickly and safely as possible. A quick and safe response can be achieved in part through good communication practices and procedures. The emergency response system is usually activated by a dispatcher who receives the call for help.

Dispatchers (also called telecommunicators) should be sufficiently familiar with the district and with field operations to communicate effectively with both callers and responding rescue personnel **(Figure 2.3)**. Since the advent of the enhanced 9-1-1 emergency phone system, if a caller is too excited to speak coherently or if the caller does not speak English fluently enough to clearly communicate the nature and specific location of the incident, the dispatcher will at least have the location of the telephone from which the call is being made. Of course, this assumes that the call is being made from a land-based telephone at a fixed location. If the call is coming from a cellular phone, the dispatcher may have to rely upon the caller to supply as much information as possible. However, improvements in global positioning system (GPS) technology are making it possible to locate cell phone callers through a system of triangulation by signal alone.

Telecommunicator — Person who works in the communications center and processes information from the public and emergency responders; also referred to as a *dispatcher.*

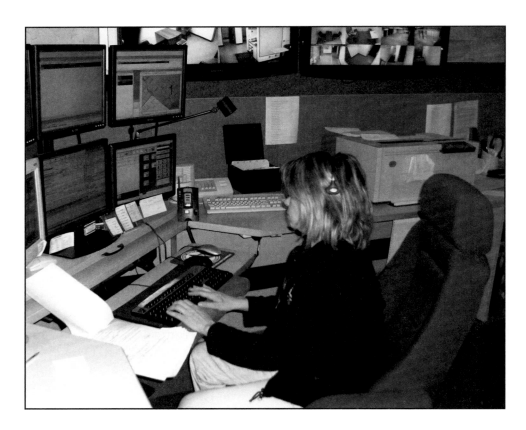

Figure 2.3 Telecommunicators serve a vital role between the general public and the emergency responders. *Courtesy of Alan Braun, University of Missouri Fire and Rescue Training Institute.*

In some cases, excited or confused callers provide incorrect information about the location of an incident, such as mistakenly describing the location to be at the intersection of two parallel streets. However, if the dispatcher knows the district, he or she should be able to recognize the discrepancy and question the caller further to get more accurate information.

Effectively handling the initial response is the first step toward efficiently organizing an extrication incident. Therefore, dispatchers must attempt to determine the nature and extent of the emergency so that the most appropriate response can be dispatched. To do this, dispatchers should follow their agency's standardized procedure, guideline, or checklist for taking information from the reporting party.

The dispatcher receiving the call should first determine the nature and extent of the problem because it may not even be an emergency. The problem may involve more than one agency, or it may not be an incident that is appropriate for an extrication agency. The next piece of essential information is the location of the problem – street address, business name, or some nearby landmark. And finally, the dispatcher should find out how many people are involved and what their status is – injured, trapped, or in immediate mortal jeopardy.

Although obtaining this information may seem to be a cumbersome and time-consuming process, it is the best way of determining the services and resources required at an incident. The dispatcher should try to get as much information as possible, giving priority to the nature of the problem and the location of the incident. The dispatcher can then use this information to dispatch emergency crews based on predetermined response levels and on what appears to be needed. For more information on this topic, refer to the IFSTA **Telecommunicator** manual.

Implementing the Response Plan

A major part of pre-incident planning is determining what the initial response for each type of extrication incident should be to any location within the district. Many emergency response organizations have predetermined responses for specific types of incidents. To the extent possible, responses to extrication calls should also be standardized so that each responding personnel knows which other resources can be expected to arrive at the scene. First-arriving personnel can use this knowledge to call for additional help or to cancel apparatus already en route. A predetermined, standardized response has many benefits and is an important step in organizing the extrication incident.

In determining the standard response for an extrication call, the resources most likely to be needed for dealing with such incidents should be included. Standardizing the response helps to ensure that all personnel and apparatus that may be needed will arrive soon enough to be used effectively. Primary elements that should be included in any extrication response are extrication capabilities, emergency medical services, fire protection, law enforcement, and any other outside agencies that could affect the outcome positively. Each of these entities should be aware of its role in the response plan and how it will be expected to participate in emergency extrication activities.

Taking Charge

Any rescuer, regardless of rank, may have to initially assume command of an extrication incident. All extrication personnel should be prepared to accept this responsibility. The major responsibilities of the incident commander (IC) are making decisions and managing resources, not the hands-on activities involved in affecting the rescue.

In addition to knowing the applicable response plan, the potential IC must also be mentally and emotionally prepared to assume command. Making decisions involving life-threatening situations can produce significant stress, and the stress is multiplied if the rescuer lacks the training and experience needed to prepare him or her for the pressures of command. Realistic drills and simulations will help rescuers develop the confidence, mental agility, and emotional stability needed to command extrication incidents. An effective leader must be able to remain calm even if there is chaos at the scene. To some, this calmness may appear to be indifference or indecision, but because anxiety and fear are contagious, it is critical that the IC exhibit a demeanor of quiet confidence.

The first decision that the IC must make is whether or not the incident is an extrication call. It may be a needless call resulting from a citizen misinterpreting what was seen or overreacting to some minor event such as a vehicle crash that involved serious property damage but no injuries or entrapments. To make this and other critical initial decisions, the IC must quickly find the answers to some basic questions about the incident. These basic questions are as follows:

- What has occurred?
- What are the conditions within the inner and outer circle surveys?
  - Outer Circle Surveys . The area beyond each vehicle. (Examples include: trees, power lines/poles, patients, other vehicles and traffic)
  - Inner Circle Surveys. The area adjacent to each vehicle. (Examples include: patients, stabilization, downed powerlines, fluids and other hazards)
- How many patients are there, where are they, and what is their status?
- Is the situation stable or getting worse?
- What is likely to occur without immediate intervention?
- What safety issues are involved?

If the answers to these questions confirm this to be an extrication incident, the IC must then make three more potentially critical decisions: (1) whether it is safe and/or feasible to attempt a rescue, (2) whether the operation should be conducted as a body recovery, and (3) whether the resources on scene or en route are sufficient to handle the incident or if additional resources need to be called.

Size-Up

Even before the first-due extrication team arrives at the scene, the officer in charge and every other member of the crew should be sizing up the incident to which they are responding. Prior to arrival, they can analyze whatever information was provided in the initial dispatch. They can also factor in any information they may remember from pre-incident planning visits to the incident location. In some cases, there may be a fully developed operational plan based on pre-incident planning information. This plan may be available to the officer in hard copy or electronically. In any case, the more information that the responding rescue crew has available en route, the better prepared it will be to make the sometimes critical initial decisions once it arrives at the incident scene.

The sections that follow describe the process of completing size-up of an incident. For the purposes of this manual, the steps are drawn out and described in detail. At real incidents, experience and training make this process very quick and decisive in most cases.

Scene Assessment

At extrication incidents, scene assessment involves observing a variety of variables and factoring them into the initial decision-making process. These variables include, but may not be limited to, the following:

- Weather
- Day of the week
- Time of day
- Emergency and nonemergency vehicular traffic approaching and at the scene
- Pedestrians in and around the scene
- Number of vehicles apparently involved
- Apparent hazards

All these variables must be considered by the first-arriving personnel when attempting to see the "big picture" – to make a general assessment of the situation and to decide whether more resources will be needed. On-scene personnel should be assigned to perform those tasks that relate to protecting everyone at the scene – themselves, pedestrians, and trapped patients.

- *Weather* — Inclement weather may have the following effects on an incident:
  — May have contributed to the incident occurring
  — May have an adverse effect on trapped victims
  — May hinder extrication operations
  — Slow the response of emergency vehicles
  — Obscure the vision of others approaching the scene and may make it more difficult for them to stop short of the scene or to proceed around it
  — Cold weather can make trapped victims more susceptible to hypothermia
  — Extremely hot weather can put victims at risk of suffering heat-related conditions and dehydration
  — Temperature extremes can also adversely affect rescue personnel
- *Day of the Week* — An incident that occurs on a weekday may be very different from one occurring on a weekend. Pedestrian and traffic patterns can vary significantly depending upon the day of the week. For example, during the week, many people are either at work or at school during the day, and relatively few are engaged in leisure and recreational activities. However,

on the weekends, the reverse may be true. These variables can seriously affect the volume of traffic to be expected in the vicinity of a particular crash scene.

- *Time of Day* — The time of day can also have a significant effect on an extrication incident. Incidents occurring during the morning or afternoon commute can be very difficult for emergency resources to reach. Traffic may be significantly affected during shift changes at industrial locations. Those incidents occurring at night have the added problems associated with darkness and limited visibility. At certain hours of the day, large numbers of school children might be expected to be walking to and from school. Likewise, heavy pedestrian traffic might be expected around shopping areas, theaters, hospitals, and sports arenas at particular times of the day or night.

- *Vehicular Traffic* — The volume and speed of both emergency and nonemergency vehicular traffic approaching and already at the scene must also be considered as part of scene assessment. While it is important for emergency vehicles to reach the scene and quickly as safely possible, excessive speed and/or overly aggressive driving by emergency vehicle operators can cause additional collisions. Regardless of how well emergency vehicle operators drive, the greater the volume of traffic, the slower the response is likely to be. These possible delays must be factored into the initial size-up.

- *Pedestrians* — Pedestrians at the scene of an incident may be curious spectators drawn to the scene or witnesses who saw the incident and can contribute valuable information during the extrication operations and/or during the subsequent investigation. They may also be occupants of involved vehicles who were able to free themselves from the wreckage. In any case, they need to be protected, and their presence needs to be factored into the initial scene assessment.

- *Vehicles Involved* — While a detailed assessment of each involved vehicle is part of a later step in the size-up process, observing the number of vehicles involved is a part of scene assessment **(Figure 2.4)**. This, too, is part of the process of seeing the "big picture." Obviously, the initial assessment will be very different if the incident involves a single automobile or one that involves multiple vehicles and/or multiple victims.

- *Hazards* — Hazards at an incident will dictate the types of responders needed such as foam application apparatus or law enforcement or haz mat teams. There are a number of possible hazards that could place those at the scene in some danger such as the following:
  - Leaking fuels and/or other flammable or combustible liquids
  - Traffic/crowd control
  - Downed power lines or broken power poles
  - Hazardous materials spilled at the scene

Vehicle/Equipment Assessment

The second step in the initial size-up of extrication incidents involves a more detailed assessment of the vehicles and equipment involved than was done as part of scene assessment.

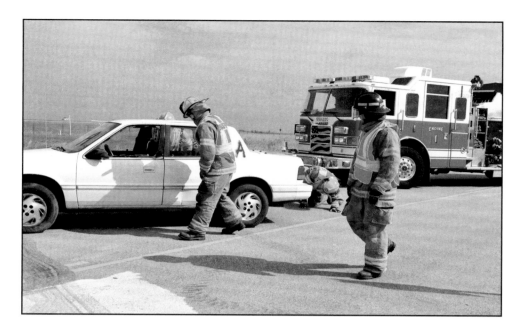

Figure 2.4 Rescuers beginning an assessment of the vehicles at an accident scene. *Courtesy of Sonrise Photography.*

As a suggested minimum, rescue personnel should attempt to determine the number of vehicles/equipment involved, the size/type of vehicles/equipment involved, and condition of each vehicle/equipment.

Each vehicle involved in the incident must be assessed in terms of its position, stability, and condition, in that order.

- *Position* — Is the vehicle or piece of equipment upright, on its side, or upside down? Is it in some other position, such as partially over or under another vehicle or object?

- *Stability* — Determination of the vehicle as stable or not; if not, what will be required to stabilize it. The following are important question to ask when considering stability:

  — Is the vehicle on a stable surface and just needs to be chocked or cribbed, or is it teetering on the brink of a cliff or other precipice?

  — Will jacks, cribbing, step chocks, and/or shoring suffice, or will ropes, chains, or webbing be required to secure it?

  — Will it require a four- or six-point crib, or will the cable from a tow truck's winch be needed?

- *Condition* — Depending upon the sizes and types of vehicles or equipment involved, the speed of impact and other variables, they may look significantly different than it did a moment before the collision. For example, a passenger vehicle accident may have the following conditions depending upon the type of impact:

  — *Front-impact collision* — may "accordion" the engine compartment and the rest of the front end straight back or to one side or the other, making it difficult to locate and disconnect the battery; may also displace the dashboard and steering column rearward into the passenger compartment, along with one or both kick panels. The doors may be jammed shut. The windshield and other windows may or may not be intact. Fuel, coolant, and hydraulic fluid may be leaking from the engine compartment.

— *Rear-end collision* — rear fenders and trunk may be crumpled, and there may be heavy fuel leaks if the tank has been punctured. The valves and piping associated with an LPG tank may have been damaged and are allowing flammable gas to leak.

— *Side-impact collision* — chassis may or may not be in one piece. The chassis may be wrapped around whatever it came into contact with. The doors on the impact side may be seriously damaged and virtually inaccessible, while the doors on the opposite side may be fully functional.

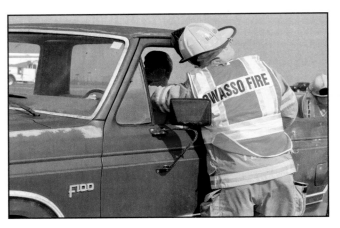

Figure 2.5 A rescuer assessing a patient.

Assessment of Patients

The next step in the initial assessment of an extrication incident involves a more detailed assessment of the trapped patients than was done during vehicle or equipment assessment. There should be a sufficient number of personnel on scene initially to allow this process to occur simultaneously with the vehicle/equipment assessment.

Depending upon the dynamics, there may be one or more patients outside of the involved vehicles. They may have been pedestrians struck by one of the vehicles, or vehicle occupants who were ejected from one of the vehicles. In any case, they must be located and assessed as soon as possible.

The initial assessment of those trapped inside a vehicle ideally should not be performed until it is stabilized **(Figure 2.5)**. This precaution is necessary to prevent sudden and unexpected movement of the vehicle as a result of rescue personnel entering and moving around inside the vehicle. A risk/benefit decision must be made for each incident based upon the conditions found. Each individual incident will dictate whether personnel enter the vehicle to perform emergency medical procedures prior to stabilization or after stabilization. To the extent possible under these circumstances, rescue personnel must attempt to determine how many victims are trapped in each vehicle and the apparent condition of each victim.

Rescuers should ask the following types of questions in order be fully informed when they engage in the final size-up step, extrication assessment:

● What do the patients' major injuries appear to be?

● Are they wedged under the dashboard and/or entangled in the foot pedals?

● Are they conscious or unconscious?

● Can they communicate, or are they dazed and disoriented?

● Are they bleeding, and if so, how profusely?

● Are they breathing, and if so, is it nearly normal or very labored?

● Are their limbs in a normal position, or are they contorted?

● Are a sufficient number of ambulances on scene or en route, or are additional ones needed?

Triage Considerations

The authority having jurisdiction should have an established policy regarding the uniform method for conducting an initial evaluation of patients during vehicle accidents, multiple casualty incidents, or disaster. Each jurisdiction should establish the emergency medical training and operational requirements for its personnel.

Generally, initial triage will be conducted by individual first responders using categories such as Immediate, Delayed, Minor, and Dead/Non-salvageable. Standardized tags that are color coded to match the four levels of care should be used during triage. One specific triage method is *Simple Triage and Rapid Treatment (START)*. START evaluates a patient's respiratory, circulatory and neurological function and then categorizes the patient in one of the four care categories. The START method is recommended for use by first-arriving responders for initial and secondary field triage. Initial triage takes precedence over any emergency treatment at the incident scene. Triage team members should limit any emergency care they provide to opening the patient's airway, controlling severe bleeding, and elevating patients' lower extremities. Personnel working in treatment areas shall perform secondary triage and annotate any additional injuries or conditions found on the patient's triage tag.

Rescue personnel should attempt to determine the following:

- Number of patients inside of the vehicles
- If patients are injured or merely trapped
- Each patient's individual medical priority
- Any additional transportation resources (additional ambulances, medevac helicopter, etc.) that may be needed

Extrication Assessment

The next step in the process of sizing up an extrication incident involves an assessment of what will be needed to safely and quickly extricate the trapped victims. This step will provide the incident commander (IC) with the final information needed to make critical decisions regarding operational priorities and how available resources can be used to best advantage.

The vehicle assessment step in the size-up process attempts to determine what actions will be needed to extricate those trapped in the vehicle. The following are just a small sampling of questions that can aid an IC in making decisions about an extrication:

- Are flammable or toxic materials leaking or spilled?
- Do the vehicle's windshield and/or windows need to be removed?
- Do the vehicle's doors need to be forced open or removed?
- Does the roof need to be flapped forward or backward or removed all together?

The IC must also assess what equipment and resources are necessary and available to properly and safely execute the extrication. Given all the information supplied by all the steps in the size-up process, the IC must determine

Simple Triage and Rapid Treatment (START) — Triage evaluation method for checking respiratory, circulatory and neurological function with the intention of categorizing patients in one of the four care categories: Immediate, Delayed, Minor, and Dead/Non-salvageable. The START method is recommended for use by first-arriving responders for initial and secondary field triage.

Incident Commander (IC) — Person in charge of the incident management system and responsible for the management of all incident operations during an emergency.

what personnel and equipment resources are needed to provide fire protection and/or hazard mitigation, victim care and management, and the needed extrication operations. If those resources are not already at the scene or en route, they must be requested immediately.

As a suggested minimum, rescue personnel should attempt to determine the following:

- How to stabilize the involved vehicles
- How to gain access to the trapped patients
- How to free the trapped patients
- Any additional resources (cutting tools/equipment, cranes, booms, air supply, lighting equipment, etc.) that may be needed

Resource Assessment

Successful resource assessment begins with a good size up. Perform your primary size up of the scene. Think to yourself what has happened. What is happening? What is likely to happen? With this information assess is the apparatus and personnel in route, or on scene going to be enough to mitigate the incident. Are the correct agencies, such as a designated rescue, an ambulance, highway maintenance department, and law enforcement responding? Good assessments are continuously ongoing during the incident.

Patient Removal Assessment

There are two basic approaches to removing a patient from a vehicle.

- Normal Extrication — Removing the vehicle and equipment away from the patient. Normal extrication may include applying a cervical spine stabilization device and a short spine board (or a vest-like immobilization system) before moving the patient. Once these are in place, the patient is then moved onto a long backboard and strapped to it. The long backboard is placed onto a stretcher and secured to the stretcher prior to moving the patient to the ambulance.

- Rapid Extrication — Removing the patient from the vehicle. Rapid Extrication is used only in emergency situations in which the lives of the patient and, possibly, the rescuers are in danger. The rescuers should apply cervical stabilization and maintain such stabilization manually until the patient is positioned on a backboard. The patient should then be strapped securely to the backboard and the backboard secured to the stretcher prior to moving the patient to the ambulance.

Outside Assistance

The IC cannot be expected to be an expert on every aspect of every extrication situation. Therefore, in the process of assessing the risk/benefit of a number of possible extrication alternatives, he or she should obtain whatever expert assistance is necessary. Following are some examples of the types of experts whose advice the IC may need during extrication incidents:

- Structural or mechanical engineers
- Chemists or hazardous materials specialists
- Railroad officials

- Farmers or agricultural extension agents
- Industrial plant maintenance or engineering personnel
- Elevator mechanics or building engineers
- Mine, cave, or tunnel rescue experts
- Heavy equipment operators
- Construction engineers
- Physicians
- Military specialists

Experts or professionals in a specialized field can be brought to the incident command post (ICP) to advise the IC. These resources may be able to better predict the consequences of a particular action and to suggest alternatives. When dealing with unfamiliar situations, an effective IC will take advantage of every resource available. In some cases, it may be advantageous to implement a unified command to more effectively manage the incident.

Incident Command Post (ICP) — Location at which the incident commander and command staff direct, order, and control resources at an incident; may be co-located with the incident base.

Incident Command/Management of Extrication Operations

The purpose of using any form of incident command/management system is to organize an emergency operation so that it can be conducted safely, efficiently and effectively. It is important that the incident command/management system be established as part of the operational routine and that it be used at every incident so that all department personnel become familiar with it. Incident command/management systems are useful to large and small departments alike, but they can be especially beneficial to smaller departments that are not accustomed to working large-scale incidents. Staffing levels, equipment availability, and standard operating procedures determine when and to what extent any command/management system will be implemented at any given incident.

In the United States, the National Incident Management System - Incident Command System (NIMS-ICS) is a mandated command structure. It is designed to be applicable to small, single-team incidents that may last only a few minutes as well as complex, large-scale incidents involving several agencies and many mutual aid responders that could possibly last much longer. IFSTA recommends this system for use in departments that respond to extrication incidents in the United States.

Many extrication organizations have established incident command/management systems that specify who is in command at all times. These generally specify that the first member on the scene, such as a rescuer or a company officer, establishes command by advising the dispatcher that the individual is "establishing (name of incident) command." For example, the officer in charge of the first-arriving emergency response vehicle calls the communications/dispatch center and transmits, "Dispatch, Battalion Seven, I am establishing Olive Street command." If more than one emergency vehicle arrives simultaneously, the senior person usually has this responsibility. The person establishing command has the full authority that goes with the position and remains in command until formally relieved or the incident is terminated.

The first rescuer or apparatus arriving on the scene of an emergency should initiate the incident command/management system. This individual is at least temporarily in command of the incident. If the size-up discussed earlier reveals that the incident management decisions required to make this a successful rescue are beyond the scope of this person's training, command should be transferred at the earliest opportunity to someone more qualified. In the meantime, the initial IC should do whatever the individual is qualified to do, such as initiating a command structure by naming the incident and announcing the location of the command post.

Incident Announcement Example

An actual incident announcement might be as follows:

"Dispatch, Engine 31."

Dispatch answers, "Go ahead, 31."

"We are at the intersection of Riverside and Park where there is a two car collision with two patients. I am establishing Riverside Command. Dispatch extrication and an ALS ambulance to the command post at the southwest corner of Riverside and Park."

Dispatch replies, "Riverside IC, Dispatch copies you need extrication and an ALS ambulance at the southwest corner of Riverside and Park."

If the company on scene is not trained and equipped to begin the extrication, members should begin to stabilize the incident to their level of qualification. This may be limited to cordoning off the area and identifying and isolating any witnesses to the accident. The IC should begin to formulate an incident action plan that reflects the following priorities:

1. Providing for extrication personnel safety and survival

2. Preventing others from becoming patients

3. Rescuing those who can be saved

4. Recovering the remains of those beyond saving

Whenever the command/management system is implemented, there should be only one incident commander, except in multijurisdictional incidents when a unified command is appropriate. Even when a unified command is used, the chain of command must be clearly defined. All orders should be issued by one person through the chain of command to avoid confusion.

If other agencies such as law enforcement are involved, each agency should be familiar with the type of system used by the host agency so they can function properly within its structure. This interagency cooperation and effectiveness can best be accomplished through regular joint-training exercises held as often as necessary, but at least annually.

Industrial Extrication Incidents

In industrial extrication incidents, company policy may dictate that a company employee, such as the facility manager, must be in charge of anything on company property. But when the expertise and resources of the extrication team are clearly needed, the manager should defer to the IC for the strategic and tactical decisions needed to mitigate the emergency. The manager can act on behalf of the company by advising the IC in the decision-making process and by authorizing the expenditure of company funds.

The IC should assemble enough resources to handle the incident and organize them in a way that will ensure that orders can be carried out promptly, safely, and efficiently. Having sufficient resources at the scene will help to ensure the safety of all involved. The organization must be structured so that all available resources can be utilized to achieve the goals of the IAP. If necessary, the IC can appoint a command staff to help gather, process, and disseminate information. Initially, establishing a formal ICP may not be necessary. However, it is recommended to at least designate the first-arriving emergency vehicle as the incident command post until it is determined whether a formal ICP is needed. If the incident involves multiple emergency vehicles and it appears that it will be a protracted operation, a formal, easily identified incident command post should be established.

All incident personnel must function according to the incident action plan. Personnel should function according to the department's SOPs, but every action should be directed toward achieving the goals and objectives specified in the plan.

Components of an Extrication Operation

Extrication incidents can be as simple as a single car accident with a trapped but uninjured patient to a multicar pileup with multiple trapped and injured patients. Depending on the nature and the scope of the incident, different levels of incident management will be needed. The entire incident command/management organization does not need to be implemented on every incident. Only the parts of the system should be used that are needed to handle that particular incident safely and efficiently and that make managing that incident easier.

When a relatively simple extrication incident occurs, a formal command/management system may not be needed to handle the incident safely and effectively. However, it is good practice for the officer in charge of the first (and perhaps only) apparatus at an incident to formally assume command as part of the initial report of conditions upon arrival. This keeps incident command/management in the forefront and makes for a smooth transition from handling a single-apparatus incident to managing a larger and more complex incident with a command/management system. The more that people practice using a command/management system on the simple day-to-day incidents, the more likely they are to use it effectively on the significant impact incident.

Not all extrication incidents will be simple, and the size and complexity of the incident organization should reflect the size and complexity of the incident.

When a relatively small incident develops into a larger and more complex one, command may have to be transferred several times as the organization grows to meet the need. It is important that the transitions be made as smoothly and as efficiently as possible. The sections that follow introduce the reader to various components that may be portions of an extrication incident.

Command and Control

After an initial size-up, the IC must decide how to deploy the available resources. Under the rescue command and control category, there are several ways in which the IC can subdivide the resources into functional groups within the chain of command. These groups may vary from incident to incident or from agency to agency, but in general, those most commonly used are as follows:

- Scene control
- Vehicle stabilization
- Patient access and disentanglement
- Medical treatment
- Extrication
- Triage/treatment
- Transportation
- Shelter and thermal control for protection of patients
- Rehabilitation of the incident responders

The typical extrication incident command chart looks similar to other incident command charts, except that the titles of some of the components are different. The system by which the functional groups and geographic divisions are organized should meet the specific needs of the particular extrication operation. The typical rescue scene organization may have to be modified according to the demands of a specific incident and to the needs, capabilities, and limitations of the agencies involved.

Within the limits of span-of-control, the IC is responsible for the actions and coordination of these groups. On relatively small incidents, the IC can and should stay in constant contact with the supervisors of the groups and make certain they are performing and interacting properly. On larger, more complex incidents, an Operations Section Chief (Ops) should be appointed to coordinate the operations of the various functional groups.

Incident Operation Groups and their Responsibilities

Effective management strategies must be employed in order to handle both small and large incidents, and the use of an incident command/management system to assign functional groups should facilitate the task. Preparation is vital in order to achieve good results. It is important that extrication personnel train and work within this system regularly so that company members become and stay familiar with it.

Each group should have one person in charge, a group supervisor, to see that all of its assigned responsibilities are completed. The group supervisor is also responsible for coordinating through the chain of command with the IC and with other group. Group supervisors, as well as the IC and all other position specialists, should be easily identifiable to personnel on the scene. Wearing colored vests (labeled with the position titles) over protective clothing and marking a specific location or vehicle as the incident command post are the generally accepted ways of promoting easy identification.

The sections that follow describe the activities associated with common operations groups that may be formed and active and extrication incidents.

Extrication Group

The responsibilities of the Extrication Group vary with the type, magnitude, and complexity of the situation. In general, its duties are as follows:

- Determine the number, location, and condition of the patient(s) both alive and otherwise
- Evaluate the resources required for the extrication of trapped patients and/or the recovery of bodies
- Stabilize the vehicle(s)
- Determine whether treatment is necessary and if it can be safely delivered on-site or if patients will have to be moved before treatment; if necessary, move patients to the triage/treatment area(s)
- Advise the IC (through the chain of command) of resource requirements
- Allocate and supervise resources assigned to the extrication function
- Perform disentanglement to extricate patients
- Report progress to the IC, and give an "all clear" signal when all of the patients have been removed
- Coordinate with other groups through the chain of command.

Medical Group

There are generally three functions that the Medical branch or group performs:

- *Triage* — Responsible for the assessment and categorizing of patients based upon the seriousness of their injuries
- *Treatment* — Provides on-scene, prehospital care
- *Transport* — Responsible for delivering patients from the scene to the appropriate medical facility

Those requiring treatment should be stabilized and continually monitored until they are transported to a medical facility. Separate areas should be set up for those with the most serious injuries (immediate treatment), those with less serious injuries (delayed treatment), and those with minor injuries (minor treatment). The Treatment Supervisor should advise the Transportation Group Supervisor (if one has been appointed) of the number of patients in the immediate-, delayed-, and minor-treatment categories so that appropriate transportation can be arranged.

The responsibilities of the Medical branch or group can be summarized as follows:

- Triage patients and continually evaluate their condition
- Determine the resources needed to treat and transport patients, and advise the IC through the chain of command

Immediate Treatment — Classification for patients with the most serious injuries at an incident and will require packaging and movement to a health care facility as soon as possible

Delayed Treatment — Classification for patients with serious but not life threatening injuries; these patients may need additional care but may not need that care immediately

Minor Treatment — Classification for patients with minor injuries; they may simply require first aid and may even be able to be transported to medical facilities in private vehicles without the care of EMS staff

- Identify and establish suitable treatment areas located near an easily accessible pickup point for immediate-, delayed-, and minor-treatment categories; advise the IC of these areas

- Assign and coordinate resources to provide suitable treatment for patients

- Determine transportation priorities and communicate this information to the Transportation Supervisor and/or the IC. If local protocols allow, patients in the minor-treatment category may be able to use public transportation or be transported by private vehicle.

- Maintain an accurate record of patients and where they are transported in the absence of Transportation

- Keep the IC informed of progress/problems

- Coordinate with other groups/sectors through the chain of command

Transportation Group

The Transportation Group is responsible for taking stabilized patients to the appropriate medical facilities. In order to do its job properly, the Transportation Group/Sector must coordinate with the Treatment Group. Generally, transportation will not be the job of the rescue unit but most likely will be handled by the emergency medical organization within the jurisdiction of the incident. This does not mean that fire/rescue personnel should not be involved in the operation of the Transportation Group. On the contrary, appropriate personnel should be assigned to this group/sector to coordinate with other groups/sectors and with those providing the transportation. The responsibilities of the Transportation Group are as follows:

- Determine transportation requirements (based on data from the Treatment Group) and the availability of ambulances and other methods of transportation

- Report progress and additional resource requirements to the IC

- Identify ambulance staging and loading areas and determine helicopter landing zones if applicable

- Verify the patient-handling capabilities of the medical facilities that are to receive the patients

- Determine the specific entry and exit locations from the triage/treatment area(s)

- Coordinate the order of patient transportation and medical facility allocation with the Treatment Group

- Notify hospitals of incoming patients and their condition

- Maintain a record of where each patient is taken

- Establish a means for transporting ambulatory patients

- Coordinate with other groups/sectors through the chain of command

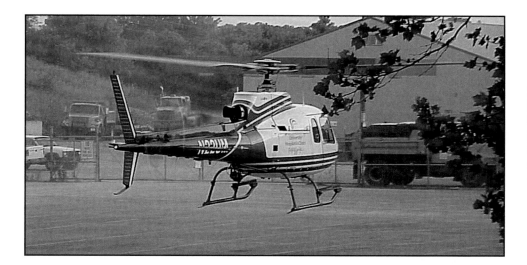

Figure 2.6 Medical evacuation helicopters save valuable time in transporting critically injured patients to medical facilities. *Courtesy of Alan Braun, University of Missouri Fire and Rescue Training Institute.*

Air Transportation

If helicopters are to be used to transport patients from the scene to medical facilities, the Transportation Group is responsible for setting up the landing zone. Personnel should locate the largest open area that is as close as possible to the scene. Appropriate sites might include parking lots, open fields, highways, or median strips. The unobstructed open area should be at least 70 x 70 feet (21 m by 21 m) during the daytime and 100 x 100 feet (30.5 m x 30.5 m) at night, with no more than a 2 percent slope. Helicopters rarely land straight down or take off straight up, so the area surrounding the landing zone should be clear of tall obstructions **(Figure 2.6)**. The landing zone should be well marked so it is clearly visible to the pilot. Any objects that will not be blown about by the downdraft and that contrast starkly with the color of the landing surface may be used for this purpose. Flares may also be used if there is no danger of them starting fires. Hand lights or vehicle headlights may be used at night.

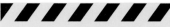

CAUTION
During night operations, personnel should never shine lights toward an operating helicopter, whether it is aloft or on the ground.

Shelter and Thermal Control

Inclement weather can be an issue at any extrication incident. In extremes of heat or cold or during heavy precipitation (rain, snow, or sleet), extended vehicle extrication operations pose a risk to rescuers and patients alike. Personnel at a vehicle accident may experience heat related stress during the summer months or suffer hypothermia or frostbite during the winter. It is important that rescuers in such situations be outfitted properly (dress appropriately for the weather conditions) and rotated into sheltered areas on a routine basis to prevent such injuries.

Large tents, canopies, gazebos, and temporary shelters often used for establishing rehab or personnel decontamination areas may also be used to provide cover and protection from the sun or precipitation. Covered trailers and air-conditioned apparatus cabs may be used to provide shelter from the elements. Portable heating and cooling units may be used to provide temperature control inside enclosed temporary structures or trailers. In the absence of portable structures, pre-existing permanent structures such as houses, storage facilities, auditoriums, barns, gymnasiums, or other structures may be used if located near the incident.

Patients may also need such protection. Whenever necessary, rescuers should make every effort to protect accident patients from inclement weather conditions. This may include using salvage covers or rapidly erected canopies to divert precipitation from the patient or to prevent direct contact by sunlight. Blankets and heating or cooling packs may be used to control the temperature directly around the patient.

The authority having jurisdiction should identify the need for such resources during pre-incident planning. If needed, these resources should be purchased and stored in such a manner that they are readily accessible for use at an incident. If it not possible to purchase these resources, every opportunity should be made to establish an aid agreement with an organization that possesses them.

Apparatus Placement

Proper placement of apparatus at emergency scenes can be an important part of safe and effective extrication operations. Vehicles that need to be closest to the operation should be positioned as such. However, a clear path of entry and egress should be left clear for additional apparatus in case needs and responsibilities during the incident change. Apparatus, such as engine companies, that do not need to be close to the rescue area should leave room for later-arriving EMS and rescue vehicles. Rescue vehicles need to be close enough to the scene to operate effectively, especially if these apparatus are used to supply electrical power or operate hydraulic tools. To some extent, those at the scene can be protected by positioning emergency response vehicles between the scene and any oncoming traffic to act as *blocking* or *shadow vehicles* (**Figure 2.7**).

To avoid the danger of being struck by oncoming traffic, rescue personnel should exercise caution when exiting apparatus upon arrival and when working around apparatus to gather tools and equipment for the extrication operation. All personnel should wear some type of reflective vest or protective clothing with reflective elements to make themselves more visible and to help motorists see them in low light conditions.

In keeping with field research and in order to avoid blinding and/or confusing oncoming drivers, many agencies have adopted a policy of shutting off all rear lights (except amber ones) on vehicles positioned in traffic lanes. Most modern fire apparatus are constructed with warning lighting intended to alert motorists to the fact that the apparatus is blocking the traffic lane. But, in all cases, vehicle drivers should follow their agency's protocols regarding emergency lights on vehicles parked at the scene.

Traffic Control

Fire and rescue personnel should be trained in the basics of traffic management and safety. Traffic control devices include signs, channeling devices (traffic cones and flares), lighting devices, and shadow/advance warning vehicles that rescue organizations and personnel should use to help control traffic near an incident (**Figure 2.8, p. 54**). *The Manual on Uniform Traffic Control Devices (MUTCD)* identifies the types of traffic control devices that should be used to establish work

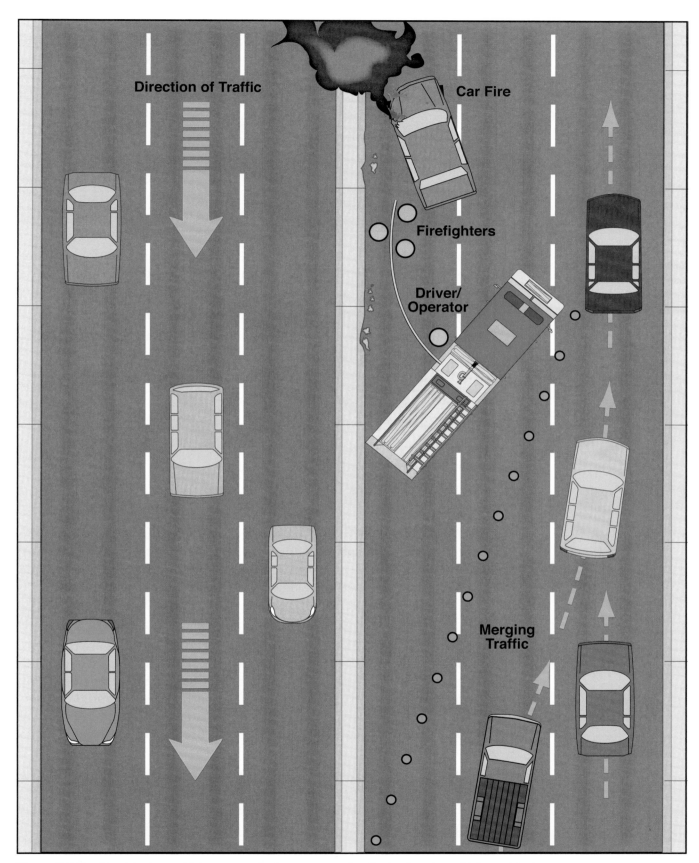

Figure 2.7 Blocking/shadow vehicles can protect rescuers and patients at motor vehicle accidents.

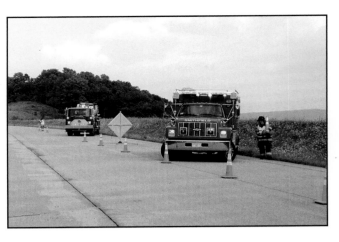

Figure 2.8 Examples of traffic control devices being setup at a motor vehicle accident.

areas and identify incident scenes as well the methods for deploying these devices. The types of traffic control devices used and the methods in which they are applied will depend on the size of the incident, the availability of personnel, and the amount of time spent mitigating the incident.

Upon arrival at a vehicle accident, the IC must determine a number of conditions and factors that will influence traffic control and scene safety. These conditions and factors include but are not limited to the following:

- Type of roadway (single lane, two lane, four lane, etc.)
- Location of the incident in relation to the road (on the road, on the median, on the shoulder, off the road)
- Number of lanes that might need to be closed and their locations
- Length of time that the incident may last
- Volume and speed of oncoming traffic
- Available line of sight leading up to the scene
- Need to restrict, detour, or stop traffic flow
- Available traffic control resources
- Weather and roadway conditions

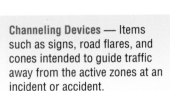

Channeling Devices — Items such as signs, road flares, and cones intended to guide traffic away from the active zones at an incident or accident.

Traffic must be routed into unobstructed lanes around the accident scene to protect rescuers and patients during extrication operations. While shutting down the roadway may be the only safe option, every effort should be made to detour traffic around the accident site, if possible.

The IC must then determine if the available resources are sufficient for the incident or if further resources from mutual aid organizations, law enforcement departments, or Department of Transportation agencies are required. After appropriately positioning responding apparatus, the IC must determine what traffic control devices and methods will be utilized. The emergency responder or responders positioning traffic control devices should wear reflective clothing or vests. While positioning these devices, these personnel should be extremely cautious and constantly observe traffic around them to prevent being struck by on-coming vehicles.

Many of the signs now used by emergency responders are of the collapsible type that are small, easy to carry, and easy to erect. Common warning signs used during vehicle extrication operations include:

- Accident/Emergency Ahead **(Figure 2.9a)**
- Right/Left Lane Closed **(Figure 2.9b)**
- Be Prepared to Stop **(Figure 2.9c)**
- The Flagger Symbol **(Figure 2.9d)**

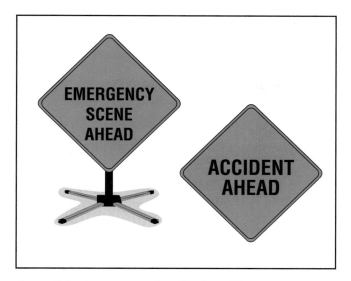

Figure 2.9a An example of an "Accident/Emergency Ahead" warning sign.

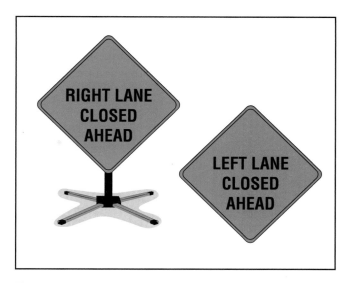

Figure 2.9b This sign lets oncoming traffic know that the "Right (or Left) Lane" is closed ahead.

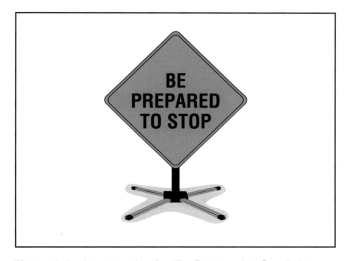

Figure 2.9c An example of a "Be Prepared to Stop" sign.

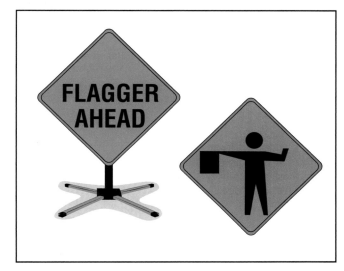

Figure 2.9d The "Flagger Symbol" sign.

These signs should be positioned well in advance of the accident site, on the right side of the roadway (no closer than 24 inches [610mm] from the road edge) facing oncoming traffic **(Table 2.1)** A combination of signs may be employed to warn oncoming traffic of the emergency ahead.

Table 2.1 Recommended Spacing Distances for Advance Warning Signs			
Type of Road	Distances Between Advanced Warning Signs**		
	A	B	C
Urban – low speed*	100 ft (30 m)	100 ft (30 m)	100 ft (30 m)
Urban – high speed*	350 ft (100 m)	350 ft (100 m)	350 ft (100 m)
Rural	500 ft (150 m)	500 ft (150 m)	500 ft (150 m)
Freeway/Expressway	1,000 ft (300 m)	450 ft (1,500 m)	2,640 ft (800 m)

*   Highway agency determines speed category.
**   **Dimension A:** Distance from transition/restriction point to first sign.
      Dimension B: Distance from first sign to second.
      Dimension C: Distance from second sign to third. The third sign is the furthest from the transition/restriction point and the first sign an oncoming driver will approach.

Based on information found in the Manual of Uniform Traffic Control Devices for Streets and Highways, 2003 edition, Part 6, Chapter 6C.

Next, a flagger or flaggers should be used to direct, slow, or stop traffic as needed. The flagger(s) may use a Stop/Slow paddle, red or orange flag, or red wand or flare to direct traffic. Flaggers should exercise extreme care during flagging operations. Some general rules for flaggers to follow include:

Flaggers — Individuals at incident sites whose responsibility it is to control the speed, direction, and flow of traffic.

● Wearing reflective protective clothing or a reflective vest

● Standing on the shoulder of the roadway where the flagger will be visible to oncoming traffic but not directly in front of such traffic

● Identifying an escape route to ensure personal safety

● Positioning the flagger based on the speed of traffic flow **(Table 2.2)**

● Using light wands or flares during darkness

● Monitoring the flow of traffic and movement of vehicles at all times

If adequate time, resources, and personnel are available, traffic channeling devices such as traffic cones, reflective triangles, flashing lights, and/or flares (if they do not pose an additional fire hazard) may be used. The devices used should be positioned in a tapered line from the edge of the roadway on the side of the accident to the edge of the clear lane or lanes of traffic. This taper establishes a transition area for on-coming traffic to move in the desired direction and transition away from the lane where the accident vehicles, responding apparatus, rescuers, and patient are. The taper should be at least 50 feet (15 m) long except on 4-lane roads with speed limits of 55 miles per hour (89 kph) or higher where the taper should be at least 100 feet (30 m) long. A minimum of six cones or reflective devices should be used. The longer the taper, the more traffic control devices should be used. The first taper cone should be placed just behind the flagger along the inner edge of the pavement or the pavement edge marker line. The next device is placed several feet closer to the accident site and a couple of feet further into the traffic lane. This process is continued until all cones are positioned forming the taper (**Figure 2.10, p. 58**).

If needed and available, warning vehicles with flashing or reflective arrows may be used to redirect traffic. Generally, these types of vehicles are highway department vehicles. Warning vehicles should be positioned well ahead of the incident scene to warn oncoming traffic of the incident.

Control Zones

Proper scene management reduces congestion and confusion around the extrication incident. The most common method of organizing a rescue scene is to establish three operating zones, commonly labeled "restricted," "limited access," and "support" (**Figure 2.11, p. 59**). Control at smaller incidents may be as simple as cordoning a particular area as the only zone where activity is happening.

Restricted (Hot) Zone

The restricted zone is where the rescue is taking place. Only personnel who are dealing directly with treating or freeing the patients are allowed in the restricted (also called the hot) zone. This limits crowding and confusion at the scene. The size of this zone may vary greatly depending upon the nature and extent of the rescue problem.

Limited Access (Warm) Zone

This zone is immediately outside of the restricted zone. Access to this zone should be limited to personnel who are not needed in the restricted zone but who are directly aiding rescuers in the restricted zone, such as firefighters preparing/staging hydraulic tool power units, providing emergency lighting, and standing by on hoselines.

Support (Cold) Zone

This zone surrounds the previously described zones. This area may include the ICP, the incident information officer's (PIO) location, and staging areas for personnel and portable equipment. Additional rescuers and other resources are staged in this zone until needed in the limited access or restricted zones. The outer boundary of this area should be cordoned off from the public. An entry/egress corridor should be established to control the movement of vehicles and personnel into and out of the controlled areas.

Table 2.2
Flagger Positioning (Traffic Speed and Stopping Sight Distances)

SPEED*		STOPPING SIGHT DISTANCE	
mph	kph	feet	meters
20	32	115	35
25	40	155	47
30	48	200	61
35	56	250	76
40	64	305	93
45	72	360	110
50	80	425	130
55	89	495	151
60	97	570	174
65	105	645	197
70	113	730	223
75	121	820	250

* Posted speed, off-peak 85th-percentile speed prior to work starting, or the anticipated operating speed.

Based on information found in the Manual of Uniform Traffic Control Devices for Streets and Highways, 2003 edition, Part 6, Chapter 6E.

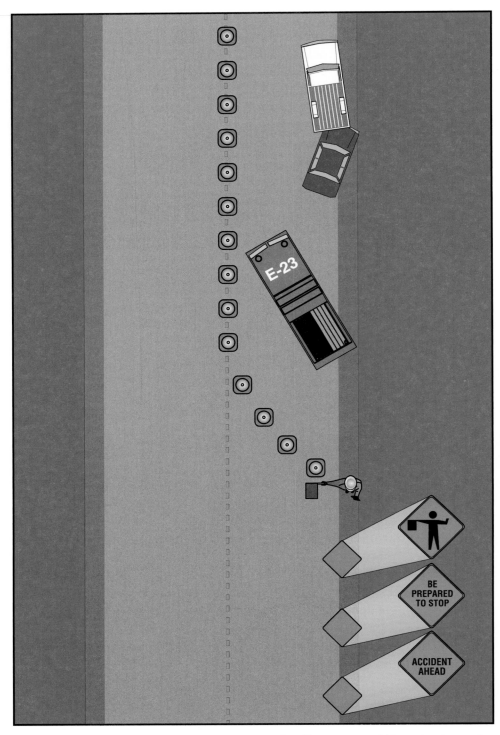

Figure 2.10 An example of how warning signs and traffic cones would be setup to create a traffic channeling taper.

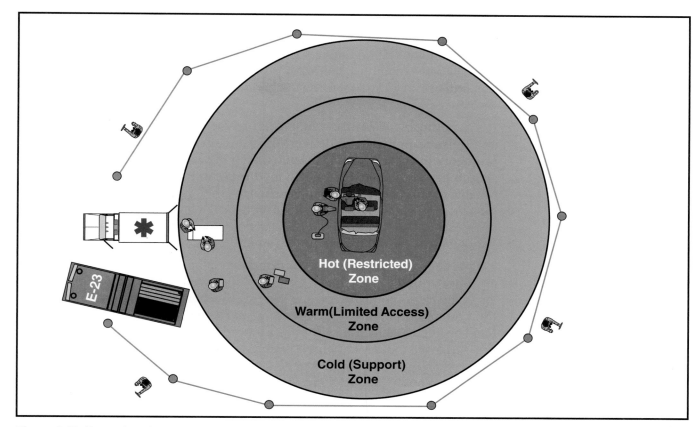

Figure 2.11 Examples of emergency control zones.

Cordoned Area

In smaller incidents where no evacuation is necessary, cordoning off the area keeps bystanders a safe distance from the scene and out of the way of emergency personnel. There is no specific distance or area that should be cordoned off. The zone boundaries should be established taking into account the amount of area needed by emergency personnel to work, the degree of hazard presented by elements involved in the incident, and the general topography of the area. Cordoning can be done with rope or warning tape tied to signs, utility poles, parking meters, or any other fixed objects readily available. However, the material used to cordon off the scene should not be tied to vehicles that may need to be moved during the incident. Once the area has been cordoned off, the boundary should be monitored to make sure that unauthorized people do not cross the line.

Crowd Control

Crowd control is essential to managing a well-organized extrication operation. This function is usually the responsibility of the law enforcement agency at the scene, but it may sometimes have to be performed by firefighters or other rescue personnel. It is the responsibility of the IC to ensure that the scene is secured and properly managed.

Evacuation Routes

At some incidents, evacuation may be necessary. Depending on the number of people involved and their condition, evacuation can be relatively simple or it can be a very complex operation. After it has been determined that evacuation is necessary, the first thing the incident commander must decide is what area needs to be cleared.

The key to a successful evacuation is pre-incident planning. The authorities and those responsible for delivering rescue service should have established protocols and procedures for various levels of evacuation. Contingency plans should be established for small-, medium-, and large-scale evacuations. A reliable means of notifying people when to evacuate should be included in the plan. Arrangements should be made with local television and radio stations to broadcast evacuation orders and instructions. Law enforcement and emergency management personnel can be extremely helpful in evacuations.

Evacuees should be given clear directions as to where they should relocate and approximately how long they will be displaced. Those who cannot evacuate themselves should be assisted in doing so. Some people may refuse to leave their homes or businesses. Depending on the reason for the evacuation and local protocols, they may either be allowed to stay or they may be placed in protective custody by law enforcement personnel and forced to leave. Where established evacuation plans exist for specific occupancies such as nursing homes, schools, industrial facilities, and hotels, these plans can be used to account for those being relocated. Whenever possible, medical monitoring should be available at each relocation site.

Vehicle Extrication Duties

The duties performed during a vehicle extrication operation are generally the same as any other emergency operation, with some possible variations. The sections that follow discuss the steps generally followed at an extrication and are organized in the order that those steps would normally be performed. However, some of these tasks may be performed simultaneously.

Recognizing and Controlling Hazards

The primary hazard at most accidents is the potential for fires though there are other hazards as well. Spilled fuels are common after crashes, and any ignition sources that might ignite those fuels should be recognized and isolated before addressing any other concerns. Open flames are obvious ignition sources and should be extinguished, for example. Others types of hazards include trip hazards, bodily fluids, hazardous materials, and bystanders **(Figure 2.12)**.

Energy sources including downed power lines, vehicle batteries, undeployed air bags, and energy-absorbing struts that may explode if overheated can all provide ignition sources for fires and are commonly found at accidents. Isolating these hazards may require any of the following:

- Identifying and cordoning off any downed wires
- Disconnecting vehicle batteries
- Deactivating undeployed air bags
- Avoiding devices like the pyrotechnic devices for seat belt pretensioners
- Protecting shock absorbers and bumper struts from excessive heat and/or physical damage

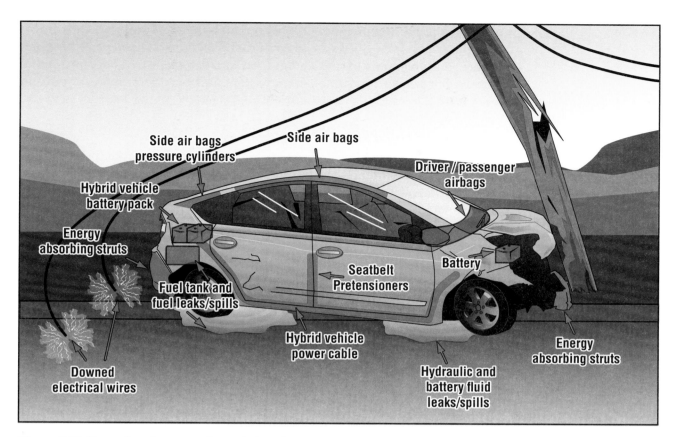

Side air bags pressure cylinders

Side air bags

Driver / passenger airbags

Hybrid vehicle battery pack

Energy absorbing struts

Fuel tank and fuel leaks/spills

Seatbelt Pretensioners

Battery

Hybrid vehicle power cable

Downed electrical wires

Hydraulic and battery fluid leaks/spills

Energy absorbing struts

Figure 2.12 Examples of common hazards found at a motor vehicle and extrication scene.

Biohazard Concerns

Body fluids or biohazards resulting from patient injuries may be encountered during extrication operations and can contaminate the interior and exterior of the vehicle involved. Rescuers should follow the agency's Blood Borne Pathogen procedures and wear appropriate protective clothing and equipment to avoid exposure to these materials. An additional biohazard procedure may be to affix biohazard warning labels to the contaminated vehicle to warn others of the potential hazard. On overturned vehicles, these labels should be affixed so that they can be read by personnel approaching the vehicle.

Given the potential for fires at vehicle crashes, establishing fire protection is almost always indicated. Fire protection can range from someone standing by with a portable fire extinguisher to a number of fully charged hoselines being deployed and foam-making capability set up. Personnel must always follow local protocols, but it is recommended that at least one 1½-inch (38 mm) hoseline be charged and ready for use by at least two firefighters equipped with full PPE including SCBA.

Planning and Performing the Extrication

After ensuring that all potential hazards have been mitigated, rescuers at the scene can complete the size-up of the incident, plan the extrication, and complete it. For the purposes of this manual, many of these quickly drawn judgment calls have been spread out into the sections that follow. With experience, making many of these judgments and decisions will become second nature, but a close description of these steps and considerations is important preparation for making decisions on a real scene.

Determining Initial Patient Considerations

As soon as it is safe to do so, rescue personnel must determine the condition of the patient or patients. The number of patients, their conditions, locations, and positions within a vehicle will have a bearing on the stabilization of the vehicle, methods and sequence of their extrication, as well as their packing and transport to medical care.

Developing the Extrication Plan

Given the information received up to this point of the incident, the command staff can develop an extrication plan for determining the safest methods for:

- Determining what tools and equipment will be needed
- Stabilizing the vehicle
- Identifying which patient should be extricated first, if there is more than one
- Packaging the patient(s)
- Providing emergency medical care during and after extrication
- Extricating the patient or patients

Stabilizing the Vehicle

Stabilizing a vehicle means preventing sudden and unexpected movement of the vehicle in any direction. In other words, keeping the vehicle from suddenly moving horizontally, vertically, or rotationally. Stabilizing a vehicle can be done using a variety of chocks, cribbing, shoring, webbing, ropes, and/or chains.

Determining and Creating Vehicle Access/Egress Points

This means surveying the vehicles in which patients are trapped to determine how best to gain access to the patients and how to remove them once they are properly packaged. This may mean deciding to remove one or more doors, remove or penetrate the roof, make entry/egress through a rear hatch, or any of several other possible actions. Once the decisions regarding where and how to gain access to trapped patients have been made, all that remains is to create those openings. This may involve the use of a variety of manual and/or electric tools, pneumatic and/or hydraulic tools, and/or thermal cutting devices.

Disentangling the Vehicle From the Patients

Once access to trapped patients has been obtained, the work of safely freeing them from entrapment can begin. This may involve manipulating and/or removing the parts of the vehicle that prevent or restrict movement by the patients. Protecting the trapped patients during the disentanglement process is key to a successful operation.

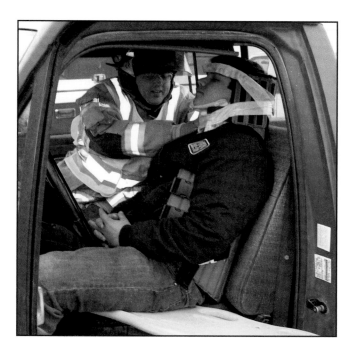

Figure 2.13 A patient being packaged for movement onto a backboard. *Courtesy of Alan Braun, University of Missouri Fire and Rescue Training Institute.*

Removing Packaged Patients

Once patients have been freed from entrapment, they can be safely removed from the wreckage provided that they have been properly packaged for movement **(Figure 2.13)**. Once packaged, patients may be turned over to EMS for transport to an appropriate medical facility.

Terminating the Incident

When all patients have been extricated and they have been treated and released or transported to a medical facility, all that remains is to terminate the incident. However, terminating an incident may be more complicated than it sounds. The objectives of terminating an incident are to restore the scene to as near normal as possible, make it safe for people to occupy, and make it safe for vehicles to drive through. Even after all patients have been dealt with, emergency responders may have to maintain control of the scene because of an ongoing investigation or hazards that have not yet been mitigated.

Restoring the Scene

Once the ranking law enforcement official releases the scene, all wrecked vehicles must be removed. If fuel or other hazardous materials have contaminated the scene, these hazards must be mitigated before the incident can be terminated. Likewise, if power lines and/or poles have been broken, utility company personnel will have to repair the damage (or at least remove the downed lines/poles) before the incident can be terminated. In some cases, such as when one or more vehicles burn during an incident, the roadway surface or other highway features may have been so badly damaged that vehicles cannot safely drive on or near them. Appropriate barricades will have to be placed so that drivers will know to avoid these areas until they can be repaired.

Picking Up and Cleaning Up

After all of these problems have been solved, emergency responders must retrieve the tools and equipment they used during the incident. They must inspect them and make sure that they are ready for use at the next incident. Returning tools and equipment to the apparatus from which they came can be made much easier if all items are clearly marked **(Figure 2.14, p. 64)**.

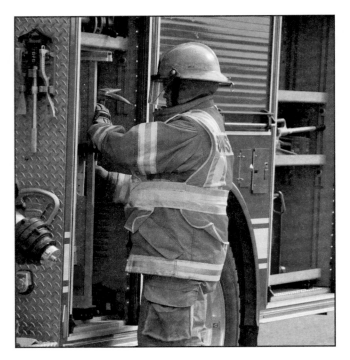

Figure 2.14 Rescuers returning extrication equipment to their emergency vehicle. *Courtesy of Sonrise Photography.*

Restoring Traffic Flow

Traffic control should not be required once the incident is terminated and all debris, damaged vehicles, and emergency vehicle have been removed from the roadway. To restore normal traffic flow through the area, the traffic control components should be removed in reverse order:

- First – Remove all traffic channeling devices.
- Second – Remove the flagger(s).
- Third – Remove the warning signs.

Restoring Operational Readiness

Following an incident, all responding emergency vehicles must be restored to full operational readiness, a process that should include all of the following:

- Reservicing the apparatus' and equipment fuel and agent tanks
- Cleaning tools and equipment
- Conducting post incident inspection, maintenance, and operational checks of tools and equipment
- Repairing or replacing damaged or expended tools and equipment
- Replacing expended extrication and medical materials

Conducting an AAR

After an emergency, the incident should be reviewed from a technical standpoint to see whether future performance can be improved because of anything learned from this incident. An after action report might be conducted prior to leaving the scene of the incident while a more formal critique should be accomplished at the station.

Conducting a Critical Incident Stress Debriefing (CISD)

Personnel who had to deal directly with patients of horrific injuries should be required to attend a professionally conducted critical incident stress debriefing session. Everyone reacts to and deals with traumatic stress in different ways — some more successfully than others. Because emergency responders must train themselves to control their emotions during emergency situations, they sometimes lack an effective way of acknowledging and dealing with the effects of especially traumatic incidents — critical incident stress. Firefighters and other emergency responders sometimes use humor to defuse stress after traumatic incidents, but this is not always effective, and the effects of such stress can build up over time. Left untreated, the effects of critical incident stress can build up over time and lead to a very serious condition known as post-traumatic stress disorder (PTSD). PTSD can produce some debilitating conditions that may be more than just career-threatening; they may be life-threatening. Finally, because firefighters and other emergency responders

Post-Traumatic Stress Disorder (PTSD) — A disorder caused when persons have been exposed to a traumatic event where they have experienced, witnessed, or been confronted with an event or events that involve actual death, threatened death, serious injury, or threat of physical injury to self or others. *Also called post-traumatic stress syndrome.*

may feel that it is a sign of weakness to seek counseling for critical incident stress, those who have had close contact with dead or seriously injured patients should attend a CISD. They should not be required to participate, but they should be required to attend.

Summary

A properly organized and managed extrication incident is a safer extrication incident. This is true for both rescuers and patients alike. Organizing a safe and effective extrication operation actually begins before the incident occurs, in the form of pre-incident planning. This planning results in the development of operational plans and standard operating procedures that help guide emergency response personnel during the incident. If all of this planning is successful, the most appropriate rescue resources will be dispatched to the scene initially, the incident will be sized up correctly, resources will be deployed effectively, and an effective incident command/management system will be used on every extrication incident. Resources invested in planning and training before an incident occurs will usually translate into minimizing injuries and the loss of life during a extrication incident. The final part of organizing an effective extrication operation is providing for incident termination and recovery, including a means of helping extrication personnel cope with the stresses associated with these incidents.

Review Questions

1. Which NFPA standards govern incident management at extrication operations?

2. What are the roles of the incident safety officer, the telecommunicator, and the incident commander in an extrication operation?

3. What assessments are part of the size-up process?

4. Who are examples of outside assistance an incident commander may call upon during an extrication operation?

5. Which document identifies the types of traffic control devices that should be used to establish extrication work areas?

6. What methods are used to deploy traffic control devices at vehicle extrication scenes?

7. What is the purpose of each control zone?

8. What are the steps for planning and performing an extrication operation?

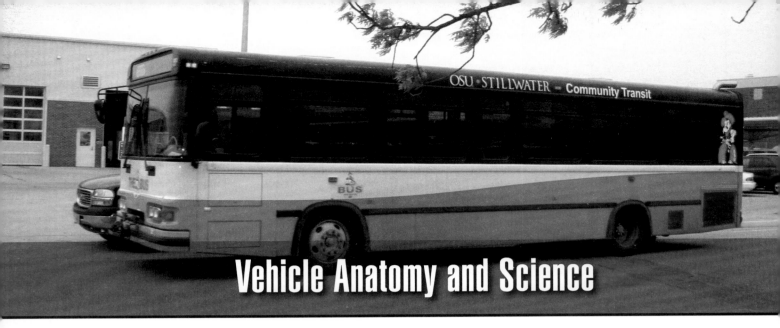

Vehicle Anatomy and Science

Chapter Contents

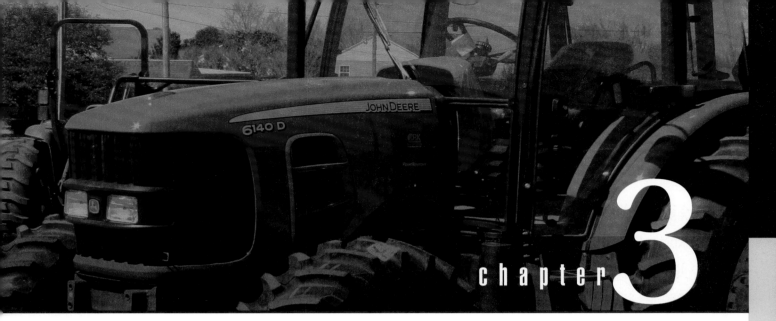

chapter 3

Key Terms

Job Performance Requirements

This chapter provides information that addresses the following job performance requirements (JPRs) of NFPA® 1001, *Standard for Fire Fighter Professional Qualifications* (2008), NFPA® 1006, *Standard for Technical Rescuer Professional Qualifications* (2008), NFPA® 1670, *Standard on Operations and Training for Technical Search and Rescue Incidents* (2009).

NFPA® 1001 JPRs

6.4.1

6.4.2

NFPA® 1006 JPRs

4.3.1	10.1.1	10.1.6
4.3.2	10.1.3	10.1.7
5.2.3	10.1.4	10.2.1
10.1	10.1.5	

NFPA® 1670 JPRs

4.1.4	8.3.4
4.5.1.1	8.4.2
8.2.3	

Vehicle Anatomy and Science

Learning Objectives

1. Describe various vehicle classifications.

2. Explain general vehicle anatomy.

3. Distinguish among the types of vehicle frames.

4. Describe supplemental restraint and rollover protection systems.

5. Identify types of materials used in modern vehicle windows.

6. Identify types of vehicle fuels and fuel systems.

7. Describe vehicle exhaust systems.

8. Identify critical components of vehicle electrical systems.

9. Describe vehicle power train systems.

10. Describe the key vehicle science concepts.

Chapter 3
Vehicle Anatomy and Science

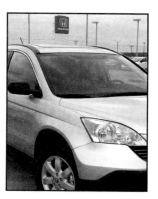

Case History

Numerous reports released in 2008 and 2009 describe a new series of challenges faced by extrication personnel. While extrication personnel strive to remain current in vehicle science and anatomy, improvements in automobile safety and construction have often seriously impacted vehicle extrication operations and techniques. Many new vehicles incorporate reinforced steel and light, strong, exotic metals. While these have resulted in greater safety and survivability for passengers involved in motor vehicles accidents, it has increased the difficulty involved in and time required to extricate patients from damaged vehicles.

Some vehicles built after 2005 are so strongly constructed that extrication times can be two or more times longer than those encountered on older model cars. Extrication tools experience heavy wear and tear during extrication operations on some newer cars. In some instances, hydraulic shears and spreaders were damaged or were unable to defeat vehicle components. Manufacturers of extrication tools and equipment are beefing up their products, but the improvements are often bulkier, heavier, and more expensive. Rescue personnel are constantly developing new techniques and approaches to remain on the "cutting edge" of extrication technology. Vehicle manufacturers are providing vital vehicle construction and safety information to extrication equipment manufacturers and emergency responders.

In order to perform vehicle extrication swiftly and safely, rescue personnel need to be thoroughly trained in vehicle anatomy and science. Vehicle extrication rescuers need to understand the type(s) of vehicle involved, what it is constructed of, and how it is constructed.

This chapter will discuss vehicle classifications, general vehicle anatomy, types of vehicle materials and construction, and vehicle integrity. It will also address supplemental restraint and protection systems, windows, and fuel, electrical, and power train systems. Finally, it will cover vehicle science as it relates to a vehicle's center of gravity and mass, as well as the kinematics of force dissipation.

Vehicle Classifications

Personnel who perform vehicle extrication need to know the different classifications of vehicles and the types of vehicles found in each classification. This knowledge will aid rescuers in determining the hazards, materials, construction, strengths, and weaknesses found in a given vehicle at a vehicle extrication incident.

Passenger Vehicles, Cars, and Light Trucks

Passenger vehicles are motorized vehicles that are designed to carry 10 people or less. This category does not include low-speed vehicles, multipurpose passenger vehicles, trucks (medium and heavy), motorcycles, or trailers **(Table 3.1)**. Light trucks are single unit vehicles with two axles and, generally, four tires that weigh 10,000 lbs (4 536 kg) or less. The passenger cars and light trucks category of vehicles include:

- Microcars
- Subcompacts
- Compacts
- Midsize
- Full size
- Station wagons
- Limousines
- Sports
- Convertibles
- Roadsters
- Kit Cars
- Pickup trucks
- Vans
- Minivans
- Sports utility vehicles (SUVs)
  (formerly called truck-based stationwagons)
- Crossover SUVs
- Utility vehicles
- Smaller motor homes

Medium and Heavy Trucks

Medium and heavy trucks are designed for hauling cargo or serve as the chassis for special vehicles such as fire apparatus and tow trucks. In the United States, medium trucks are defined as weighing between 13,000 lbs (6 300 kg) and 33,000 lbs (15 000 kg). In the United Kingdom the cutoff weight is 7.5 tonnes (16,535 lbs). Common local delivery and garbage trucks are generally medium trucks. Heavy trucks are defined in the US as weighing more than 33,000 lbs (15 000 kg). The axle assemblies of heavy trucks may include two or more axles some of which are powered. Medium and heavy trucks include straight trucks, truck/semitrailer combinations, and specialty trucks **(Table 3.2, p. 73)**.

Straight Trucks

Straight trucks are those trucks in which all of the vehicle's axles are attached to one frame. These vehicles usually have two or three axles some of which are powered and some of which are retractable.

Table 3.1
Examples of Passenger Vehicles, Cars, and Light Trucks

Types	Example	Type	Example
Microcars shown: Smart Fortwo		**Station Wagons** shown: Dodge Magnum Station Wagon	
Subcompacts shown: Honda Fit		**Limousines** shown: Springfield Coach Body on a Mercury Lincoln Town Car Chassis	
Compacts shown: Ford Focus		**Sports** shown: Chevrolet Corvette	
Midsize shown: Honda Accord		**Convertibles** shown: Chrysler PT Cruiser	
Full size shown: Chevrolet Impala		**Roadsters** shown: Pontiac Solstice	

Continued on page 72

Types	Example	Type	Example
Kit Cars **shown:** Locust 7		**Crossover SUVs** **shown:** Dodge Journey	
Pickup Trucks **shown:** Ford F-150		**Utility Vehicles** **shown:** Mitsubishi Mini Truck	
Vans **shown:** Chevrolet Express (15-passenger)		**RV** **shown:** Four Winds RV Body on Ford E350 Chassis	
Minivans **shown:** Dodge Grand Caravan			
Sports Utility Vehicles (SUV's) (formerly called truck-based station wagons) **shown:** Honda Pilot			

Table 3.2
Examples of Medium and Heavy Trucks

Type	Example	
Straight trucks	Straight trucks are those trucks in which all of the vehicle's axels are attached to one frame. These vehicles usually have two or three axles some of which are powered and some of which are retractable.	
Truck/semi trailer combinations	Truck/semi trailer combinations (also called semi-trailer trucks, tractor-trailors, 18-wheelers, semis, or big-rigs in the US; articulater lorries, artics, or truck and trailers in the UK, Ireland and New Zealand; and semis in Austrailia and Canada) are articulated vehicles composed of a motorized tractor designed to pull one or more trailers.	
Specialty trucks	Fire apparatus, Military vehicles, Logging trucks, Large motor homes, Bookmobiles, Medical treatment vehicles, Highway repair vehicles.	

Truck/Semitrailer Combinations

Truck/semitrailer combinations (also called semitrailer trucks, tractor-trailors, 18-wheelers, semis, or big-rigs in the US; articulated lorries, artics, or truck and trailers in the UK, Ireland, and New Zealand; and semis in Australia and Canada) are articulated vehicles composed of a motorized tractor designed to pull one or more trailers. A fifth wheel device, mounted on the truck tractor vehicle, serves as the attachment point for a semitrailer and allows the tractor and trailer to articulate. In some countries, truck tractors may pull more than one trailer.

Specialty Trucks

Specialty trucks are those designed for specific purposes and include but are not limited to the following:

- Fire apparatus **(Figure 3.1)**
- Military vehicles **(Figure 3.2)**
- Logging trucks
- Large motor homes **(Figure 3.3)**
- Bookmobiles
- Medical treatment vehicles **(Figure 3.4)**
- Highway repair vehicles **(Figure 3.5)**

These types of vehicles may be straight trucks or truck/semitrailer combinations.

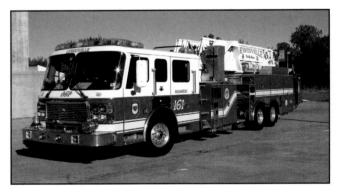

Figure 3.1 Fire apparatus such as this aerial apparatus are an example of one type of specialty truck.

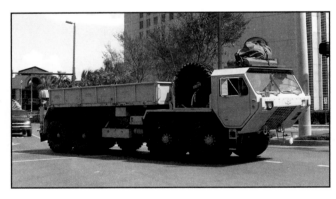

Figure 3.2 This military vehicle is another type of specialty truck. *Courtesy of District Chief Chris Mickal, New Orleans (LA) FD Photo Unit.*

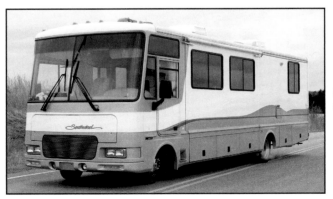

Figure 3.3 Specialty trucks also include large recreational vehicles (RVs).

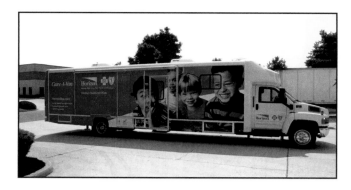

Figure 3.4 This medical treatment van is an example of a specialty truck. *Courtesy of LaBoit, Inc. Special Vehicle Manufacturer.*

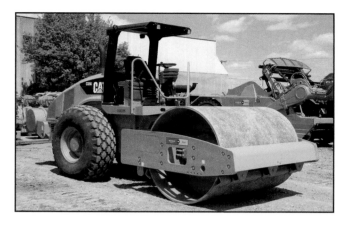

Figure 3.5 Specialty trucks also include highway repair vehicles.

Agricultural Equipment

Rescue personnel need to be familiar with the types of agricultural equipment in their communities, how these vehicles are constructed, and how to perform extrication procedures for each type of vehicle **(Table 3.3, p. 76)**. Examples of common agricultural equipment include but are not limited to:

- Agricultural tractors
- Combines
- Forage harvesters
- Skid steer loaders
- Telehandlers
- Windrowers
- Logging skidder

Buses

Buses are useful in transporting large numbers of people locally and regionally. These vehicles are used to provide rural, city, intercity, and tourism transportation for transporting children to school, people from their homes to work and shopping, and people traveling from city to city. Buses may be straight or articulated. In North America there are four types of school buses, types A, B, C and D. There are also transit, commercial, and specialty buses **(Table 3.4, p. 79)**.

Heavy Equipment and Machinery

Heavy equipment and machinery are used in warehouses, as well as in building and highway construction site work **(Table 3.5, p. 80)**. The massive size, extreme weight, and heavy-duty construction of these vehicles provide additional challenges to extrication operations involving them. This category includes vehicle, such as the following:

- Backhoes
- Bulldozers
- Cement trucks
- Cranes
- Dumpers
- Excavators
- Graders
- Fork lifts
- Loaders
- Scrapers
- Skid steer loaders
- Haul trucks

Table 3.3
Examples of Agricultural Equipment

Type	Example
Agricultural tractors	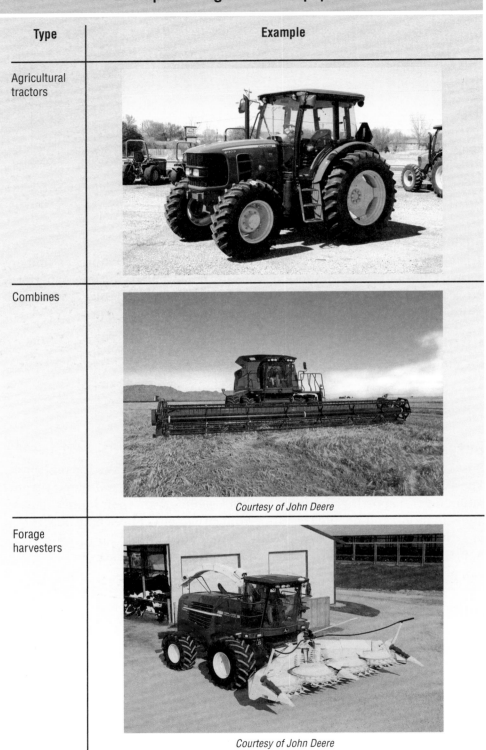
Combines	*Courtesy of John Deere*
Forage harvesters	*Courtesy of John Deere*

Continued on next page

Table 3.3 (Continued)
Examples of Agricultural Equipment

Type	Example
Skid steer loaders	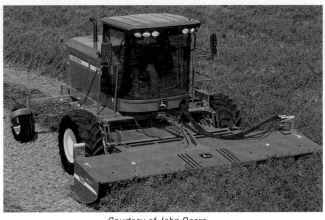 *Courtesy of John Deere*
Telehandlers	
Windrowers	*Courtesy of John Deere*

Continued on next page

Table 3.3 (Continued) Examples of Agricultural Equipment	
Type	**Example**
Logging skidder	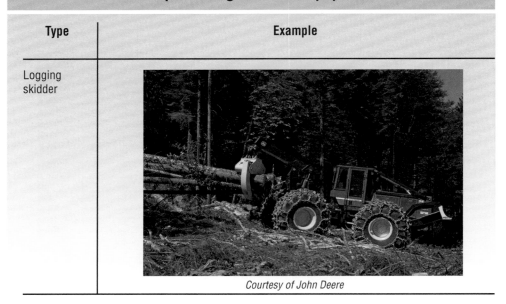 *Courtesy of John Deere*

General Vehicle Anatomy

In order to perform vehicle extrication safely and effectively, rescuers should have a thorough understanding of the materials used in constructing vehicles and various vehicle aspects (or sides) and components. The following sections will serve as an introduction to these topics.

Common Vehicle Terminology

Common terminology is useful, particularly during emergency situations where confusion must be avoided **(Figure 3.6, p. 84)**. From an extrication standpoint, every vehicle can be considered to have eight sides with which rescuers must be concerned. Regardless of the type or size of vehicle, rescuers must observe, evaluate, and deal with all aspects or "sides." The following are common terms used to describe various areas of a vehicle:

- *Roof* — Depending upon how the vehicle came to rest, the roof may be oriented toward one side or may be what the vehicle is resting on. The roof is always called the roof no matter how the vehicle rests. Regardless of which part of the vehicle is facing up, rescuers must be aware of what it means in terms of ease or difficulty of gaining access to the passenger compartment.

- *Undercarriage* — The undercarriage contains the chassis or frame, drive train, and the floor pan.

- *Driver's Side* — The driver's side is always the side with the steering wheel. More often than not, after a vehicle crashes there is someone in the driver's seat, so this is the first place to look for vehicle occupants.

- *Passenger Side* — The passenger side is found opposite of the steering wheel.

Table 3.4
Examples of Bus Types

School Bus Type	Example	Type	Example
A		Transit	
B	No driver's door on left side	Commercial (Charter bus)	
C		Specialty	
D			

Table 3.5
Examples of Heavy Equipment and Machinery

Type	Example
Backhoes	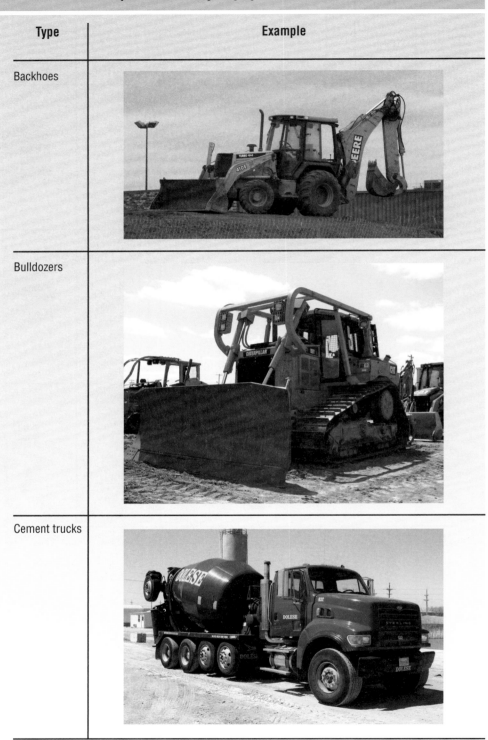
Bulldozers	
Cement trucks	

Continued on next page

Table 3.5 (Continued)
Examples of Heavy Equipment and Machinery

Type	Example
Cranes	
Dumpers	
Excavators	

Continued on next page

Table 3.5 (Continued)

Examples of Heavy Equipment and Machinery

Type	Example
Fork lifts	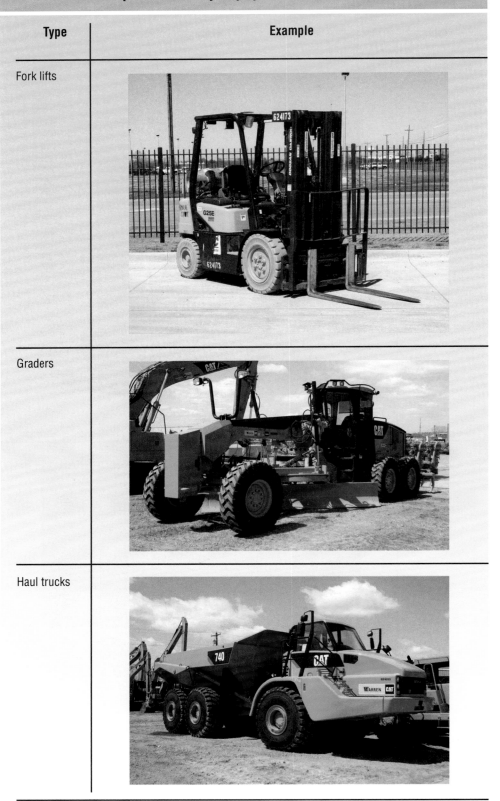
Graders	
Haul trucks	

Continued on next page

Table 3.5 (Continued)
Examples of Heavy Equipment and Machinery

Type	Example
Loaders	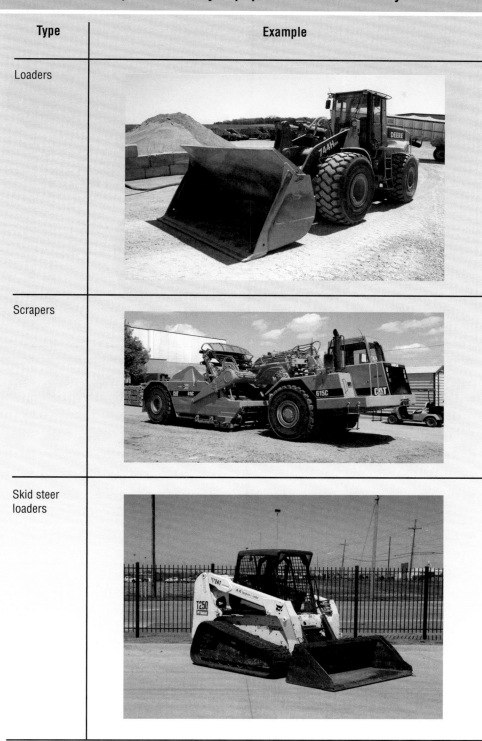
Scrapers	
Skid steer loaders	

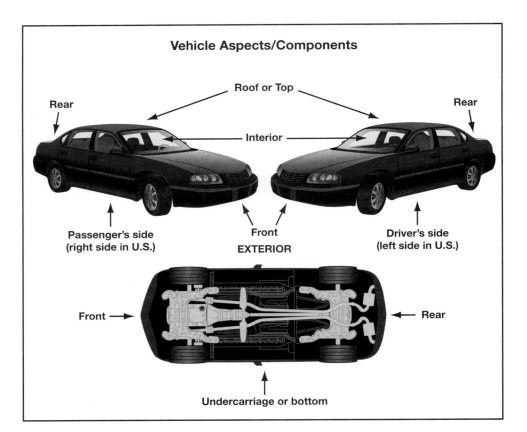

Figure 3.6 The terms used to describe various vehicle aspects or components.

- **Front** — The front of the vehicle is generally defined by the direction the driver faces during normal travel or operation. Generally indicated by the headlights.

- **Rear** — Opposite end of the vehicle from the front. Usually indicated by the taillights.

- **Interior** — The interior of a vehicle is composed of the passenger compartment and may contain, depending on the vehicle, the storage compartment.

- **Exterior** — All of the features of the outside of a vehicle. The exterior is composed of the vehicle's body panels, glass, bumpers, and other components.

In addition, individual vehicle components are commonly described by specific terms. It is important that extrication personnel use the same terms for the door/roof posts and various other vehicle components. Terms for specific components are as follows:

- **Door/Roof Posts** — Also called pillars, these are the structural members that surround the doors and support the roofs of vehicles. Door/roof posts are normally identified alphabetically from front to rear **(Figure 3.7)**. For example, the correct term used to describe the front pillar is the A pillar.

- **Fenders** — While the term quarter panel is used to describe the auto body material that surrounds the area of rear tire, the term fender or front fender describes the body material that surrounds the front tires. The fender starts at the front of the vehicle, proceeds around the front tire and ends at the fire wall.

Door/Roof Posts

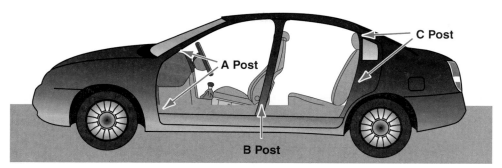

Figure 3.7 This illustration shows how door/roof posts are identified.

- ***Quarter Panels*** — The rear sections of the vehicle's body shell which include the rear fender and the C-post. In most modern car bodies, the rear fender is one piece and blends smoothly into the rear panel and the bottom of the rear window frame.

- ***Firewall*** — The firewall is a partition between the engine compartment and the passenger compartment of a vehicle. It is designed to protect vehicle occupants from the engine and its associated hazards.

- ***Rocker Panels*** — These are the usually rounded narrow body panels on each side of an automobile below the doors and between the kick panel and the quarter panel.

- ***Kick Panels*** — These are vertical panel walls that are enclosed by several structural members. An example of this would be the side panel in front of the A-pillar that runs up to the sides of the bulkhead on top and to the floorpan at the bottom end.

Types of Vehicle Materials and Construction

What a vehicle is constructed of and how those materials are used in the vehicle's construction can have an impact on vehicle extrication operations. An amazing number of materials are used in modern automobile construction such as steel, aluminum, magnesium, copper, plastics, composite materials, alloys, and glass to name a few **(Figure 3.8, p. 86)**. These materials are used in a variety of automobile components:

- ***Steel*** — Vehicle frame, body components, and I-beam safety components

- ***Aluminum*** — Vehicle bodies and engines, frames

- ***Magnesium*** — Tire rims, engine components, transmission housings, steering columns, frame support members, and dash boards

- ***Copper*** — Electrical system wiring

- ***Plastics*** — Light covers, vehicle body components, exterior/interior panels, dashboards, and seats

- ***Composite materials*** — Various vehicle components

- ***Alloys*** — Engines and vehicle body components

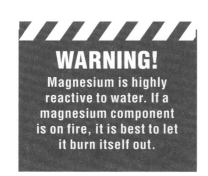

WARNING!
Magnesium is highly reactive to water. If a magnesium component is on fire, it is best to let it burn itself out.

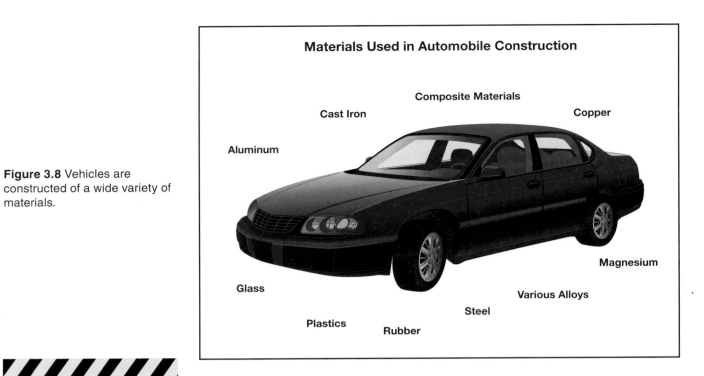

Materials Used in Automobile Construction

Composite Materials
Cast Iron
Copper
Aluminum
Magnesium
Glass
Various Alloys
Steel
Plastics
Rubber

Figure 3.8 Vehicles are constructed of a wide variety of materials.

Kevlar® — The trademarked name of a lightweight, very strong para-aramid synthetic fiber. It is used in many products to include bicycle tires, sails, body armor, and armor components for vehicles.

Armormax® — A combination of numerous synthetic fibers used to form an opaque composite ballistic armor.

Lightweight Transparent Armor® **(LTA®)** — Polycarbonate bulletproof glass sheets bonded together to form windows and windshields for armored vehicles and structures.

- *Glass* — Windshields, windows, lights, and light covers
- *Rubber* — Tires and electrical wiring insulation
- *Cast iron* — Agricultural and construction equipment bodies

An increasing number of vehicles equipped with armor and ballistic protection are operating on the roads **(Figure 3.9)**. These vehicles are popular with government officials and agencies, industrialists, corporate executives, religious leaders, and celebrities. The materials used to protect the passengers from attack can also hinder vehicle extrication efforts. Opaque armor may consist of layers of high-hardened ballistic steel plating, composite materials such as Kevlar® and Armormax®, and/or ballistic nylon armor. These materials are used in the vehicle body (roof, sides, and floor) to absorb the impact of projectiles and concussive forces. Transparent armor for windshields and windows are constructed of polycarbonate bulletproof glass such as Lightweight Transparent Armor® (LTA®) glass.

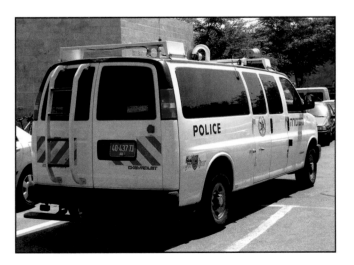

Figure 3.9 A vehicle equipped with armor and ballistic protection.

Armored or ballistic protected vehicles often have armored batteries; ballistic wrapped fuel tanks; special heavy duty shocks, struts, and brakes; ram bumpers, and bulletproof or "run flat" tire systems. These devices provide additional protection against battery acid and fuel explosions and support the vehicle's continued operation during and after an attack upon it.

Special training and equipment are needed for conducting vehicle extrication operations on armored or ballistic protected vehicles. Armored vehicle manufacturers should be contacted by the rescue organization to determine equipment needs and training opportunities and locations.

Vehicle Integrity

The structural integrity of a vehicle is how strong the vehicle's chassis remains after a collision. A vehicle's frame provides the basic structural foundation or integrity of the vehicle. As of the publication of this manual, there are three basic types of frames used in modern vehicles: full or rigid frames, unibody, and space frames. Additional specialty frames such as the monocque do exist and may be found **(Figure 3.10)**.

Monocque — Construction technique in which an object's external skin supports the structural load of the object.

The structural integrity of full or rigid frame vehicles may be less affected by a collision than that of vehicles with unibody or space-frame construction. Also, the structural integrity of rigid frame vehicles is less affected than vehicles with unibody construction when rescuers remove doors and/or the roof of the vehicle. Older vehicles tend to retain more of their structural integrity because they contain more steel and less aluminum, magnesium, and plastic in their construction.

NOTE: When rescue personnel remove a vehicle's doors, roof, and side panels, the chassis is weakened to a greater or lesser degree. When the chassis is weakened, it tends to collapse in on itself. This creates unwanted and perhaps dangerous movement that must be prevented if rescuers and those trapped in the vehicle are to be protected.

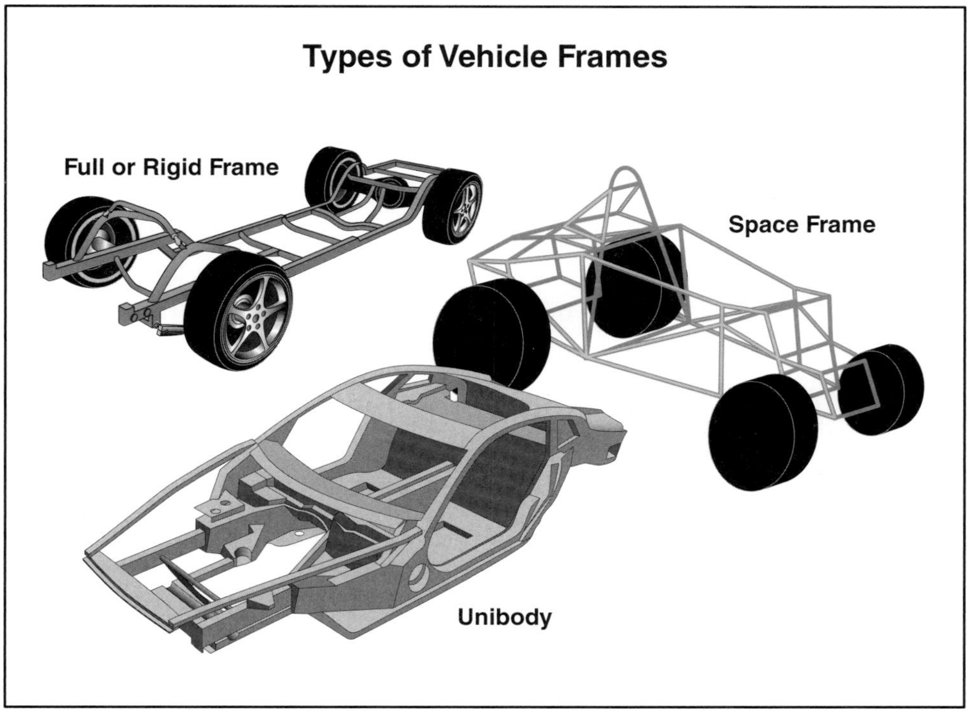

Types of Vehicle Frames

Full or Rigid Frame

Space Frame

Unibody

Figure 3.10 Examples of full (rigid), unibody, and space frames used in vehicle construction.

Modern Windshields

Modern automobiles rely on more than just the vehicles frame and body for structural integrity. Modern windshields are a key component of a vehicle structural, helping to prevent the roof from caving in during a rollover as well as providing a support for the deployment of the passenger side airbag. In some vehicles, the windshield can provide up to 80% of the passenger compartment's structural integrity.

Full or Rigid Frame

Full or rigid frames used in automobile construction have been around since the creation of vehicles. Early automobiles had frames made of wood but steel has been the material of choice. This type of automobile construction is known as body-on-frame construction. An advantage to body-on-frame construction is that it allows frequent changes to body styles and types without having to make changes to the chassis.

To form a chassis, a steel ladder frame is constructed using two parallel beams that run along the long axis of the vehicle. Cross members are bolted and welded between these beams to provide rigidity and support. This chassis then supports the powertrain and the vehicle body is bolted to the frame. While smaller autos and even some SUVs have begun using unitized or unibody construction, manufacturers still use full or rigid frames on larger automobiles and trucks, particularly heavy duty vehicles that carry or pull heavy loads.

Unibody (Unitized Body)

As the price of aluminum dropped in the 1920s and 1930s, automobile manufacturers began to look at the use of unitized body (also called unibody or integral frame) construction that was becoming common in the aviation industry. In unibody construction, a vehicle's stress bearing elements and sheet metal body parts are built together as one unit instead of attaching the vehicle's body to a frame as in body-on-frame construction. Unibody construction became more common following World War II and today, spot welded unibody construction is the dominate automobile construction technique.

Space Frame

Space frames are aluminum skeletons that are similar to aircraft frames upon which the aluminum, plastic, or composite skin of the vehicle's body is attached. The internal structure of these space frames provides the structural support for the vehicle while the skin provides aerodynamics, styling, and protection from the elements. Space frames are designed to support the entire load of the vehicle even if the skin of the vehicle is damaged. Because they are constructed of aluminum, these frames may weigh as much as 50% less than conventional steel or aluminum unibody frames.

Lighter vehicles built on space frames can be more fuel efficient and, in smaller production runs, less expensive to build than the more common steel or aluminum unibody vehicles. Current examples of vehicles that exploit aluminum space frame technology include the Plymouth Prowler and the Audi A8.

Supplemental Restraint and Rollover Protection Systems

Increased collision protection for vehicle occupants is provided by a variety of restraint and protective systems such as Supplemental Restraint Systems (SRS), Side Impact Protection Systems (SIPS), Head Protection Systems (HPS), knee bolsters, seat belt pretensioners, and Rollover Protection Systems (ROPS). Because restraint system technology is evolving so rapidly, all rescue personnel are encouraged to make every effort to stay current on what systems are being installed in new vehicles. One of the best ways to do this is to frequently visit the NHTSA web site listed in Chapter 1.

Although these systems have saved many lives, they have also added a potential safety hazard for both rescuers and vehicle occupants — accidental activation of one or more of these systems during extrication operations. Some modern vehicles have multiple systems whose locations may not be readily identified. For their own safety and that of the trapped occupants, rescue personnel must know where these systems may be located and the possible procedures to mitigate them.

Supplemental Restraint Systems (SRS)

Over the past years there have been many improvements to the restrain systems on vehicles. The windshield is the major restraint in a vehicle, boasting in some vehicles up to 80% of the vehicles A-post integrity. Air bag systems prevent passengers from striking the steering wheel, dashboard, windshield, side windows, and door frames. Seat belts are used to keep the passengers upright in the seat. Seat belt pretensioners assist the airbags by preloading the seat belt just before the air bag deploys to set the passengers upright. The airbags are to help reduce passenger injuries. With the introduction of "Smart Systems" in the late 90s, the restraint systems are helping reduce injuries much more successfully. The following sections will cover Supplemental Restraint Systems.

Front Impact Air Bags

Front-impact air bags are called supplemental systems because they are intended to supplement seat belts, not replace them **(Figure 3.11)**. Children under the age of 12 should not ride in the front seat of vehicle with a passen-

> **WARNING!**
> Air bags can deploy at speeds of up to 200 mph (322 km/h) and exert a tremendous force — potentially lethal under the right conditions.

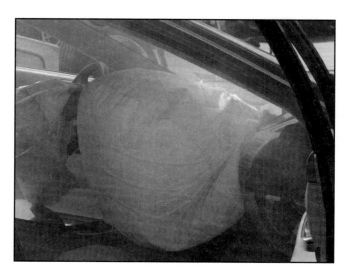

Figure 3.11 Front air bags immediately following deployment.

ger-side airbag that is armed. Electrically operated restraint systems receive their energy from the vehicle's battery. They are designed to activate through a system of inertia switches located forward of the passenger compartment and by microelectronic controls that may be located under the front seats or in the console between the front seats. These systems have a reserve energy supply that is capable of deploying an air bag even if the battery is disconnected or destroyed in the collision. When the battery is disconnected, the reserve energy supply will eventually drain away, disarming the restraint system. Vehicle manufacturers list different time estimates on how long it takes for the reserve to deplete entirely. These estimates range from as little as 1 second to as much as 30 minutes. Many pick-up trucks have features that allow the passenger air bag to be disarmed.

Side-Impact Protection Systems (SIPS)

Some side-impact protection systems are mechanically operated and do not require power from the vehicle's electrical system to activate. Therefore, these air bags may deploy even if the battery has been disconnected. In mechanical systems, isolating or preventing air bag deployment may require that the connection between the sensor and the air bag inflation unit be cut. How and where this is done is specific to each vehicle make and model. Electronically activated SIPS will need to be isolated by isolating the battery. This process will vary from vehicle to vehicle.

Head Protection Systems (HPS)

A growing number of vehicles have head protection systems (HPS) installed. On vehicles equipped with side-impact collision, these air bags deploy from a narrow opening between the headliner and the top of the door frame (**Figure 3.12**). Unlike SRS and SIPS that deflate immediately after deployment, HPS bags remain rigidly inflated after activation. However, they are easily removed by cutting the nylon straps or deflated by being punctured with a sharp object or being cut with a knife. A slightly different type of HPS curtain is inflated by a high-pressure cylinder. This curtain deflates automatically shortly after deployment. The two types of head protection systems are inflatable tubes and window curtains.

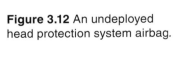

Figure 3.12 An undeployed head protection system airbag.

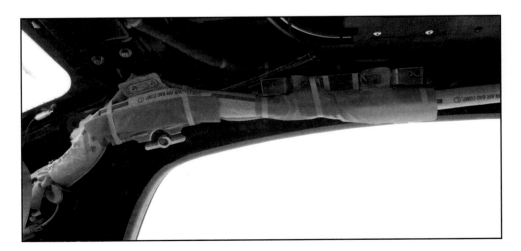

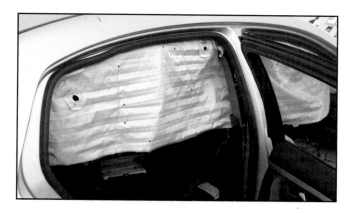

Figure 3.13 An example of a deployed window curtain.

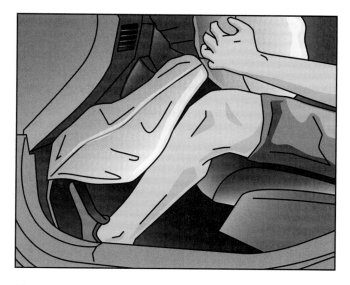

Figure 3.14 This illustration shows how a knee bolster deploys to protect a driver's legs.

- **Inflatable Tubes** — When inflatable tubes are activated, they instantly inflate. This shortens them and snaps them down into place across the side window. Unlike other air bags, inflatable tubes remain inflated after deployment. They are easily deflated by being punctured with a sharp tool or being cut with a knife.

- **Window Curtains** — When window curtains are activated, they instantly inflate also. However, unlike inflatable tubes, window curtain head protection devices quickly deflate automatically **(Figure 3.13)**.

One danger with both of these systems is that if a rescuer is working through the window opening, he is in the deployment path of the air bag. This danger can be mitigated by a complete roof removal. However, when cutting the posts for roof removal, rescuers must be careful not to cut into high-pressure cylinders.

Knee Bolsters

Some vehicles are equipped with restraint devices that are intended to protect the lower legs of the driver **(Figure 3.14)**. They are also intended as "antisubmarine" devices — that is, they are intended to help prevent the driver from sliding forward and becoming wedged under the dashboard. The same precautions apply as with other front-impact restraints.

Antisubmarine Device — Any device designed to prevent a driver from sliding forward and become wedged or trapped beneath the dashboard of a vehicle.

Seat Belts and Seat Belt Pretensioners

Since the late 1960s, all passenger vehicles manufactured in the United States have had to be equipped with passive restraint systems, also called seat belts. These systems consist of a belt that attaches across the wearer's lap and extends across the upper torso **(Figure 3.15, p. 92)**. They are intended to restrain the wearer in his seat and keep him from bolting forward in a front-impact collision. More importantly, they are designed to keep the wearer inside the vehicle if the doors come open. Following a collision, these restraints can easily be removed by releasing the buckle or by cutting the belt.

Both testing and experience have made it clear that seat belts are most effective when they are pulled tightly across the wearer's body. But because this can be rather uncomfortable, few vehicle occupants tighten their belts as snugly as they should. Therefore, some manufacturers have added seat belt pretensioners to their vehicles. These devices are activated when the front-impact air bags activate, and they instantly tighten (pretension) the seat belts so that the wearer receives maximum benefit of the belts when the crash energy reaches him.

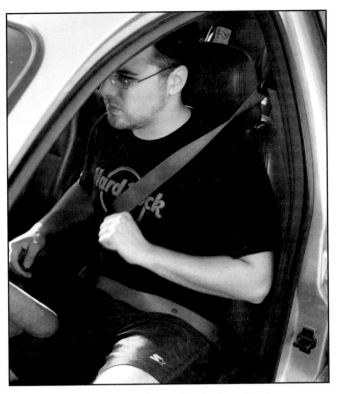

Figure 3.15 A driver wearing a standard seat belt.

Most vehicles are equipped with seat belt pretensioners. Because seat belts are most effective when they are adjusted tightly across the torso of the people wearing them, pretensioners have been added to tighten the belts as the front-impact air bags deploy. These pyrotechnic devices are operated by the ignition of nitrocellulose that drives a piston to instantaneously eliminate any slack in the belt. In some cases, the belts may be tightened to the point that they restrict the wearer's ability to breathe normally. Simply releasing or cutting the seat belts will relieve this pressure.

Because the pyrotechnic activating devices for seat belt pretensioners are usually located inside the B-post next to the seat, rescuers must be careful about cutting these posts **(Figure 3.16)**. To avoid accidentally activating the pretensioner, cuts into the B-post must be made well above or well below the

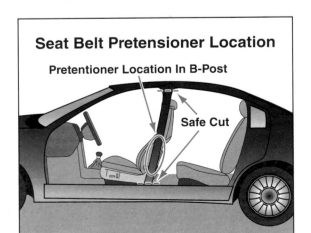

Figure 3.16 The approximate location of a seat belt pretensioner in a vehicle's B-post.

external seat belt retractor. Another way of handling those situations where the pretensioners are located in the B-post is to cut the seat belt and remove the buckle and excess belt so that they cannot strike anyone if the system suddenly activates. If the pretensioners are located between the front seats, all that should be necessary is to unbuckle or cut the belts. If heated during a vehicle fire, pretensioners can explode, creating a fireball and shrapnel. Some automobile manufacturers enclose pre-tensioners within steel caissons or casings inside the B-post to protect them from being cut.

Child Safety Restraint Devices

For years, child safety seats had to be purchased separately and fastened securely into the backseat of most automobiles. Because of the wide range of child seat sizes and securing mechanisms, as well as the equally wide range of rear seat belt configurations, some installations were not as safe as intended.

Many new automobiles are being manufactured with child safety restraint devices and integrated child safety seat as original factory equipment **(Figure 3.17)**. An integrated child safety seat is normally located at the center of the rear seat and folds down to form a child seat complete with seat belts. It may be necessary for rescuers to extricate an infant or toddler from one of these devices at an emergency scene. Knowledge of these systems will assist rescuers with maintaining the safety of the young patient.

Energy-Absorbing Features

Many automobiles are equipped with shock absorbing components designed to absorb the force of side, front, and rear collisions. Since the early 1970s, automobiles manufactured in North America have been equipped with energy-absorbing bumpers. Many cars and light trucks have also been equipped with reinforced door and dashboard structures to increase side impact protection. All these features are intended to reduce the monetary and human costs of vehicle collisions. However, they also add some potentially lethal hazards for emergency response personnel, and they can increase the difficulty of performing vehicle extrication.

Crushable Bumpers

A number of different designs were used by vehicle manufacturers to meet federal standards intended to reduce the monetary costs of low-speed collisions — those at 5 mph (7.5 km/h) or less, later reduced to 2.5 mph (3.75 km/h). The first most prevalent design for energy-absorbing bumpers are crushable bumpers.

Some crushable bumpers are made of polystyrene foam molded into an egg crate structure, covered by a flexible rubber shell. Others are made of synthetic rubber molded into a honeycomb structure covered with a flexible shell **(Figure 3.18, p. 94)**. These bumpers are designed to absorb energy by flexing when struck. Unlike the bumpers with gas-filled struts discussed next, crushable bumpers are not a hazard in a fire — until the fire is out. As these bumpers cool after being exposed to the heat of a fire, beads of a clear liquid form on the surface of the bumper. This liquid may appear to be water but it is actually concentrated hydrofluoric acid (HF), a highly corrosive substance.

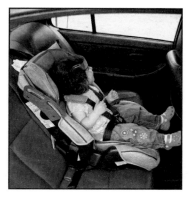

Figure 3.17 Child safety seats like this one save many lives.

WARNING!

Avoid skin contact with the clear liquid (hydrofluoric acid [HF]) that forms on the surface of crushable bumpers after a fire. Hydrofluoric acid is absorbed through the skin and contact could be fatal. Flush these bumpers with copious amounts of water.

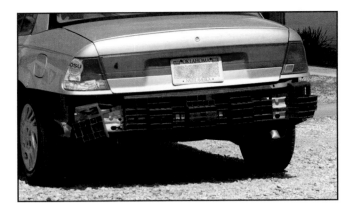

Figure 3.18 A crushable bumper system minus the flexible rubber shell.

Struts

In addition to crushable bumpers, many automobiles are equipped with energy-absorbing bumper struts. These struts make the vehicle less vulnerable to damage in low-speed collisions. Two struts are mounted between the front bumper and the vehicle frame or chassis, and two more are mounted in the rear of the vehicle **(Figure 3.19)**. Similar to conventional shock absorbers, these sealed units contain hydraulic fluid and compressed gas. When these struts are exposed to the heat of a fire, they can explode with tremendous force. If both struts attached to a bumper explode simultaneously, they can launch the bumper and/or the struts 100 feet (30 m) or more from the vehicle. If only one strut explodes, the other acts as a pivot point and the bumper can swing in an arc across the front or rear of the vehicle. Obviously, anyone in the path of a bumper attached to an exploding strut is in serious jeopardy. Therefore, when the front or rear bumper of an automobile is exposed to heavy flame impingement, all personnel should stay out of the danger zone — directly in front of the bumper and to each side a distance equal to the length of the bumper.

Another hazard of which firefighters should be aware are the gas-filled struts used to support the hoods and hatchbacks (when open) on some vehicles. When exposed to the heat of a fire, these struts can explode and launch parts many yards

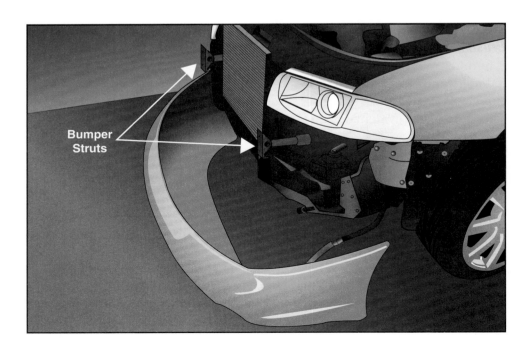

Bumper Struts

Figure 3.19 An illustration of a bumper strut system.

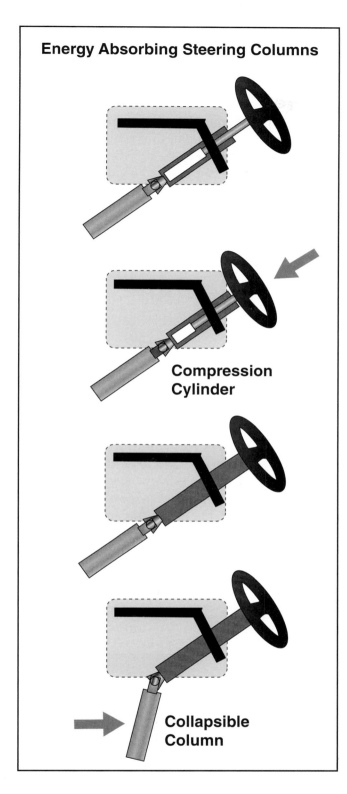

Energy Absorbing Steering Columns

Compression Cylinder

Collapsible Column

Figure 3.20 Types of energy absorbing steering columns.

(meters) from the vehicle at speeds sufficient to cause fatal injuries. Firefighters have been impaled when these struts have exploded and forcibly ejected strut components from the vehicle.

Yet another strut system on vehicles is the suspension system. Some front suspensions are equipped with a shock absorber that is mounted directly below the coil spring. Struts are also used in some independent, rear-suspension systems that have a shock-absorber strut assembly on each side. Piston rods are composed of a plated rod that is attached to the piston of the shock-absorber and usually extend up to the top of the shock to attach to the vehicle.

Steering Columns

Introduced in the late 1960s, the energy absorbing steering column has proven effective in saving lives and limiting injuries during front-end crashes **(Figure 3.20)**. These devices, along with driver-side airbags, protect the driver by absorbing the force of the driver's forward movement during a collision. With the introduction of tilt and combination collapsible/tilt steering columns, it is no longer recommended that the steering column be pulled.

Crumple Zones

Another energy absorbing mechanism utilized on modern vehicles is the crumple zone. Certain body and frame components at the front and rear of a vehicle provide adequate structure support for normal vehicle operations and usage but are designed to give way or compress in a calculated manner during a collision **(Figure 3.21)**. Crumple zones lengthen the time a vehicle takes to come to a complete stop during an accident, thus reducing the force of deceleration upon the vehicle's passengers.

Side-Impact Beams and Bars

Because a great number of all vehicle injuries and fatalities are the result of side-impact collisions, passenger cars manufactured in North America have been equipped with side-impact beams since the late 1960s. Early designs were several layers of ordinary mild steel formed into a corrugated beam about 7 inches (178 mm) wide and about 2 inches (50 mm) thick, installed across each side door. Because mild steel has a tensile strength of about 20,000 to 23,000 psi (140 000 kPa to 161 000 kPa), these beams were relatively easy to cut with hydraulic shears. However, newer designs have made two major changes — the construction of the door beams and the addition of a dashboard support beam.

Newer designs of side-impact protection incorporate stronger materials such as high-strength low-alloy (HSLA) steel and micro-alloy (MA) steel **(Figure 3.22)**. HSLA steel has a tensile strength of 40,000 to 70,000 psi (280 000 kPa to 490 000 kPa). MA steel has a tensile strength of 110,000 to 215,000 psi (770 000 kPa to 1 505 000 kPa). Often these are long bars running horizontally or diagonally within a door. These new alloys may be too hard for the blades of available power shears. If this is the case, rescuers may have to make relief cuts above and below the bar and use a power spreader to move the end of the bar. These bars may embed themselves into the A-, B-, or C-posts when the vehicle is compressed front to back creating a "deadbolt lock."

These new alloys add significantly to the structural integrity of any vehicle, and reduce the likelihood of the vehicle folding in the middle when struck from the side. They are also used in the construction of some dashboard support beams. These collision beams span the width of the vehicle from A-post to A-post.

> **Collision Beams** — Structural member within a vehicle door designed to prevent the door from collapsing inward if struck.

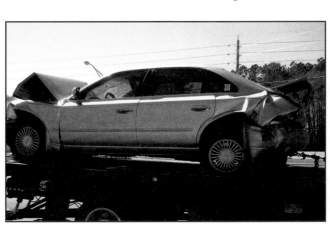

Figure 3.21 This photo shows the effectiveness of crumple zones in protecting the passenger compartment. *Courtesy of Heather and James Cripps.*

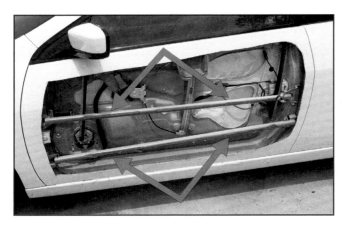

Figure 3.22 Examples of side impact bars inside a vehicle door.

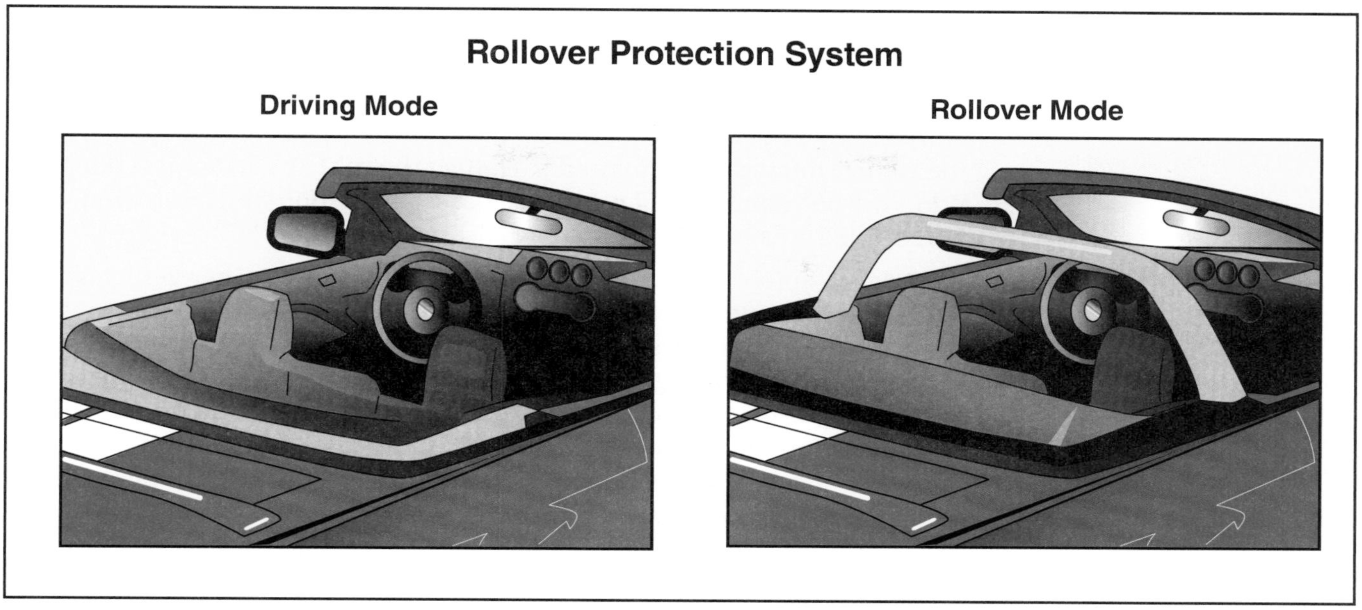

Figure 3.23 An illustration showing an active rollover protection system in the driving mode and rollover mode.

Rollover Protection Systems (ROPS)

Many convertible automobiles and open body vehicles that lack the C-post of hardtop vehicles are equipped with roll bars **(Figure 3.23)**. Roll bars are made of tubular steel that and are anchored to the vehicle body or frame. They extend up behind the passenger cabin. Usually made of hardened tubular steel stock, these roll bars are intended to protect the vehicle occupants in rollover crashes. All other passenger vehicles are now required to have roof supports (commonly called "roll cages") that will withstand a force equal to 1.5 times the weight of the vehicle without the roof collapsing in a rollover crash. Even though roll bars and cages are designed to withstand significant impact without collapsing, they are not indestructible and can collapse onto the occupants, pinning them in their seats. Roll bars and cages can add to the challenge for rescuers in extrication situations.

Some manufacturers provide an extendable roll bar system on some of their newer models. This "pop up style" roll system activates and extends up behind the passengers rapidly when the vehicle exceeds 23 degrees from the horizontal, a lateral angle limit of 62 degrees, or a longitudinal angle of 72 degrees. Additionally, these systems can deploy if the vehicle experiences a 3G acceleration force, or becomes weightless for at least 80 milliseconds. While these devices allow better visibility to the rear of the vehicle and a more esthetic appearance while maintaining rollover protection, they pose a significant safety hazard to rescuers when they deploy.

NOTE: Roll bars should NOT be confused with anti-roll bars which are stabilizer bars that designed to prevent a vehicle from rolling over.

Windows

The windows of a vehicle are designed to do more than simply maintain the internal environment and to protect the occupants from being struck by insects or flying objects. Vehicle windows also serve to help keep the occupants inside the vehicle during accidents and can affect the vehicle's structural integrity. Windows on vehicles can be made of glass, polycarbonates, laminated, tempered, and transparent armor materials.

Early automobiles were open compartment, fair weather vehicles with windshields as optional equipment. As time passed and passenger compartments began to be enclosed, windshields and windows of regular glass became more common. Regular glass was used in vehicles manufactured prior to 1927 when the laminated safety windshield was introduced. The trend towards safer glass for automobiles continued with the developments of improved laminated safety glass, enhanced performance glass (EPG), tempered glass, and now polycarbonates and transparent armor.

Laminated

Laminated safety glass consists of two sheets of glass bonded to a sheet of plastic sandwiched between them **(Figure 3.24)**. This type of glass is most commonly used for windshields and some rear windows. Impact produces many long, pointed shards with sharp edges. The plastic laminate sheet holds most of these shards and fragments in place. When broken, the glass remains attached to the laminate and moves as a unit which makes windshield removal easier.

Some manufacturers have laminated an additional layer of plastic to the passenger side of the windshield for added protection. Some laminated glass side windows are more than 1/3-inch (9 mm) thick. Many laminated windshields and rear windows are now held in place with polyurethane glue. These windows can be identified by the black shading around the perimeter of the window, designed to protect the glue from sun damage.

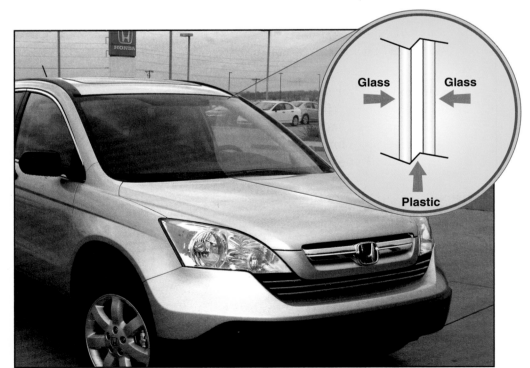

Figure 3.24 Laminated glass is required in passenger vehicle windshields.

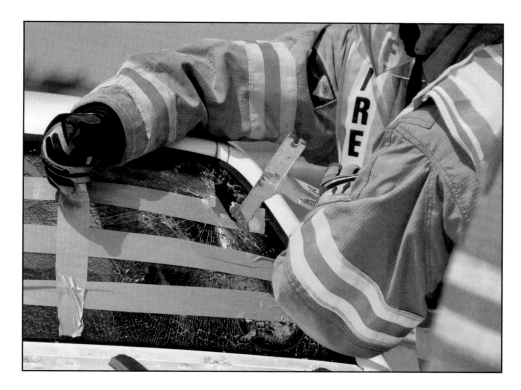

Figure 3.25 Rescue personnel preparing to break and remove tempered glass. *Courtesy of Sonrise Photography.*

Tempered

Tempered glass is most commonly used in side windows and some rear windows (**Figure 3.25**). Tempered glass is designed to spread small fracture lines throughout the plate when struck. This results in the glass separating into many small pieces, decreasing the hazards of long, pointed pieces of glass. However, new problems are created such as small nuisance lacerations to unprotected body parts and the possible contamination of open wounds and the eyes with tiny bits of glass.

Polycarbonate

Advancements in the plastics industry have made the use of polycarbonate window glazing over glass for side and rear windows more prominent common place. These window systems provide greater scratch resistance, reduced weight, and a wider variety of window shapes. Some disadvantages of polycarbonate glass are its cost and the difficulty involved in penetrating it.

Transparent Armor

Transparent armor or ballistic glass and plastic are commonly made of sheets of polycarbonate material sandwiched between sheets of glass (**Figure 3.26, p. 100**). Heat and pressure are used to laminate these materials together to form a ballistic glass capable of absorbing the impact of bullets or shrapnel and preventing them from piercing the glass.

Fuel Systems

Modern vehicles use a variety of different fuel systems. Most vehicles are still powered by conventional fuels such as gasoline (also called petrol in some countries) or diesel (also called petrodiesel). Others are powered by alternative fuels such as propane, liquefied natural gas (LNG), auxiliary fuel cells, alcohol/gasoline blended mixtures (such as ethanol), hydrogen, biodiesel, and JP-8.

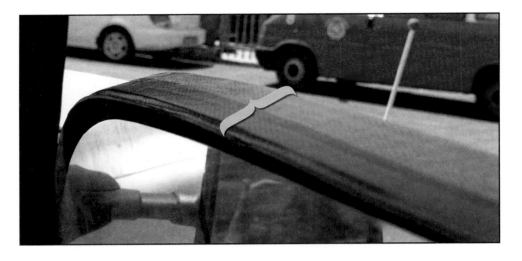

Figure 3.26 This photo demonstrates the thickness of transparent armor or ballistic glass.

Conventional Fuels

The two most common fuels used in automotive vehicles are gasoline and diesel. Both of these are hydrocarbon based fuels derived from petroleum. These fuels can be ignited easily and, during extrication operations, rescue personnel must ensure that gasoline or diesel leaks from the tanks of accident vehicles are controlled and ignition sources are isolated to prevent fires. Fire protection must be established during extrication operations to ensure these fuels are not ignited or, if ignited, the fires should be extinguished rapidly.

Hybrid Vehicles

In the ongoing effort to economize on fuel consumption and protect the environment, automobile manufacturers have been developing and constructing increasing numbers of hybrid vehicles. Hybrid vehicles are powered by multiple propulsion systems such as gasoline-electric hybrids which have internal combustion engines and electric motors **(Figure 3.27)**. Regenerative braking is also used to collect electrical power to be stored in the hybrid vehicle's batteries until needed for motive power.

The danger associated with hybrid vehicles is the high voltage stored within the batteries and running through wiring connected to the vehicle's electric motor. These wires can carry as much as 650 volts of DC current. Rescue personnel attempting to isolate the motive electrical power system and batteries

Regenerative Braking — A mechanical system that reduces the speed of a vehicle by converting part of the vehicle's kinetic energy into another type of energy that can be fed back into a power system or stored for future use.

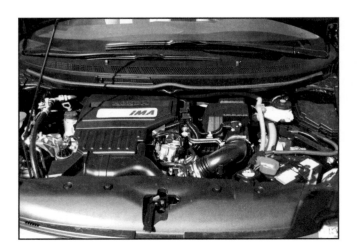

Figure 3.27 The gasoline engine and electric motor of a hybrid vehicle. *Courtesy of Alan Braun, University of Missouri Fire and Rescue Training Institute.*

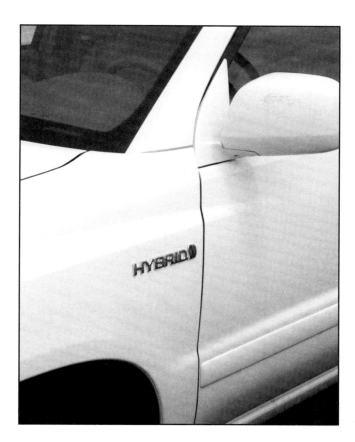

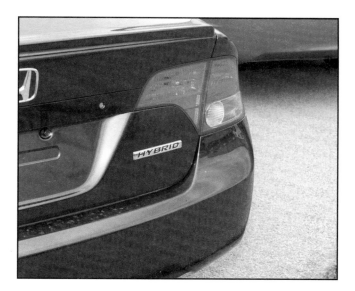

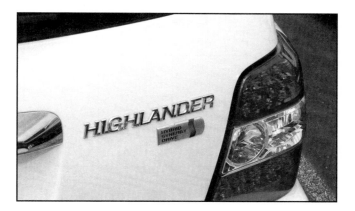

Figure 3.28 Examples of some of the "hybrid labels" used by different automobile manufacturers on their vehicles.

are exposed to the danger of electrical shock. To help rescuers and emergency responders to recognize the power wires and cables for this system are color coded orange and covered with orange shielding or orange tape.

There currently is no standardized means to identify a hybrid vehicle by sight upon approach. Manufacturers currently use different symbols and different wording placed in different locations on the vehicles to identify them as hybrids **(Figure 3.28)**. One organization is trying to encourage automobile manufacturers in the U.S. to adopt a proposal to construct hybrid vehicle air bags out of an orange colored material to provide one means of identifying hybrid vehicles. However, rescuers would need to rely upon the air bags deploying during a vehicle accident to assist them with this means of identification.

Rescue organization members are encouraged to monitor the development and production of hybrid cars by automobile manufacturers. **Table 3.6 (p. 102)** contains a partial list of manufacturers and the hybrid vehicles they produced at the time this manual was developed. Some manufacturers post information on their company websites for emergency responders to use in dealing with their vehicles during an emergency. The NHSTA website is a resource for gathering further information regarding hybrid vehicles. Another site is www.firegraphics.org that has emergency response guides for a variety of hybrid vehicles.

Table 3.6
Examples of Hybrid Cars (by automobile manufacturer)

Manufacturer	Model Name	External Identification	HV Battery Locations	High Voltage (HV)	HV Cable Route	HV Isolation Methods
Ford/Mercury	Escape / Mariner	Ford Hybrid Green Leaf on fenders and tailgate	Cargo area under carpet	300+ volts Orange Cables	Under the vehicle from the right side near the rear axle to just off-center behind the front axle	Turn off ignition key, remove key from ignition, and place on dash. Disconnect negative cable on the 12 volt battery. Place high voltage service disconnect switch into service position, if possible.
General Motors	Chevrolet Silverado / GMC Sierra	"Hybrid" badge located on vehicle's doors and 120v outlets in bed	Under the rear seat	42 volts (intermediate voltage) Blue Cables	Under the vehicle from beneath the rear seat to the center behind the front axle	If 120 VAC APO indicator is on, depress the APO button, turn off ignition key, remove key from ignition, and place on dash. Disable the 42 volt battery pack using the service disconnect switch behind the lower right corner of the battery unit. Disconnect the 12 volt battery.
	Saturn VUE Green Line	"Vue" and "Hybrid" badges on lift gate and "Hybrid" badge on front doors	Under rear cargo floor	36 - 42 volts (intermediate voltage) Blue Cables	Under the vehicle from beneath the rear cargo floor to the center behind the front axle	Turn off ignition key, remove key from ignition, and place on dash. Disconnect both negative cables on the 12 volt battery. If ignition key can't be reached, remove the 30 amp ignition maxi fuse in engine compartment.
Honda	Accord / Civic	Word "Hydrid" on rear of vehicle	Behind the rear seat	144 volts Orange Cables	Under the vehicle from the right side near the rear axle to just off-center behind the front axle	*Best method:* Turn off ignition key, remove key from ignition, and place on dash. *Second best method:* Remove main fuse and disconnect both negative cables on the 12 volt battery.
	Insight	Word "Hydrid" on rear of vehicle rear "wheel pants"	Behind the passenger seats and below the cargo area	144 volts Orange Cables	Under the vehicle from the left side near the rear axle to just off-center behind the front axle	*Best method:* Turn off ignition key, remove key from ignition, and place on dash. *Second best method:* Remove main fuse and disconnect both negative cables on the 12 volt battery.
Lexus	GS450h	Lexus GS450h logos on rear trunk and "Hybrid" logos on rear door moldings	In the trunk behind the rear seat.	288 volts Orange Cables	Under the vehicle from the center near the rear axle to the right side behind the front axle	**Procedure 1:** Turn off ignition key, remove key from ignition, and place on dash. If key cannot be removed, disconnect the 12 volt battery. **Procedure 2 (If ignition key can't be reached):** Disconnect the 12 volt battery and remove IGCT No. 4 fuse relay in engine compartment. *Power remains in the HV system for 5 minutes after disabling.*

Continued on next page

Table 3.6 (Continued)
Examples of Hybrid Cars (by automobile manufacturer)

Manufacturer	Model Name	External Identification	HV Battery Locations	High Voltage (HV)	HV Cable Route	HV Isolation Methods
Lexus (continued)	RX400h	Lexus RX400h logos on rear hatch	In the passenger compartment under the rear seat	288 boosted to 650 volts at engine. Orange Cables	Under the vehicle from the right side near the rear axle to just off-center behind the front axle	**Procedure 1** **(If READY indicator is on):** Push POWER button once. **(If READY indicator is not on):** Do NOT push POWER button. Keep SMART KEY at least 16 feet (5 m) from vehicle. If SMART KEY cannot be located, disconnect the 12 volt battery. **Procedure 2 (If POWER button can't be reached):** Disconnect the 12 volt battery and remove IGCT No. 1 fuse in engine compartment. Pull all fuses if unable to identify correct fuse. **Procedure 3 (If POWER button and engine compartment can't be reached):** Remove RH J/B-B fuse trunk. Pull all 3 fuses if unable to identify correct fuse. Then disconnect the 12 volt battery ***Power remains in the HV system for 10 minutes after disabling.***
Toyota	Camry	Camry and "Hybrid Synergy Drive" logos on trunk lid. "Hybrid" logos on front fenders	In the trunk behind the rear seat	245 volts Orange Cables	Under the vehicle from the right side near the rear axle inboard to center line to just above center of the left front axle	**Procedure 1** **(If READY indicator is on):** Push POWER button once. **(If READY indicator is not on):** Do NOT push POWER button. Keep SMART KEY at least 3.3 feet (1 m) from vehicle. If SMART KEY cannot be located, disconnect the 12 volt battery. **Procedure 2 (If POWER button can't be reached):** Disconnect the 12 volt battery and remove IGCT No. 2 fuse in engine compartment. Pull all fuses if unable to identify correct fuse.
	FCHV (Hydrogen is stored in the vehicle's cylinder for at up to 5,000 psi [34 474 kpa])	FCHV Fuel Cell Hybrid Vehicle labels on the hood, both rear doors, and on right side of rear door	Cargo area under carpet	274 volts Orange Cables	Under the vehicle on the right side from just forward of rear axle inboard to just off-center right in the engine compartment	Turn off ignition key, remove key from ignition, and place on dash. Disconnect the 12 volt battery. ***If unable to reach ignition key:*** Disconnect the 12 volt battery and remove the IGCT and IGCTFC fuses in engine compartment. ***Power remains in the HV system for 5 minutes after disabling.***

Continued on next page

Table 3.6 (Continued)
Examples of Hybrid Cars (by automobile manufacturer)

Manufacturer	Model Name	External Identification	HV Battery Locations	High Voltage (HV)	HV Cable Route	HV Isolation Methods
Toyota (continued)	Prius	Toyota Hybrid and Prius logos on trunk	In the trunk behind the rear seat	274 volts Orange Cables	Under the vehicle from the left side near the rear axle to just above the left front axle	Turn off ignition key, remove key from ignition, and place on dash. Disconnect the 12 volt battery. *If unable to reach ignition key:* Disconnect the 12 volt battery and remove the IGCT relay in engine compartment. *Power remains in the HV system for 5 minutes after disabling.*
	Highlander	Toyota Highlander "Hybrid Synergy Drive" logos on rear hatchback door	In passenger compartment under second row seat	288 volts Orange Cables	Under the center of the vehicle from under the second row seat to the engine compartment	Turn off ignition key, remove key from ignition, and place on dash. Disconnect the 12 volt battery. *If unable to reach ignition key:* Disconnect the 12 volt battery and remove the IGCT No. 4 fuse in engine compartment. If unable to identify the correct fuse, pull all 4 fuses. *Power remains in the HV system for 5 minutes after disabling.*

The information for this table was gathered from emergency response guides produced by the manufacturers for these vehicle models. The information was accurate at the time this manual was written.

Alternative Fuels

For fuel economy and environmental protection, a variety of alternative fuels are used to power modern vehicles. Rescuers need to keep in mind that they may encounter these alternative fuels and the hazards associated with them at an extrication operation. Alternative fuels include but are not limited to:

- Propane and Liquefied Natural Gas (LNG)
- Auxiliary Fuel Cells
- Alcohol/Gasoline Blended Mixtures
- Hydrogen
- Biodiesel
- JP-8

Propane and Liquefied Natural Gas (LNG)

Some passenger vehicles are equipped with a fuel selector that allows the engine to run on either gasoline, propane or other liquefied petroleum gas (LPG. Propane, also known as Liquefied Petroleum Gas [LPG or LP-Gas]) in the U.S., is often used to power buses, forklifts, and taxis, and can also be found used as a fuel for heating and cooking in campers and recreational vehicles **(Figure 3.29)**. When used as a vehicle fuel in other countries, propane is called autogas. Propane is actually a byproduct of petroleum refining and natural gas production.

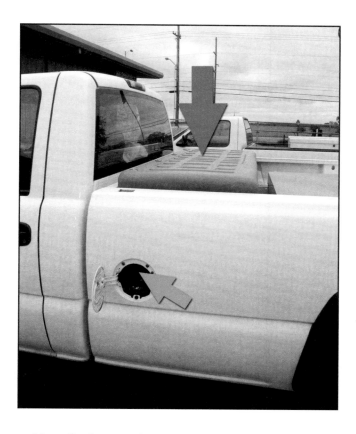

Figure 3.29 The LPG tank in this light truck is located in the plastic box in the bed of the truck while the fill point is located near the gasoline tank fill point.

Liquefied natural gas is produced from oil and natural gas fields around the world. Because LNG burns cleaner and produces fewer greenhouse gases than petroleum fuels, it is viewed as an environmentally friendly fuel.

Should a propane or LNG tank leak or rupture during an accident, the fuel released will vaporize and could be ignited by an ignition source. Fire department personnel need to be standing by to provide fire protection during extrication operations.

Auxiliary Fuel Cells

In essence, fuel cells are electrochemical energy conversion devices that produce electricity while converting hydrogen and oxygen into water. Because the electrical output of a single fuel cell is quite limited, a bank or stack of fuel cells is used to generate sufficient DC current to power electrical motors in vehicles.

The production of hydrogen does result in a net loss of energy. Currently hydrogen is not readily available for automotive use and the storing of hydrogen for fuel cell usage is difficult. Because of hydrogen's very low density storage, storing it in cryogenic storage tanks or as a liquid in pressurized tanks simply doesn't store enough energy for extended driving. Some fuel cells use reformers to draw the hydrogen for the cells to use from gasoline, methane, or ethanol. Because hydrogen is highly flammable, caution must be taken around hydrogen storage tanks during extrication operations to prevent the release and ignition of this fuel.

Alcohol/Gasoline Blended Mixtures

Alcohol/gasoline blended mixtures such as E85 (85% ethanol and 15% gasoline) are becoming more commonplace in the United States and in other countries. E85 is about 35% less costly to purchase than gasoline but in vehicles manufactured in 2002 and before they are less fuel efficient. In newer, flexible fuel engines, E85 runs more efficiently.

Hydrogen

Hydrogen can also be burned in internal combustion engines to produce motive power for vehicles. Again, the problems associated with using hydrogen as a fuel include:

- Limitations in hydrogen production and storage.
- Flammability.
- High pressure compressed gas storage.

Biodiesel

Biodiesel is a fuel like diesel that is derived from animal fats or vegetable oils such as corn and soy. It is non-toxic, biodegradable, and produce fewer emissions than petroleum based diesels during the combustion process. Biodiesel is classified as a non-flammable liquid with a flash point of 320° F (160° C).

Jet Propellant - 8 (JP-8)

Beginning in the 1990s, the U.S. military and North Atlantic Treaty Organization (NATO) have been converting to JP-8, a kerosene derivative, as a single fuel to power diesel and turbine engines in land-based vehicles as part of a "single fuel concept". While JP-8 is primarily used as an aircraft fuel, military forces have begun using it as a fuel for land based vehicles such as Humvees, heavy military trucks, military fire apparatus, and other tactical military vehicles.

Fuel Tanks

Terne Coated Steel — Cold rolled sheet steel that has hot-dip coated with a lead-tin alloy. This dull gray coating provides corrosion protection from contact with petroleum fuels.

Historically, vehicle fuel tanks were constructed of aluminum or terne coated steel. Older tanks tend to corrode, weigh more than plastic tanks, and are more expensive to produce than modern plastic fuel tanks. One hazard that plastic tank manufacturers have had to overcome was the flammability of the tank materials themselves when the tank became involved in fire. Recent advances in the plastics industry has led to the development of less flammable materials.

Plastic tanks can be punctured easily during an accident or rapidly fail in the event of a fire. Rescue personnel should always "read-the-wreck" upon arrival and determine the presence of or the potential failure of the fuel tank. Fuel that is released from a failed reservoir can pose a very serious risk to rescue members, the victims, and the environment.

Exhaust Systems

Modern automobile exhaust systems are designed to carry the exhaust gases away from vehicle occupants, reduce noise, improve performance, and improve fuel consumption (**Figure 3.30**). Because these gases are hot when they leave

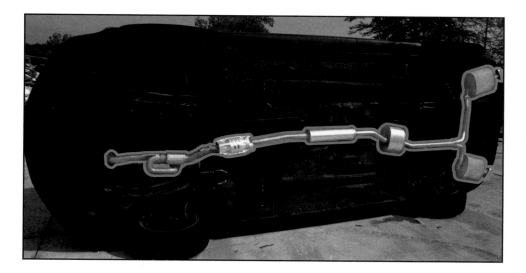

Figure 3.30 The exhaust system of a modern automobile.

the engine, the exhaust system piping and components tend to be hot as well. The heated piping and components can be dangerous for rescuers to touch because of the risk of getting burned.

- **Exhaust Piping** — Exhaust piping is generally constructed of stainless steel or zinc-plated steel. This piping channels the exhaust gases from the engine exhaust manifolds to the catalytic converter (if so equipped), from the catalytic converter to the muffler, and from the muffler to the outside air.

- **Catalytic Converters** — Catalytic converters (sometimes simply a "catalyst") are stainless-steel canisters that are integrated into a vehicle's exhaust system that convert vehicle exhaust emissions into less harmful materials. Each catalytic converter is composed of a thin layer of catalytic material (composed of platinum, rhodium, and palladium) arranged over inert supports. Highly efficient three-way catalysts are available in vehicles that employ a feedback fuel-air ration control system to produce a precise combustion control.

- **Mufflers** — Mufflers reduce the volume of noise produce by the engine and carried by the exhaust gases.

Electrical Systems

The electrical system of a vehicle is designed to store and deliver the electricity needed to start the engine and to power and operate the various electrical components of the vehicle. A typical vehicle electrical system is composed of the battery which stores the electricity, an alternator which produces the electricity, wiring, fuses that protect the electrical system, and the lights, fans, and other ancillary equipment (air conditioning, radios, stereos, mobile phones, power windows and seats, etc.).

Vehicle electrical systems include any of the systems and subsystems that comprise the automobile wiring harnesses. The starting, charging, and lighting systems are all parts of a vehicle's electrical system.

Most vehicle electrical systems are either 12 volt or 24 volt systems. Passenger vehicles and light trucks are usually 12 volt systems while larger trucks, recreational vehicles, and military vehicles operate on 24 volt systems.

At extrication operations, one key safety task that must be performed is the isolation of the electrical power to the vehicle(s) or piece(s) of equipment involved. Part of this process is to unplug the connections from the vehicle's or equipment's electrical system from the source of electricity such as the battery or batteries. When isolating the battery, the negative terminal should be disconnected first.

Multiple Battery Systems

An automobile battery serves as the storage device for the electrical energy needed to start the vehicle or may serve as the power supply for electrical vehicles. Automobile batteries used in ignition systems are generally of the lead-acid type. Battery packs used to power electrical or hybrid vehicles include lead-acid, absorbed glass mat, nickel cadmium (NiCd), nickel metal hydride (NiMH), zinc-air batteries, lithium ion (Li-ion), and lithium ion polymer (Li-poly) **(Figure 3.31)**. Each of these battery systems can impart heat energy to various parts of a wrecked vehicle which increases the risk of shock, spark, and ignition of spilled fuels/hydraulic fluids. It is very important that rescuers are extremely cautious with these batteries and avoid touching them unless absolutely necessary.

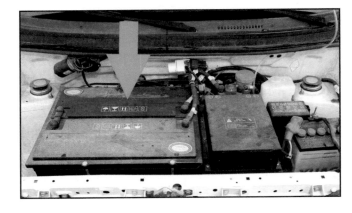

Figure 3.31 A battery pack for an electric car.

Multiple Battery Locations

The battery in passenger vehicles and light trucks may be found in the engine compartment, in the passenger compartment, or in the trunk. In some vehicles it may be covered by a retaining bar, a cover made of plastic or some other material, or the windshield washer fluid reservoir. In larger vehicles, the battery or batteries are usually in a special compartment separate from the engine compartment. Rescuers should turn on the vehicle's headlights or dome light to determine if the battery system has been isolated.

Electric Engine Cooling Fans

Most vehicles have an engine cooling fan run by the electrical system that provides additional cooling for the engine during vehicle operations **(Figure 3.32)**. Some vehicles have an auxiliary or supplemental electric engine cooling fan that is used to assist in maintaining the engine coolant temperature. These fans are controlled by the engine's computer or by a thermostat that turns them on and off based up on the coolant temperature. Because these fans are electrically driven, rescue personnel should exercise caution while working near them. The battery power must be isolated to prevent them from coming on and creating an additional hazard at the scene of an accident.

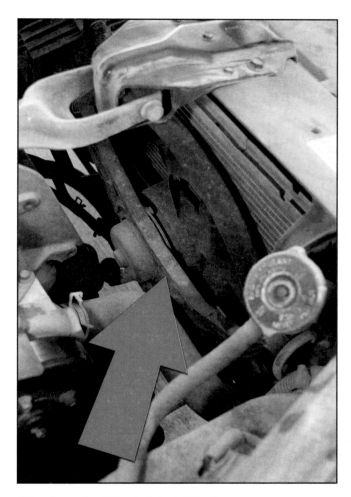

Figure 3.32 An example of an electric cooling fan.

Electronic Windshield Defoggers

Some vehicles are equipped with electronic windshield defoggers. Because of the amperage carried by these devices, rescuers should ensure the electrical power to the vehicle has been isolated to prevent shocks or the production of sparks when removing the windshield or displacing the dashboard.

Power Train Systems

Rescuers need to understand how power is transmitted to a vehicle's wheels to ensure that a wrecked vehicle is properly safetied to prevent vehicle movement and potential injury to passengers and rescuers alike. A vehicle's power train (sometimes called the drive train) includes all of the parts that create and transfer power to the road. These components include the engine/motor, transmission, drive shafts, differentials, and the drive wheels or tracks. Depending upon the number of wheels that transfer power to the surface, vehicles may be 2-wheel, 4-wheel, or all wheel drive **(Figure 3.33, p. 110)**.

- *2-wheel drive* — In 2-wheel drive vehicles, power is transferred to one axle, either in the front or rear of the vehicle, which then transfers this power to the surface.

- *4-wheel drive* — Four wheel drive (also called 4x4 or 4WD) vehicle have power sent to two axles that permits all four wheels to receive power. An advantage of 4WD is the greater traction and transfer of power when the

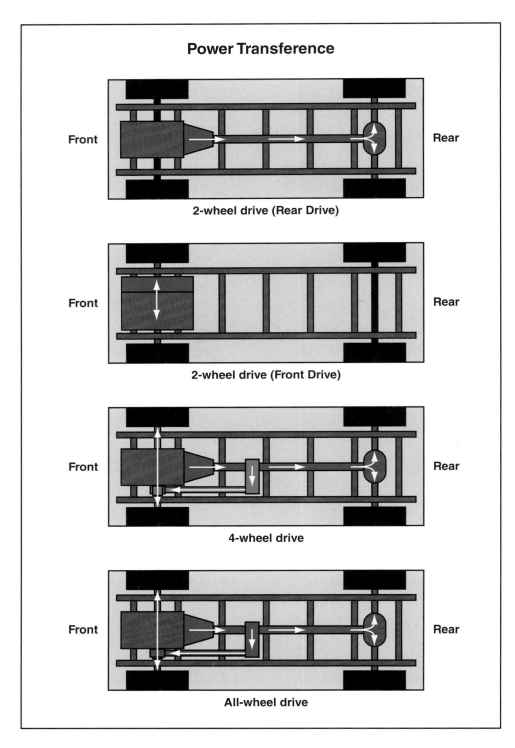

Figure 3.33 This illustration shows how power is transmitted from the engine through the drive train for 2, 4, and all-wheel drive.

vehicle is operating in areas of low traction such as gravel, mud, ice, and snow. Many such vehicles are equipped to shift (manually or automatically) between 2-wheel drive and 4-wheel drive as necessary.

- **All wheel drive** — Modern all wheel drive (AWD) vehicles normally run in 2-wheel drive mode and shift into all wheel drive automatically mode as necessary to maintain traction.

Vehicle Science

From a scientific perspective, vehicle anatomy refers to the condition of a particular vehicle after a collision. The anatomy of each vehicle involved in an incident must be assessed in terms of its center of gravity and the kinematics involved in the accident.

Center of Gravity

Whether a vehicle is upright, on its side, on its roof, or teetering on the edge of some precipice, its stability is greatly affected by its center of gravity. In general terms, half the total weight of a vehicle is on each side of its center of gravity. A vehicle's center of gravity acts as a pivot point around which the vehicle will move unless prevented from doing so **(Figure 3.34)**. The higher a vehicle's center of gravity, the more susceptible the vehicle is to rolling over. Therefore, the essence of vehicle stabilization is to support the vehicle on all sides of its center of gravity to prevent any movement.

When most automobiles and light utility vehicles are empty, the center of gravity is slightly forward of the front door in the center of the vehicle. However, given fuel in the fuel tank, objects in the trunk, and occupants inside, the center of gravity is likely to be somewhere aft of that point. Determining exactly where the center of gravity is on a particular vehicle may be especially difficult if the vehicle was significantly deformed by the collision. Therefore, every vehicle in which there are injured and trapped occupants should be stabilized to prevent any further movement.

The mass and weight of a vehicle also affect its stability after a collision. The heavier the vehicle, the greater its tendency to settle toward the stability of the ground. When a vehicle has come to rest on a slope, its mass makes it susceptible to sliding or rolling down slope. Therefore, the challenge for rescue personnel is to safely and effectively counteract this potential movement.

Kinematics — One branch of the study of dynamics that defines the motion of objects without addressing mass and force or the factors that lead to the motion. In terms of accidents, kinematics describe the effects of collisions on vehicles.

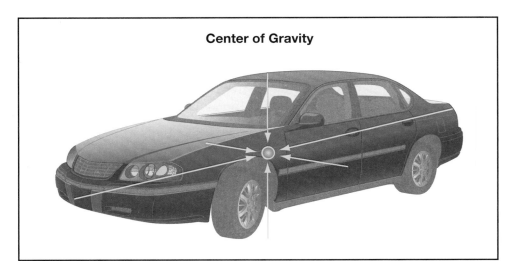

Center of Gravity

Figure 3.34 An illustration showing the approximate location of a vehicle's center of gravity.

Kinematics of Injury

The types of injuries suffered by vehicle occupants vary with the types of collisions. The point, direction, and speed of impact will dictate what injuries are most likely to be produced by any given collision. Knowing what types of injuries are produced by front-impact, rear-impact, and side-impact collisions, as well as rollovers, underrides, overrides, and rotational can help rescuers function more effectively at these incidents **(Figure 3.35)**.

Front-Impact Collisions

Some of the worst injuries to vehicle occupants are produced by front-impact collisions. Inertia forces the driver and any passengers forward as the vehicle is recoiling rearward in the split second following impact. Depending upon the speed of impact, as the front of the vehicle collapses, the dashboard and steering column may be displaced rearward into the passenger compartment.

As the vehicle recoils, if the occupants are unrestrained, the driver's chest and face collide violently with the steering wheel and steering column, causing severe facial, head, spinal, and chest trauma. The driver's hands fly forward and strike the dashboard, and if the driver's legs were stiffened in the moment before impact, they are likely to be broken. An unrestrained front seat passenger will violently collide with the dashboard, perhaps breaking both arms and suffering massive facial, head, spinal, and chest trauma. He will either be propelled over the dashboard and into the windshield (and perhaps through it), or under the dashboard to become wedged there. One or both legs may be broken in the process. As the front of the vehicle collapses further, the kick panels, firewall, and tilt steering columns may collapse and enfold the feet, legs, and any other body parts wedged under the dashboard. One or both front doors may fly open allowing those inside to be thrown out — or the doors may crumple and jam.

Unrestrained rear seat passengers will also be at the mercy of inertia. They may be propelled forward into the backs of the front seats, perhaps slipping between the front seats and colliding violently with the dashboard. The G-forces generated by their weight impacting the backs of the front seats will be added to the already tremendous forces acting on those in the front seats.

However, if the vehicle was equipped with air bags, and the occupants were wearing their seat belts, the results could be dramatically different. Depending upon the speed of impact, a properly belted driver may survive the crash virtually unscathed or with only minor injuries. If one of the driver's hands were in the 12 o'clock position at the top of the steering wheel when the air bag deployed, the force of the inflation could push that hand back into the driver's face. This may result in a broken nose, and perhaps facial lacerations if the driver were wearing glasses. If a knee bolster air bag protects the driver's lower legs as the front of the vehicle collapses, there may be little if any injury.

Front seat passengers could expect similar protection if they were buckled up in a vehicle equipped with passenger air bags. Their extremities may flail about until the vehicle comes to rest, but any resulting injuries are likely to be relatively minor. Rear seat passengers may also flail about some, but any resulting injuries are also likely to be relatively minor.

Types of Collisions

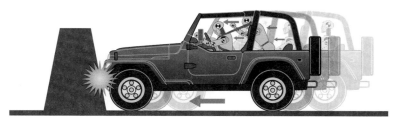

Front Impact

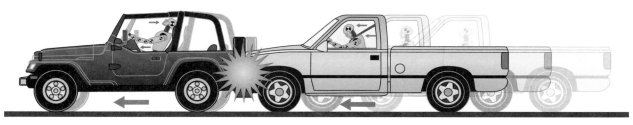

Rear Impact

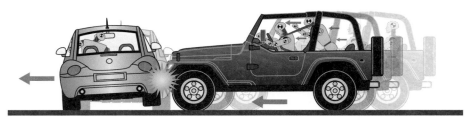

Side Impact

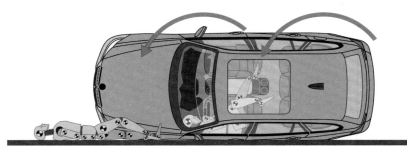

Rollover

Figure 3.35 Common types of collisions.

Types of Collisions

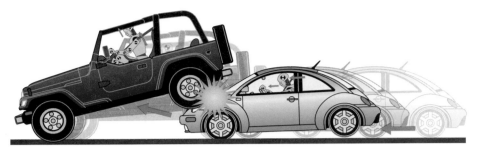

Underride

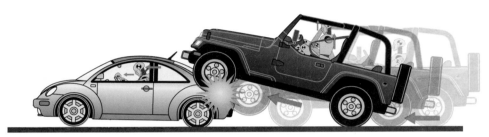

Override

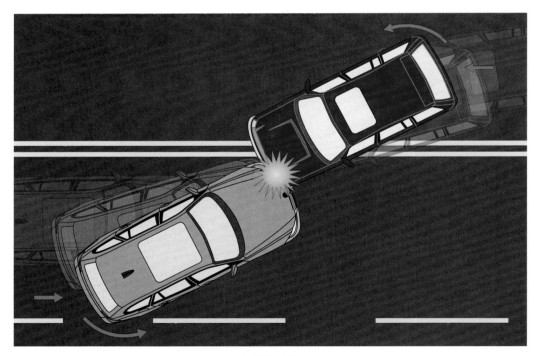

Rotational

Figure 3.35 (Continued) Common types of collisions.

Rear-Impact Collisions

Again, depending upon the speed of impact, rear-impact collisions can create their own unique problems for vehicle occupants and rescuers. In relatively low speed impacts, the rear-end structure of large sedans and station wagons can act as a crumple zone softening the impact on those inside. In higher speed impacts, those inside are susceptible to whiplash trauma resulting in spinal injuries. Unrestrained and improperly restrained occupants can also be thrown upward making violent contact with the roof of the vehicle. Additionally, the impact can cause the seatbacks to collapse complicating the injuries sustained by the occupants. Also, since the rear of most passenger vehicles is lighter than the front end, a rear-end collision can raise the rear of the vehicle off the ground while the vehicle is being pushed forward. This can result in the rear-ended vehicle rolling over. When this happens, the physical effects of being thrown about inside the passenger compartment are added to any other rear-impact injuries.

Side-Impact (Lateral) Collisions

Side-impact collisions can also produce some very serious injuries to the vehicle occupants. Whether the impact is the result of a so-called T-bone collision by another vehicle, or if the vehicle slid sideways into a tree or other solid object, the results are often the same. T-bone collisions can also result in the struck vehicle rolling over. Regardless of how the collision occurs, a vehicle that is struck in the side tends to fold itself around the point of impact. If the speed of impact is high enough, side-impacted vehicles sometimes tear completely apart leaving them in two separate pieces. Obviously, this does not bode well for anyone inside the vehicle.

While side-impact injuries can be prevented or reduced by side-impact air bags and head protection systems, many passenger vehicles still do not have these safety features. The result is that vehicle occupants on the side that is impacted suffer head, spinal, chest, abdominal/pelvic, and lower extremity injuries when they are thrown into the doors and windows by the force of the collision. They can also suffer injuries to the arm and leg on the impact side.

Rollovers

This very common type of incident can also produce a variety of serious injuries to those inside vehicles that roll over one or more times. The most common type of rollover involves a vehicle rolling sideways — that is, rolling onto its side and perhaps continuing to roll onto its roof, its other side, and back onto its wheels. Depending upon the speed at which the vehicle was traveling, the terrain and other variables, a vehicle may roll from one to several times before coming to rest. If the vehicle occupants are properly restrained by their seat belts, they may survive a sideways rollover with relatively minor injuries — provided that the roof does not collapse. If the occupants were not wearing their seat belts and/or the roof of the vehicle collapses on them, the injuries are likely to be much more serious, perhaps fatal. In addition to being tumbled over and over inside the vehicle, unrestrained occupants can be thrown out of the vehicle openings.

Less common, although not rare, are incidents involving a vehicle rolling end-over-end. To generate the force necessary to cause a vehicle to flip end-over-end repeatedly, it must be traveling at a very high rate of speed. However, the environment in which the rollover occurs can be a major contributor to this type of incident. For example, if a vehicle traveling at normal highway speed plunges down a steep slope and strikes a boulder or other solid object, inertia may cause it to flip once and the effects of gravity and the angle of the slope may cause it to continue to flip until it reaches the bottom of the slope. Because the roof of a vehicle involved in this type of incident is very likely to collapse, the occupants may suffer head and spinal injuries even if they were properly restrained.

Underride and Override

Underride occurs when a striking vehicle collides with another vehicle and comes to rest under the vehicle being struck. This often results in the roof of the striking vehicle being crushed or torn off. Passengers in such vehicles normally receive severe trauma to the head or are decapitated.

Override occurs when a striking vehicle collides with another vehicle and comes to rest on top of the vehicle being struck. The force of impact and weight of the upper vehicle can remove or collapse the roof of the lower vehicle as well as prevent the vehicle's door from opening. Passengers in the over-ride vehicle can receive injuries to the head, neck, arms, torso, and legs.

Rotational

Rotational collisions are caused by off center front or side impacts that force-fully turn the impacted vehicle horizontally inducing a spin to one or more of the accident vehicles. Collisions of this nature occur when a vehicle strikes a stationary object (such as a tree, guardrail, or post) or is struck by another vehicle. Generally, the types of injuries associated with rotational collisions are similar to those in front-, rear-, and side-impacts.

Summary

This chapter provided an overview of common types of vehicles. It also described general vehicle anatomy to include common vehicle terminology, vehicle construction, and materials used. The three types of vehicle frames and the relationship of modern windshields to a vehicle's structural integrity were discussed.

The types and roles of supplemental restraint systems and energy-absorbing vehicle features in protecting a vehicle's passenger during an accident by providing restraint, keeping them in the passenger compartment, and absorbing the energy of the impact were described. Next, various vehicle systems and the hazardous they present in an accident were discussed. Finally, the chapter covered basic vehicle science relating to center of gravity, mass, and the kinematics of injury.

Review Questions

1. What are the five main classifications of vehicles?

2. What are some common materials used in vehicle construction?

3. Which vehicle frame type has the body and frame created as one piece?

4. What hazards are posed by Supplemental Restraint and Rollover Protection Systems?

5. Describe each type of vehicle glass.

6. List types of vehicle fuels and fuel systems.

7. What are the hazards associated with various vehicle electrical system components?

8. Describe the three common power train system configurations.

9. What types of injuries are associated with each type of vehicle collision?

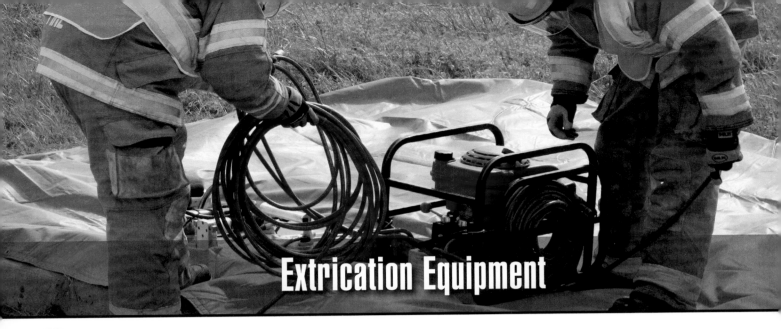

Extrication Equipment

Chapter Contents

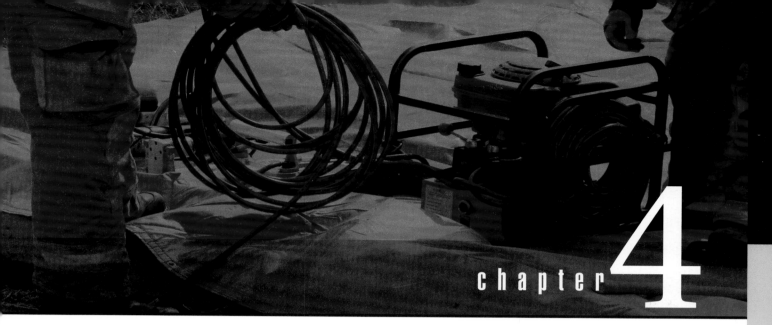

Key Terms

Job Performance Requirements

This chapter provides information that addresses the following job performance requirements (JPRs) of NFPA® 1001, *Standard for Fire Fighter Professional Qualifications* (2008), NFPA® 1006, *Standard for Technical Rescuer Professional Qualifications* (2008), NFPA® 1670, *Standard on Operations and Training for Technical Search and Rescue Incidents* (2009).

NFPA® 1001 JPRs

6.4.1

6.4.2

NFPA® 1006 JPRs

4.3	5.2.3	10.1.4	10.1.10
4.3.1	5.4.1	10.1.5	10.2.2
4.3.2	5.4.2	10.1.7	10.2.4
5.2.1	5.5.1	10.1.8	10.2.5

NFPA® 1670 JPRs

4.1.4	4.4.2.1	4.4.2.4	4.5.1.2
4.4.1.1	4.4.2.2	4.4.2.4.1	4.5.1.3
4.4.1.2	4.4.2.3	4.4.2.4.4	

Extrication Equipment

Learning Objectives

1. Identify personal protective equipment used at extrication operations.
2. Describe universal precautions to be taken against blood borne pathogens.
3. Describe equipment to be used to provide head, eyes, and face protection.
4. Identify basic facts about equipment to be used to provide hearing, body, foot, and hand protection.
5. Describe various specialized protective equipment.
6. Identify basic facts about caring for personal protective equipment.
7. Describe each type of rescue vehicle.
8. Describe different types of rescue vehicle body construction.
9. Identify basic facts about rescue vehicle chassis.
10. Identify basic facts about special rescue vehicle equipment and accessories.
11. Identify types of extrication tools and equipment.
12. Identify basic facts about the functions and purposes of various extrication tools and equipment.
13. Describe the importance of routine operational checks and maintenance.

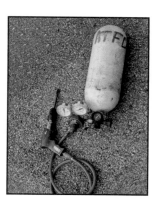

Chapter 4
Extrication Equipment

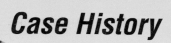

Case History

A rescue engine and paramedic unit were dispatched to a motor vehicle accident with entrapment. The first arriving officer assumed command then established and assessed the scene. Each vehicle contained one patient requiring extrication and medical treatment. A second rescue unit arrived and set up a tool cache for extrication operations. The personnel of the rescue engine stabilized the vehicles and began roof removal on Vehicle #1. Hydraulic tools were used to remove the vehicle doors, create relief cuts, and perform a dash roll. A reciprocating saw was used to perform a "third door conversion" along the driver's side to allow rescuers more space to access and remove the driver. Patient #1 was stabilized, packaged, and transferred to an ambulance for transport. Rescue personnel were equally successful in gaining access into Vehicle #2 and to patient #2. Both patients were transported to local medical facilities.

Some extrication tools and equipment have remained virtually unchanged since their introduction. However, as in every other field of rescue technology, many have continued to evolve. Personal protective equipment and a number of traditional hand tools and power tools have been greatly improved, or new ones introduced, in recent years. Likewise, auxiliary equipment, such as generators, floodlights, and air compressors that had to be added to rescue vehicles in the past are now standard equipment on most new vehicles.

This chapter discusses the personal protective clothing and equipment that rescuers need in order to perform extrication safely. Also discussed are various types of rescue vehicles and a variety of manually operated and power driven tools used in extrication incidents. Finally, routine operational checks and maintenance are outlined.

Personal Protective Equipment

Because rescuers work in hazardous environments, they should be provided with the best personal protective equipment (PPE) available. In many agencies, SOPs specify the most appropriate type and level of PPE to be used based on the hazards present, temperature and humidity, and other environmental factors. During an incident, the Incident Safety Officer (ISO) enforces the applicable SOPs and dictates any changes in the type and level of PPE as necessary. The ISO should ensure that all personnel working in the action area are wearing proper and appropriate PPE. Coveralls, street clothing, station uniforms, or even brush fire fighting jackets worn without additional PPE are usually not acceptable at extrication incidents.

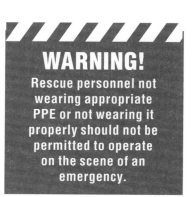

WARNING!
Rescue personnel not wearing appropriate PPE or not wearing it properly should not be permitted to operate on the scene of an emergency.

For most extrication incidents, standard structure fire turnout gear is sufficient **(Figure 4.1)**. Special operations, such as extrication in a body of water or over a steep cliff, may require specialized personal protective equipment. In the sections that follow, the basic types of turnout gear are described as well as other equipment that may be required.

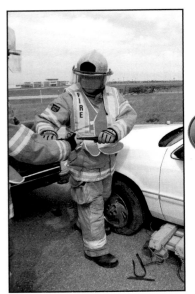

Figure 4.1 A rescuer wearing standard firefighter turn-outs, helmet, gloves, boots, and safety glasses.

Care of Personal Protective Equipment

Proper care and maintenance of personal protective equipment is vital to maintaining its reliability. After each time protective equipment is used, it should be cleaned and inspected for defects that may limit its effectiveness during its next use. Care and maintenance for all equipment — from protective clothing to breathing apparatus — should be conducted according to the manufacturer's recommendations. Test breathing apparatus regularly. For more in-depth information on respiratory protective equipment, consult the IFSTA **Respiratory Protection for Fire and Emergency Services** manual.

Head, Eyes, and Face Protection

At all extrication incidents, proper protective headgear must be worn. Helmets protect the skull from flying objects, bumps into protruding objects, and head injuries due to falls or slips. All helmets should meet the requirements set forth by NFPA® 1971, *Standard on Protective Ensemble for Structural Fire Fighting.* Helmet flaps should be pulled down over the ears to protect the ears from flying sparks or glass fragments **(Figure 4.2)**.

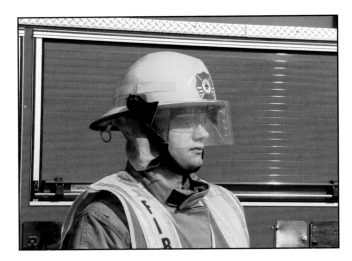

Figure 4.3 A rescuer wearing safety glasses with the helmet shield in the down position.

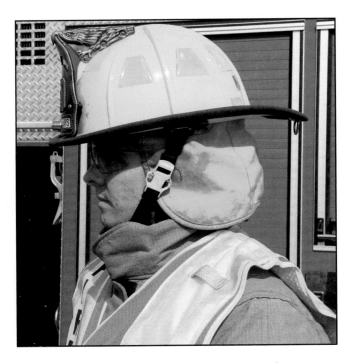

Figure 4.2 Helmet flaps prevent foreign objects from striking the wearer's ears or neck.

The face and eyes must be protected from flying objects and spraying liquids such as battery acid or hydraulic fluid that may cause severe injury. Unprotected, the eyes provide a pathway for infectious organisms. One of the most commonly used types of protection for the face is the protective shield of the helmet. The standard sizes of shields are 4 and 6 inches (100 mm and 150 mm). Generally, the 6-inch (150 mm) shield is more desirable for extrication personnel because it covers a larger portion of the face.

NOTE: NFPA® 1500 requires that helmet goggles or safety glasses be worn in addition to the helmet faceshield when performing tasks such as those involved in extrication **(Figure 4.3)**.

When agencies select head protection, fire-resistant, protective hoods should be considered. These hoods provide excellent heat protection for the neck, ears, head, and sides of the face **(Figure 4.4)**. In addition to providing protection against radiant heat and direct flame impingement, they provide warmth during cold weather. They may also prevent some cuts and scratches caused by brushing against sharp objects. These hoods are recommended on all vehicle extrication operations.

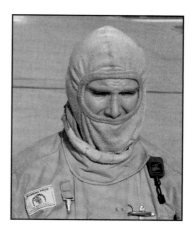

Figure 4.4 Flash hoods provide another layer of protection for rescuers.

Hearing Protection

Vehicle extrication operations can be extremely noisy. There may be generators, hydraulic power units, and power tools in use. The operators of these tools, and anyone nearby (including trapped patients), should wear appropriate hearing protection. This protection may be in the form of ear plugs inserted into the ear canal or external "ear muffs" worn along with all the other required PPE **(Figures 4.5a and b)**. Sound level surveys should be conducted during extrication training exercises to determine decibel levels. Hearing protection should be selected that is appropriate for the decibel levels measured.

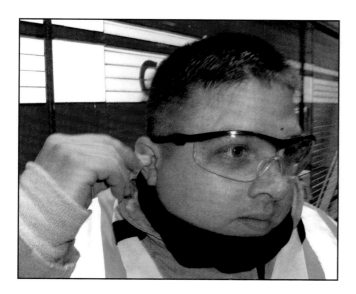

Figure 4.5a A rescuer inserting ear plug type hearing protection into his ear. *Courtesy of Alan Braun, University of Missouri Fire and Rescue Training Institute.*

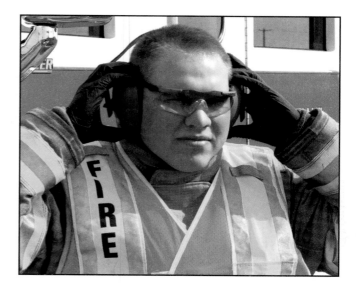

Figure 4.5b "Ear muffs" are another type of hearing protection .

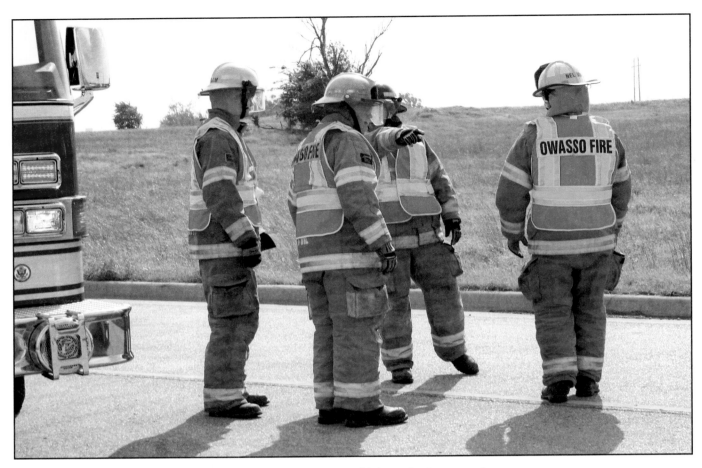
Figure 4.6 Reflective vests make rescuers more visible during vehicle extrication operations.

Body Protection

As mentioned earlier, appropriate protective clothing must be worn at all extrication incidents. Rescue company members should be in complete gear upon arrival at the scene. If turnout gear is worn, it should conform to the standards set forth by NFPA® 1971, *Standard on Protective Ensemble for Structural Fire Fighting.* In addition to providing protection against fire products, turnout gear protects rescuers from sharp objects, protruding or flying objects, and many other hazards found on the extrication scene. This protection reduces the chance of injury.

Rescue personnel must be visible on the incident scene. Regardless of color, both pants and coats should have adequate reflective striping. NFPA® 1971 gives specific requirements for the amount of striping necessary. Helmets can also be outfitted with reflective strips or patches. At a minimum, emergency response personnel who are not working in the action areas at a vehicle extrication operation should wear ANSI/DOT approved safety vests to increase their visibility to drivers passing the incident area **(Figure 4.6)**.

Foot Protection

Vehicle collision scenes are often strewn with broken glass and other potential hazards to the feet; therefore, adequate foot protection is essential. Foot protection should be selected that provides the best protection against likely hazards rescuers will encounter: heat, punctures, and impact. All footwear should meet ANSI Z41-1991, *American National Standard for Personal Protection - Protective Footwear*, as well as NFPA® 1971. Because a proper fit is important in reducing foot fatigue and in preventing blisters or other sores, appropriate footwear should be provided to each rescuer **(Figure 4.7)**.

Hand Protection

Gloves are an important part of personal protective equipment. The type of gloves worn by rescuers will vary with the job they are doing and the type of protection required. If rescue personnel are fighting fire, they should be wearing gloves that meet the standards set forth by NFPA®1971. However, when personnel are performing extrication functions that do not involve fire, this type of glove may be too bulky and restrictive to allow for the needed dexterity.

When performing most extrication functions, rescuers need gloves that protect their hands but allow freedom of movement. Therefore, in most situations, rescuers should wear close-fitting leather gloves or gloves that are specifically designed for use at vehicle extrication incidents. In addition, gloves should be thin enough to allow dexterity but sturdy enough to protect hands from cuts, punctures, and abrasions **(Figure 4.8)**. NFPA®1500 requires that rescue personnel who are likely to come in contact with blood or other bodily fluids wear medical exam gloves inside their leather gloves or wear emergency medical work gloves. These gloves must meet the requirements of NFPA® 1999, *Standard on Protective Clothing for Medical Emergency Operations.*

Universal Precautions Against Blood Borne Pathogens

Because rescue personnel must often work in close proximity to badly injured vehicle occupants, they must protect themselves from contact with blood and other bodily fluids. In addition to the other parts of the protective ensemble previously discussed, rescue personnel should wear any other items necessary to isolate them from these substances. Additional items that may be necessary include medical exam gloves worn under their leather gloves, appropriate respiratory protection, and Tyvec® gowns or sheets over their regular protective clothing.

Respiratory Protection

Although oxygen-deficient atmospheres are uncommon in vehicle extrication incidents, hazardous vapors, fumes, smoke, and dust are often present. Therefore, rescuers (and in some cases, trapped patients) often require respiratory protection. Rescue personnel should be well trained in the operation, use, capabilities, and limitations of all types of respiratory protection available to them. Achieving and maintaining this level of proficiency requires regular training and periodic testing. Rescue personnel typically use either of three types of breathing equipment —self-contained breathing apparatus (SCBA), supplied air respirators (SAR), and air-purifying respirators (APRs).

Self-Contained Breathing Apparatus (SCBA)

All self-contained breathing apparatus must be of the positive-pressure type and should meet the requirements of NFPA®1981, *Standard on Open-Circuit Self-Contained Breathing Apparatus for Fire and Emergency Services*

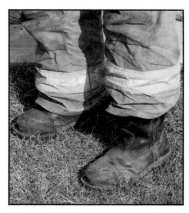

Figure 4.7 A rescuer wearing approved footwear.

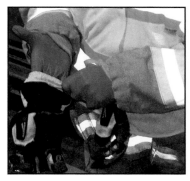

Figure 4.8 Rescue gloves may be worn over latex gloves.

Blood Borne Pathogens — Pathogenic microorganisms that are present in the human blood and can cause disease in humans. These pathogens include (but are not limited to) hepatitis B virus (HBV) and human immunodeficiency virus (HIV).

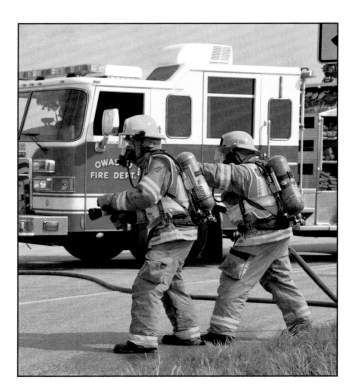

Figure 4.9 Rescuers wearing SCBA at an automobile accident. *Courtesy of Sonrise Photography.*

(Figure 4.9). Because facial contours vary from person to person, facepieces are designed in different sizes in order to obtain a proper fit. *29 CFR 1910.134* requires that each rescuer be issued a personal facepiece that is fit-tested at the time of issue and annually thereafter **(Figure 4.10).** NFPA® 1500 expressly prohibits beards, long sideburns, or other facial hair that would interfere with the facepiece seal or the operation of the unit. This restriction is based upon a 1990 ruling by OSHA which stated that anything that interferes with the facepiece seal is in violation of 29 CFR 1910.134.

Figure 4.10 A rescuer undergoing a test to ensure a proper facepiece fit. *Courtesy of Alan Braun, University of Missouri Fire and Rescue Training Institute.*

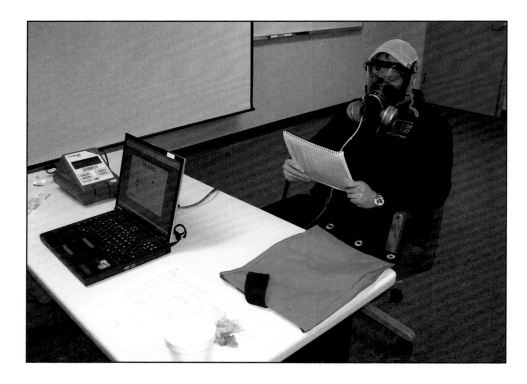

SCBA have either a 30-minute, 45-minute, or 60-minute rating. These ratings are frequently misunderstood and personnel can be put in danger if the ratings are taken literally. These ratings are determined by timing a number of average, healthy individuals breathing at a relaxed, normal respiratory rate. When each person consumes the amount of air in the cylinder or unit, the time is recorded, the average is taken, and a rated time is assigned to the apparatus. The time-related ratings of SCBA cylinders represent the maximum amount of time the air supply will last under ideal circumstances.

The actual "duration of support" depends on the individual wearer's physiological and psychological conditioning. Protective breathing apparatus training should be frequent enough and of sufficient duration to allow personnel to become comfortable with having their faces covered by their masks and to overcome any tendency they may have toward claustrophobia. Given this type of training, rescuers who know their jobs well and who are in good physical condition can remain calm during emergencies and make maximum use of the air supply in each cylinder. Further information on self-contained breathing apparatus is available in the IFSTA **Respiratory Protection for Fire and Emergency Services** manual.

Supplied-Air Respirator (SAR)

Another form of breathing apparatus is the supplied-air respirator (SAR). Air is supplied to the users by high-pressure hoses up to 300 feet (90 m) long from a bank of larger air supply cylinders or an air compressor. Rescuers using airline equipment wear a body harness to which the regulator and mask are attached. Also attached is a five- or ten-minute emergency breathing support system (EBSS) to give the wearer an emergency air supply should the airline fail. Some fire departments have adapted the breathing air systems on their aerial devices to airline systems. The same can be done to cascade systems on rescue vehicles or other apparatus.

While airline systems are most often used in the rescue of those overcome by toxic gases, fumes, or mists inside large industrial tanks, tank cars, and other confined spaces, it is possible that some extrication incidents may make the use of these systems necessary. If the scene has been or may be contaminated with airborne hazards, personnel may need to be provided with this type of air supply. Further information on supplied-air respirators is available in the IFSTA **Respiratory Protection for Fire and Emergency Services** manual.

Air-Purifying Respirators (APR)

APRs contain an air-purifying filter, canister, or cartridge that removes specific contaminants found in ambient air as the air passes through the air-purifying element. Based on what cartridge, canister, or filter is being used, these purifying elements are generally divided into the three following types:

- Particulate-removing APRs
- Vapor-and-gas-removing APRs
- Combination particulate-removing and vapor-and-gas-removing APRs

Air-Purifying Respirator (APR) — Respirator with an air-purifying filter, cartridge, or canister that removes specific air contaminates by passing ambient air through the air-purifying element; may have a full or partial facepiece.

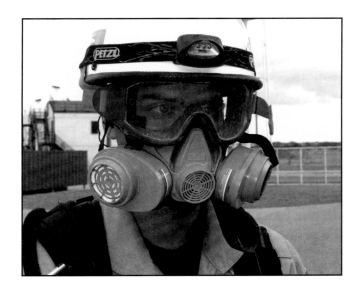

Figure 4.11 A rescuer wearing an APR.

APRs may be powered (PAPRs) or nonpowered. APRs do not supply oxygen or air from a separate source, and they protect only against specific contaminants at or below certain concentrations.

Respirators with air-purifying filters may have either full facepieces that provide a complete seal to the face and protect the eyes, nose, and mouth or half facepieces that provide a complete seal to the face and protect the nose and mouth **(Figure 4.11)**. Disposable filters, canisters, or cartridges are mounted on one or both sides of the facepiece. Canister or cartridge respirators pass the air through a filter, sorbent, catalyst, or combination of these items to remove specific contaminants from the air. The air can enter the system either from the external atmosphere through the filter or sorbent or when the user's exhalation combines with a catalyst to provide breathable air.

APRs should be worn only in controlled atmospheres where the hazards present are completely understood and at least 19.5 percent oxygen is present. If oxygen contents are lower than prescribed, positive pressure SCBA or SAR must be worn during emergency operations. As with chemical protective clothing (CPC), no single canister, filter, or cartridge protects against all chemical hazards. Responders must know the hazards present in the atmosphere in order to select the appropriate canister, filter, or cartridge. Responders should be able to answer the following questions before deciding to use APRs for protection at a haz mat incident:

- What is the hazard?
- Is the hazard a vapor or a gas?
- Is the hazard a particle or dust?
- Is there some combination of dust and vapors present?
- What concentrations are present?

Furthermore, first responders should know that APRs do *not* protect against oxygen-deficient or oxygen-enriched atmospheres. The three primary limitations of an APR are as follows:

- Limited life of its filters and canisters
- Need for constant monitoring of the contaminated atmosphere
- Need for a normal oxygen content of the atmosphere before use

Take the following precautions before using APRs or PAPRs:

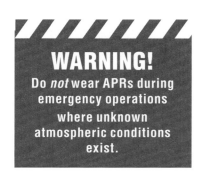

WARNING!
Do *not* wear APRs during emergency operations where unknown atmospheric conditions exist.

- Know what chemicals/air contaminants are in the air.

- Know how much of the chemicals/air contaminants are in the air.

- Ensure that the oxygen level is between 19.5 and 23.5 percent.

- Ensure that atmospheric hazards are not immediately dangerous to life and health (IDLH) conditions.

Special Protective Equipment

In a small number of extrication incidents, the IC may have to call in technical rescue personnel who are specially trained and equipped to operate in extremely hazardous environments. The special protective equipment that these teams wear may include hazardous materials suits, proximity or entry suits, body armor, and wet suits **(Figures 4.12a and b)**. However, if the trapped patients have been without benefit of respiratory protection in an extremely toxic atmosphere for some time, the IC must consider whether to conduct the operation as a rescue or as a body recovery.

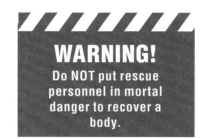

WARNING!
Do NOT put rescue personnel in mortal danger to recover a body.

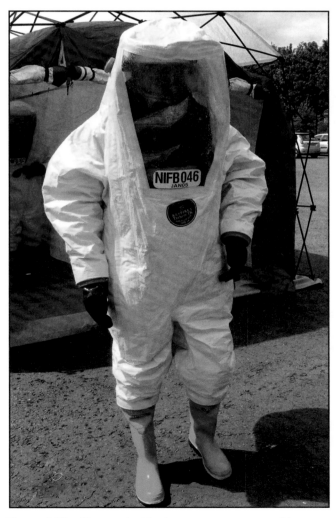

Figure 4.12a At some incidents, rescuers may need to wear hazardous materials suits.

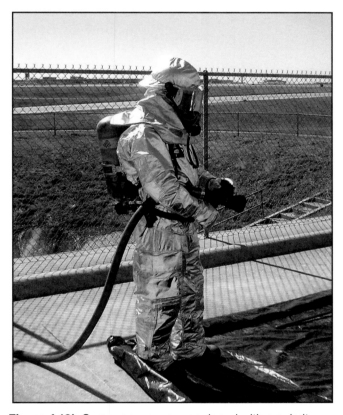

Figure 4.12b Some rescuers are equipped with proximity suits. *Courtesy of Brian Canady, DFWIA Department of Public Safety.*

More information on special protective equipment may be found in the IFSTA **Fire Service Search and Rescue** and **Hazardous Materials for the First Responder** manuals.

Rescue Vehicles

Fire departments and emergency response organizations use a wide variety of rescue vehicles and call them by a variety of names. For the purposes of clarity, rescue vehicles in this manual are referred to by the following classifications:

- Light rescue vehicles
- Medium rescue vehicles
- Heavy rescue vehicles
- Rescue engines
- Standard engines
- Ladder trucks

Light Rescue Vehicles

Light rescue vehicles are designed to handle only basic extrication and life-support functions; therefore, they carry only basic hand tools and small equipment. Often, a light rescue unit functions as a first responder unit that attempts to stabilize the situation until more appropriate equipment arrives. The standard equipment carried by many ladder and engine companies also gives them light rescue capabilities.

Light rescue vehicles can be built on a 1-ton or 1½ -ton chassis. The rescue vehicle's body resembles a multiple compartment utility truck although they may be configured out of SUV style vehicles **(Figure 4.13)**. A light rescue vehicle can carry a variety of small hand tools, such as saws, jacks, and pry bars, as well as smaller hydraulic rescue equipment and a small inventory of emergency medical supplies.

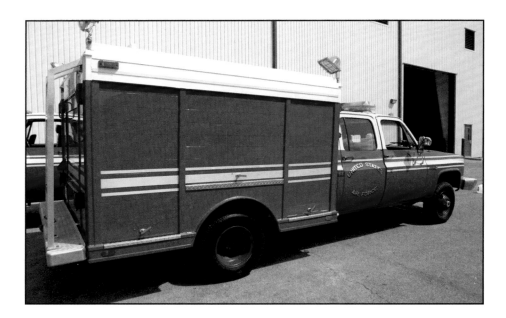

Figure 4.13 An example of a light rescue truck.

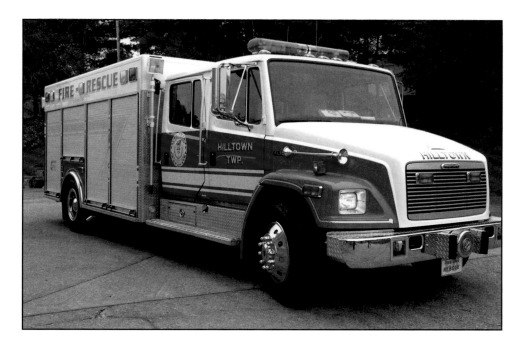

Figure 4.14 An example of a medium rescue truck.

Medium Rescue Vehicles

Medium rescue vehicles are designed to have a wider range of capabilities than the light rescue vehicles. Medium rescue units are capable of handling the majority of vehicle rescue incidents because they often carry a variety of fire fighting equipment, making them dual purpose units **(Figure 4.14)**. In addition to basic hand tools, medium rescue vehicles may carry any of the following equipment:

- Powered hydraulic spreading tools and cutters
- Pneumatic lifting bags
- Power saws
- Acetylene cutting equipment
- Ropes and rigging equipment

Specialized units may often be considered medium rescue vehicles. Specialized units have specific uses, but they may carry generalized equipment that can be used in other types of incidents. Some types of specialized units include the following:

- Hazardous materials units
- Water rescue and recovery units
- Bomb disposal units
- Mine rescue units
- Technical rescue units
- Lighting/power units.

Heavy Rescue Vehicles

Heavy rescue units must be capable of providing the support necessary to extricate patients from almost any entrapment. As their name implies, heavy rescue vehicles carry more and heavier equipment than do smaller vehicles. Additional types of equipment carried by the heavy rescue unit include the following:

- A-frames or gin poles
- Cascade systems
- Larger power plants
- Trenching and shoring equipment
- Small pumps and foam equipment
- Large winches
- Hydraulic booms
- Large quantities of rope and rigging equipment
- Air compressors
- Ladders

Some modern heavy rescue vehicles are equipped with extendable light tower systems or hydraulic cranes mounted to the apparatus. Other specialized equipment may be carried according to the responsibilities of the rescue unit and the rescue exposures identified within the response district. Heavy rescue units are sometimes oriented more toward fire fighting than smaller units because they have more space available for fire fighting equipment.

Rescue Engines

A rescue engine is a multipurpose apparatus designed to perform both the functions of a structural fire fighting pumper and a rescue vehicle **(Figure 4.15)**. As a result, this apparatus is useful at almost any type of incident and has sufficient rescue equipment to handle common extrication incidents. However, this versatility does not come without a price. Because they are dual-purpose units, they generally cannot provide the same level of service in either fire fighting or rescue as can the same size unit dedicated to one discipline or the other.

Rescue engines vary in size. Some fire departments use minipumpers or midipumpers (initial attack fire apparatus) with light rescue capabilities. Other departments use full-size engines that have been custom designed with extra-large compartments or other modifications for carrying rescue equipment. These larger apparatus are usually equipped with Class A fire pumps and large water tanks.

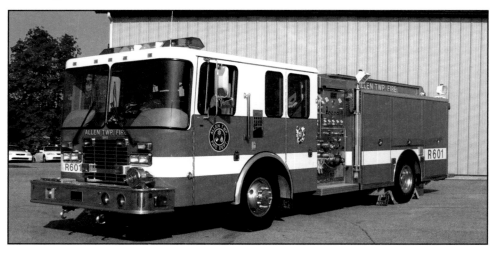

Figure 4.15 Some departments use rescue engines to respond to extrication incidents.

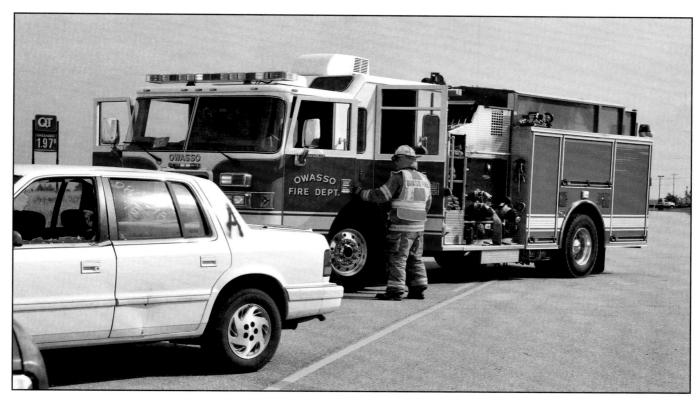

Figure 4.16 A fire pumper arriving at the scene of an automobile accident. *Courtesy of Sonrise Photography.*

Standard Engines

In some departments, engine companies are expected to provide certain extrication services. Using the equipment carried on most standard engines, company personnel are able to perform many vehicle extrication tasks **(Figure 4.16)**. In some cases, the first-arriving engine company can perform extrication before other specialized equipment arrives. In other cases, the engine company can establish a perimeter, set up fire protection, and provide additional personnel to rescue companies working the incident.

Ladder Trucks

In many fire departments, ladder companies are better equipped to perform extrication operations than are engine companies. Most ladder trucks carry a greater quantity and variety of equipment than engines. Forcible entry tools and equipment carried on ladder trucks can often be used for vehicle extrication purposes **(Figure 4.17, p. 134)**. On large-scale incidents, ladder company personnel can be used to supplement rescue personnel when additional help is needed but additional rescue companies are not readily available.

In departments whose fiscal constraints preclude the establishment of a dedicated rescue service, ladder companies normally carry a full complement of rescue equipment, and they routinely do most of the extrication work. Because aerial apparatus typically have a large amount of compartment space, they lend themselves to carrying additional extrication equipment. Personnel who are already trained in ladder company operations are often cross-trained to perform extrication operation.

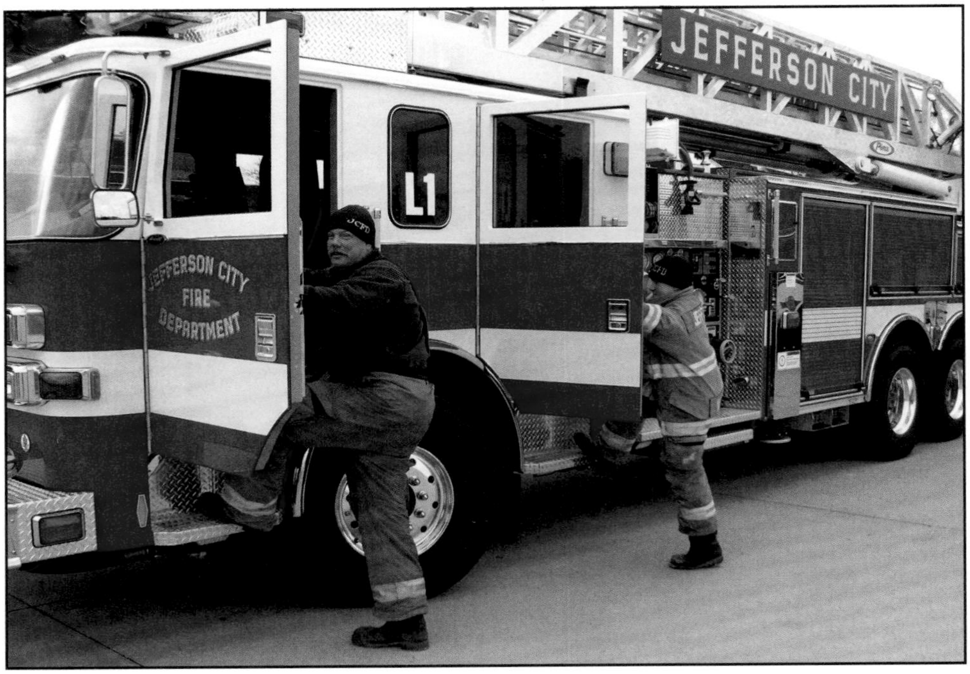

Figure 4.17 Some departments respond aerial apparatus (truck) companies to extrication incidents. *Courtesy of Alan Braun, University of Missouri Fire and Rescue Training Institute.*

Rescue Vehicle Compartmentation

Rescue vehicles are designed to transport rescuers and tools and equipment to emergency scenes. The bodies of rescue vehicle can be divided into the passenger compartment and the tool/equipment compartments. The passenger compartment of a rescue vehicle is much the same as other fire and emergency apparatus. The compartments for carrying the rescue tools and equipment vary from vehicle to vehicle but generally fit into the following three types:

1. Exclusive exterior compartmentation

2. Exclusive interior compartmentation

3. Combination compartmentation

Exclusive Exterior (Non-Walk In) Compartmentation

Exclusive exterior compartmentation is most commonly found in smaller rescue units, although some larger units are also set up in this manner **(Figure 4.18)**. These vehicles offer no walk-in/walk-through area or interior storage. Tools and equipment are only accessible from outside the vehicle.

Exterior compartmentation is advantageous because personnel do not have to enter the vehicle to access needed equipment. However, there are also disadvantages to this design. One disadvantage is that the compartment doors must have enough room to swing open which can be a problem in situations where space is limited. Vehicles equipped with roll-up compartment doors offer an alternative design that eliminates this problem. Regardless of the style of doors on the vehicle, exterior exclusive vehicles cannot transport as many personnel to an incident as other vehicles can.

Exclusive Interior (Walk In) Compartmentation

Vehicles with exclusive interior compartmentation have all of their storage in an interior walk-in/walk-through area. Some find this arrangement convenient because the entire inventory is accessible from the inside of the vehicle and out of the weather.

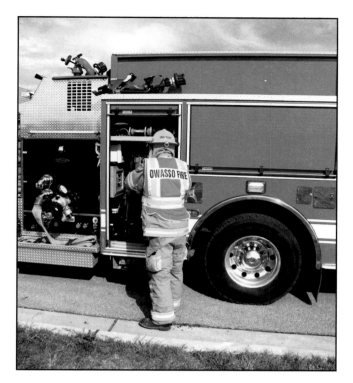

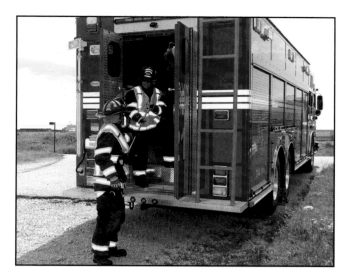

Figure 4.19 This rescue vehicle has both external and internal compartments in which equipment is stored. *Courtesy of Lake Ozark Fire District (MO).*

Figure 4.18 Equipment is carried in external compartments on this apparatus.

Vehicles designed with an interior walk-through area can sometimes transport more personnel inside the vehicle than vehicles with only exterior compartmentation. However, having to enter the vehicle for tools and equipment may slow procedures at an emergency scene. In addition, having to carry heavy tools and equipment from the walk-through level down to the ground level and back again can make the process more difficult.

Combination Compartmentation

Perhaps the most functional style of rescue vehicle body is one with a combination walk-in/walk-through area and both exterior and interior compartmentation **(Figure 4.19)**. Vehicles with this type of body offer the advantages of each design, and if equipped with roll-up compartment doors, few of the disadvantages of the less versatile designs. Having large compartments on the exterior promotes better ergonomics by allowing bulky and heavy pieces of equipment to be carried in a position where they are easily accessed. Likewise, protective clothing, medical supplies, and similar items can be carried inside out of the weather.

Rescue Vehicle Chassis

Just as there are a number of different vehicle bodies, there are also different types of rescue vehicle chassis. The two primary types of vehicle chassis are commercial and custom. Each has certain advantages and disadvantages.

Commercial chassis are built by commercial truck manufacturers **(Figure 4.20, p. 136)**. These truck chassis are typically used for commercial vehicles, such as plumber's trucks, garbage trucks, dump trucks, and delivery trucks.

Chassis — Basic operating system of a motor vehicle consisting of the frame, suspension system, wheels, and steering mechanism but not the body.

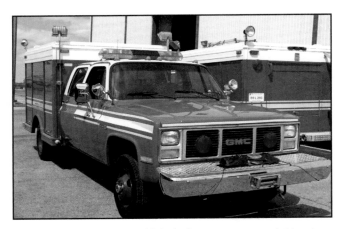

Figure 4.20 A rescue vehicle built on a commercial truck chassis.

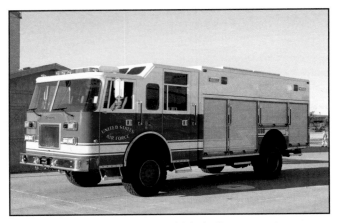

Figure 4.21 A larger rescue vehicle built on a custom chassis.

Commercial chassis are also the most commonly used chassis for rescue vehicles. All light and medium chassis units and a large percentage of heavy rescue chassis units are commercial chassis.

Custom chassis are built by manufacturers who specialize in fire apparatus chassis, so they are designed to withstand the heavy use of the emergency service **(Figure 4.21)**. Custom chassis often incorporate special design features specified by the agency purchasing them.

Special Rescue Vehicle Equipment and Accessories

Depending upon the topography within the response district and the availability of specialized apparatus from neighboring agencies, many emergency response organizations require special equipment and accessories to be incorporated into their rescue vehicles. Some of the most common of these special features include the following:

- All-wheel drive capability
- Vehicle mounted winches
- Gin poles and A-frames
- Hydraulic cranes
- Stabilizers
- Air supply systems
- Electrical Equipment

All-Wheel Drive

The nature of the response area will determine the need for this capability. Rough terrain within the district, or the likelihood of snow and ice in the winter, may necessitate that rescue vehicles be equipped with all-wheel drive capability. All-wheel drive allows safer, more reliable vehicle operation during extreme conditions. Mountainous areas and large areas under cultivation are other examples of areas where off-road capability may be necessary.

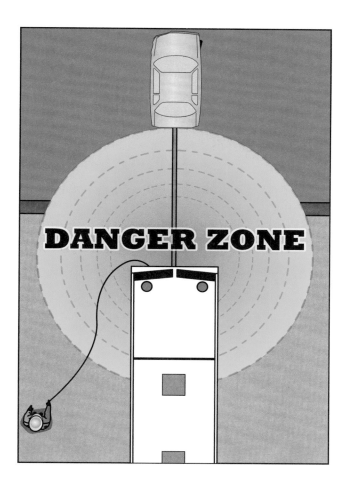

DANGER ZONE

Figure 4.22 When operating a vehicle mounted winch, rescuers should stay outside of the danger zone.

Vehicle Mounted Winches

Many rescue vehicles, especially those that are designed as multipurpose vehicles, are equipped with winches. A winch uses cable wound onto a rotating drum that is geared to give maximum pulling power. Winches may be powered by the apparatus engine or an electric motor. Most vehicle-mounted winches are operated with controls located adjacent to the winch, or remotely by means of a long electrical cord. Remote controls allow the operator to get a better view of the operation and, more importantly, allow the operator to remain outside of the winch danger zone. The winch danger zone is a circle around the winch with a radius equal to the length of cable or chain from the winch to the load **(Figure 4.22)**. Staying outside of this circle protects the winch operator in case the cable or chain breaks.

A drum brake prevents the drum from overrunning when the winch clutch is disengaged and the cable is being unwound. Some are designed on "cradles" that allow them to be placed in receiver mounts in different locations around the vehicle body. If a winch-equipped vehicle is not available or adequate at an extrication incident, private sector providers may be able to provide the necessary equipment.

The rated capacity of winches varies; however, the winch is rated at its capacity when the first layer of cable is still on the drum. A vehicle-mounted winch should never be used in an attempt to move any object that is beyond the rated capacity of the winch. Winch and cable strength are strongest on the first wrap around the drum. As more cable is wrapped around the drum and the cable becomes layered, the strength decreases. As more cable is taken off the drum, the strength capacity increases. For safety reasons, the last layer of cable should not be removed from the drum.

In operation, the winch should be positioned as close to the load as possible in order to limit the length of cable or chain between the winch and the load. This minimum distance reduces the size of the danger zone and, therefore, reduces the chances of a broken chain or cable striking the operator or anyone else.

Like all other extrication tools and equipment, winches should be periodically inspected and after each use to ensure that they are in proper working condition. Inspecting the cable or chain for wear or damage and following the manufacturer's recommended preventive maintenance schedule should be all that is necessary.

Gin Poles and A-Frames

Gin poles and A-frames are vertical lifting devices that may be attached to the front, rear, or side of an apparatus **(Figure 4.23)**. Some of these devices have lifting capabilities in excess of 3 tons (2 721 kg). Both gin poles and A-frames have a pulley at the working end that is used with a vehicle-mounted winch when lifting capability is needed. A gin pole consists of a single pole that is supported by guy wires to both sides of the vehicle. A-frames consist of two poles attached some distance apart on the apparatus roughly forming the letter A. Stabilizers, when provided, should be used to steady the rescue vehicle whenever A-frames are used.

Gin poles and A-frames are not designed to withstand lateral (sideways) stress. Guy wires or guide ropes may be used to increase lateral stability. When gin poles or A-frames are used, it is important not to exceed the rated weight the apparatus chassis is designed to carry. Exceeding the gross vehicle weight limit may result in damage to the axles, chassis frame, or both. A gin pole system or A-frame should be engineered to work with the vehicle for safety factors and working range.

Hydraulic Cranes

Cranes can generate great power for lifting and pulling during extrication operations. Some rescue organizations have access to cranes through other agencies while others have opted to add hydraulically operated cranes to

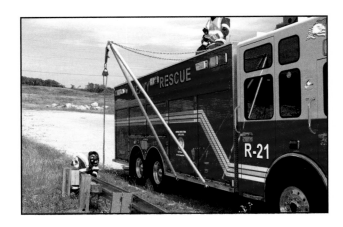

Figure 4.23 An A-frame rig attached to a rescue vehicle. *Courtesy of Lake Ozark Fire District (MO).*

their heavy rescue units, although this is rare. A hydraulic crane can be quite helpful in vehicle stabilization, removal of heavy vehicle components, and raising and lowering personnel and equipment. Some of these devices have lifting capabilities of up to 18 tons (16 329 kg) or more. Rescue vehicles that are equipped with a crane must use stabilizers that are extended to stabilize the rescue vehicle while the crane is in use. Three disadvantages to adding a crane to a heavy rescue unit are the initial cost of the crane itself, the additional maintenance required, and the loss of space for other tools because of the crane's size.

Stabilizers

Also known as stabilizing jacks or outriggers, stabilizers are used to steady the rescue vehicle when a gin pole, A-frame, or hydraulic crane is employed. Stabilizers reduce strain on the vehicle's suspension system when heavy loads are lifted and help to prevent the vehicle from rolling over when parked on a slope. Generally, there are two types of stabilizer systems: hydraulic, which are set using lever controls, and manual, which resemble a screw-type jack and are set by hand.

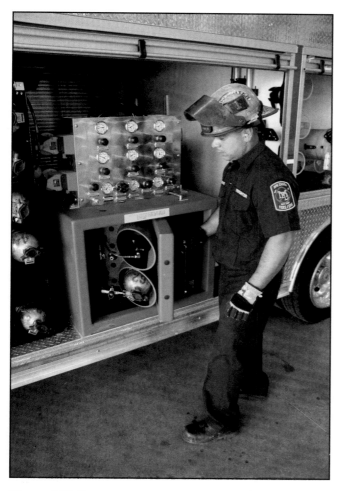

Figure 4.24 Some rescue apparatus are equipped with air bottle reservicing cascade systems.

Air Supply Systems

Rescue vehicles may be equipped with various systems to provide air for equipment and personnel. Air supply may come from tanks carried on the vehicle or be transferred from ambient air using air compressors. Three common air supply systems on rescue vehicles are cascade systems, breathing air compressors, and nonbreathing air compressors.

Cascade Systems

Some rescue vehicles are equipped with a bank of large capacity air tanks called cascade systems **(Figure 4.24)**. Most cascade systems consist of three to twelve 300-cubic-foot cylinders that are interconnected by high-pressure tubing.

Cascade System — Three or more large air cylinders, each usually with a capacity of 300 cubic feet (8 490 L), that are interconnected and from which smaller SCBA cylinders are recharged.

Their primary use is to refill SCBA tanks during an emergency operation and to refill tanks used to operate pneumatic tools such as air chisels. For more information on operating cascade systems, see the IFSTA **Respiratory Protection for Fire and Emergency Services** manual.

Breathing Air Compressors

Some rescue vehicles are equipped with air compressors that can generate breathing-quality compressed air. Air from these units can be used to fill cascade or SCBA tanks, to supply airline equipment in confined spaces, or for purging areas of nonflammable, oxygen-depleting gases. When operating, these compressors must be located in a clear atmosphere to avoid drawing contaminated air into the units and supplying it to the users. Generally, these units are placed upwind of any emergency scene to avoid such contamination.

Nonbreathing Air Compressors

Compressors that produce nonbreathing air are used to operate pneumatic equipment. Because of the many styles and sizes, as well as their relatively low cost, nonbreathing air compressors are found on many rescue vehicles. These compressors do not require a clear atmosphere for operation as do breathing air compressors. They may be commercial construction style compressors or a simple utilization of the vehicles engine compressor.

Electrical Equipment

Electrical equipment extends both to power generating equipment and the equipment that uses the power such as lighting. Power is needed to run electrical equipment, such as saws and other electric tools. Power-producing equipment are usually either inverters or generators. When agencies select power-producing equipment, they should be certain that the equipment will produce sufficient power for the tools and appliances that are to be used during extrication operations.

In addition to power-producing equipment, electrical lighting is frequently needed to illuminate the scene during nighttime operations is obviously important for safety and efficiency. Two types of lighting equipment - portable and stationary - are most often used in extrication incidents. The sections that follow describe power-producing equipment, lighting equipment, and auxiliary electrical systems.

Inverters

Also called alternators, inverters are used on rescue vehicles and ambulances when large amounts of power are not necessary (**Figure 4.25**). Inverters are step-up transformers that convert the vehicle's 12- or 24-volt DC current into 110- or 220-volt AC current. Inverters are fuel efficient and produce little or no noise during operation; however, they have limited power-producing capacities and limited range from the vehicle.

Generators

Generators can be either portable or permanently mounted on an apparatus (**Figures 4.26**). They are the most common power sources used on emergency vehicles. Portable generators are powered by small gasoline or diesel engines

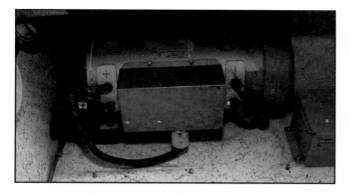

Figure 4.25 A power inverter built into a rescue vehicle compartment.

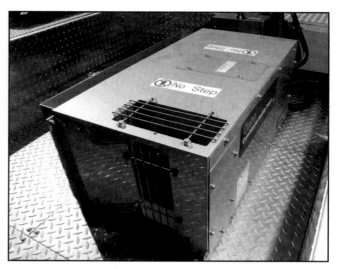

Figure 4.26 A vehicle mounted electrical generator. *Courtesy of Pat McAuliff.*

and generally have 110- and/or 220-volt capacities. Most portable generators are designed to be carried by either one or two people — a two-person carry is recommended for safety. Portable generators are extremely useful when electrical power is needed in an area that is not within reach of the vehicle-mounted system.

Vehicle-mounted generators usually have a larger capacity than portable units. In addition to providing power for portable tools and equipment, vehicle-mounted generators provide power for the floodlighting system on the vehicle. Vehicle-mounted generators can be powered by gasoline, diesel, or propane engines or hydraulic or power take-off systems. Switch-controlled floodlights are usually wired directly to the generators, and outlets are also provided for other equipment. These power plants generally have 110- and 220-volt capabilities with capacities up to 50 kw and occasionally greater. Vehicle-mounted generators tend to be noisy during operation making it difficult to communicate near them. In addition, their exhaust fumes may contaminate the scene if they are not positioned downwind.

Portable Lights
Portable lights are used when the scene is beyond the effective reach of stationary lights or when additional scene lighting is necessary. Portable lights generally range from 300 to 1,000 watts. They may be supplied by a cord from the power plant or may have an attached power unit. *29 CFR 1910.306* requires that all such cords be equipped with ground fault circuit interrupters. The lights usually have handles for safe carrying and large bases for stability. Some portable lights are mounted on telescoping stands.

Stationary Lights
Stationary lights are mounted on a vehicle using telescoping poles that allow them to provide overall lighting of the incident scene. The telescoping poles can be raised, lowered, or rotated to provide the best possible lighting. Some dedicated lighting units have hydraulically operated booms with banks of lights with capacities ranging from 500 to 1,500 watts per light. Scene lighting

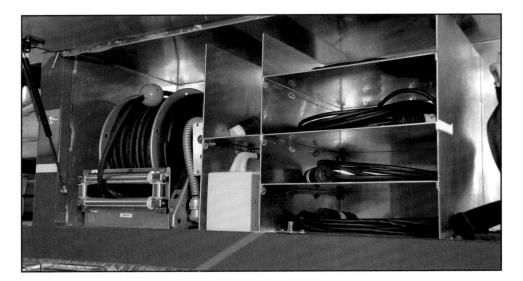

Figure 4.27 Portable electrical power reels, cords, and adapters. *Courtesy of Pat McAuliff.*

should not exceed the rated capacity of the power plant. Overtaxing the power plant will provide poor lighting, may damage the power generating unit, and will cause electric tools to not function as designed.

Auxiliary Electrical Equipment

A variety of other equipment may be used in conjunction with power plants and lighting equipment **(Figures 4.27)**. Electrical cables or extension cords are necessary to conduct electric power to portable equipment. The most common size cable is a 12-gauge, 3-wire type. The cord may be stored in coils, on portable cord reels, or on vehicle-mounted automatic rewind reels. Twist-lock receptacles provide secure, safe connections. Electrical cable must be adequately insulated, waterproof, and have no exposed wires.

Junction boxes may be used when multiple connections are needed. The junction is supplied by one inlet from the power plant and has several outlets. Many junction boxes have a small light on top that stays on as long as power is being supplied to the unit.

In areas where automatic or mutual aid operations are common, some agencies may have different sizes or types of receptacles (for example, one has two prongs; the other three). Adapters should be carried so that equipment can be interconnected when necessary. Adapters should also be carried to allow rescuers to plug their equipment into conventional electrical outlets.

Extrication Tools and Equipment

Acquiring the knowledge, skills, and abilities required to perform safe and effective vehicle extrication begins with learning the capabilities and limitations of the tools and equipment available. The tools and equipment procured by the response agency will depend upon the nature and extent of the rescue problems identified in the survey of the district required by NFPA® 1670. The sections that follow discuss the tools and equipment most commonly used in vehicle extrication incidents.

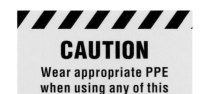

CAUTION
Wear appropriate PPE when using any of this equipment.

Stabilization Equipment

One of the first and most important steps in performing vehicle extrication safely — for the rescuers and patients alike — is stabilizing the vehicle. As mentioned earlier, any sudden and unexpected movement of the vehicle while rescuers and patients are inside can be dangerous, even fatal. Therefore, rescuers must know how to use the resources available at the scene to quickly but securely stabilize the vehicle. The means used to stabilize vehicles most often include the application of the following:

- Cribbing
- Step chocks
- Struts
- Shoring
- Rigging

Cribbing

In addition to the wooden cribbing that has been used in extrication operations for many years, some cribbing and other shoring devices available today are made of plastic while others are made of steel. Each type of cribbing has certain advantages and disadvantages, as well as certain capabilities and limitations.

Wooden Cribbing. Much of the cribbing used in vehicle extrication is made of wood that is solid, straight, and free of major flaws such as large knots or splits. Various sizes of wood can be used, but the most common is 4- x 4-inch (100 mm x 100 mm) wood timbers (pine recommended). The length of the pieces may vary, but 18 to 24 inches (450 mm or 550 mm) is average. The ends of the pieces may be painted different colors for easy identification by length. Other surfaces of the cribbing should be free of any paint or finish because the finish can make the wood slippery, especially when it is wet. Cribbing pieces may have a hole through one end and a loop of rope or webbing tied through the hole to form a handle. Cribbing can be stacked in a compartment with the grab handles facing out for easy access, or it can be stored on end inside a plastic crate or other box **(Figures 4.28a and b, p. 144)**.

Plastic Cribbing. A growing number of emergency response agencies are using cribbing made of recycled plastic **(Figure 4.29, p. 144)**. Plastic cribbing has the advantage of being impervious to oil, gasoline, and other substances that can soak into and contaminate wooden cribbing.

Cribbing Applications. The most common application for cribbing in vehicle extrication is called a box crib. This cribbing arrangement is so named because of the box that is formed when the pieces are set. On a flat, level base, two pieces are set parallel approximately 13 inches (330 mm) apart. Two more pieces are then laid at right angles atop and across the first two pieces letting the ends of each board extend slightly beyond the crosspieces. This process is continued until the desired height is reached **(Figure 4.30, p. 144)**. To maintain the stability of a box crib, the height of the cribbing stack should not exceed one and one-half times the length of the cribbing pieces being used.

Another common application of the box crib is as a base for a pneumatic lifting bag. In this application, the top tier of cribbing must be solid — that is, with several pieces laid side by side so that there is no opening in the middle

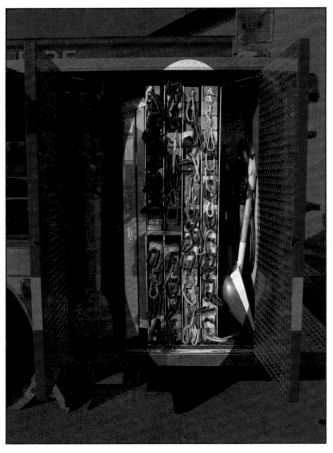

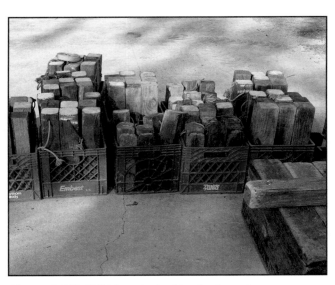

Figure 4.28b Cribbing stacked in plastic crates.

Figure 4.28a Cribbing stacked in an apparatus compartment.

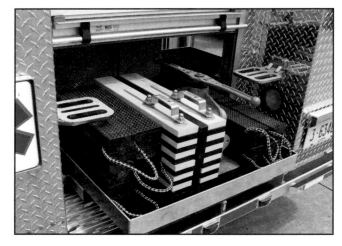

Figure 4.29 Examples of plastic cribbing made from recycled plastic.

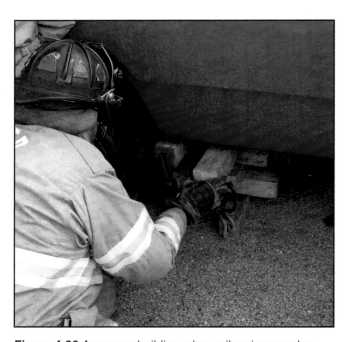

Figure 4.30 A rescuer building a box crib using wooden cribbing.

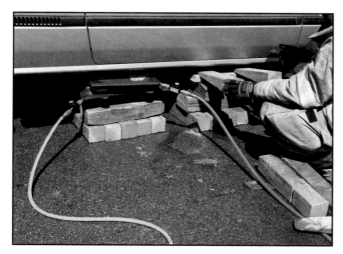

Figure 4.31 A solid crib is used to provide a stable base for air bag deployments.

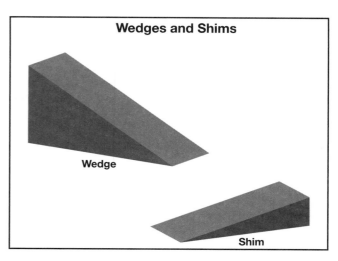

Figure 4.32 An example of a wedge and a shim.

(Figure 4.31). Leaving an opening in the middle would allow the lifting bag to bulge into the opening, reducing its lifting efficiency and perhaps damaging the bag. The inflating bag might also push the top pieces off the side of the stack. To reduce the possibility of the pneumatic bag shifting atop the cribbing stack, some agencies place a mat made of foam rubber or belting material on top of the cribbing and under the lifting bag. However, regardless of the application, constructing box cribs can be a time-consuming process; therefore, it is usually faster to use ready-made steel cribbing or step chocks.

Wedges and shims are used to supplement cribbing to stabilize vehicles **(Figure 4.32)**. Wooden wedges are usually 4- x 4- x 18- or 2- x 4- x 12-inch material cut from corner to corner. The usual application for wedges is for two of them to be driven in from opposite sides to tighten cribbing or shoring. Shims are essentially of the same shape as wedges but may be cut from smaller stock. In addition, shims are used singularly to take up space between cribbing and the object being supported.

A stack of cribbing seldom completely fills the space between the base and the underside of the vehicle to be stabilized, but it is important that the cribbing fit that opening tightly to prevent any movement of the vehicle. Therefore, the gap between the top of the cribbing stack and the vehicle must be filled by driving a wooden shim into the gap atop each of the top cribbing pieces or by driving the shims beneath the stack. The shims are driven in until the fit is tight **(Figure 4.33, p. 146)**. Properly constructed, a box crib is a very stable support.

Step Chocks

Like box cribs, step chocks are so named because of the series of steps that are formed when they are fabricated. Some step chocks are made of recycled plastic; others are made of wood **(Figure 4.34, p. 146)**. Regardless of whether an agency purchases manufactured step chocks and other shoring materials or fabricates their own, they are advised to test these devices under controlled conditions that will allow them to identify the capabilities and limitations of each. Following testing, SOPs can be developed for the safe and effective application of these devices.

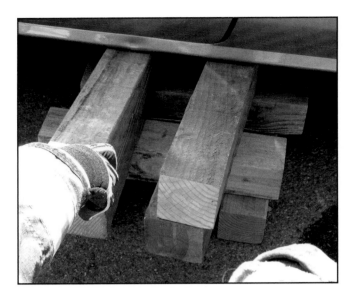

Figure 4.33 A rescuer sliding a wedge into position in a box crib.

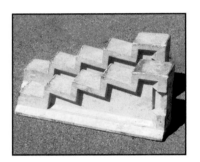

Figure 4.34 Examples of plastic step chocks.

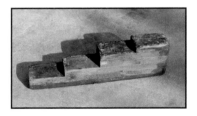

Figure 4.35 A wooden step chock made of varying lengths of 2- x 6-inch (50 mm x 150 mm) boards.

Plastic step chocks have the advantage of being impervious to fuel, oil, and other liquids that tend to soak into wood. They also do not produce splinters like wooden step chocks. However, like wooden step chocks, plastic step chocks have certain disadvantages and limitations. Brand new or nearly new plastic step chocks and other shoring devices will be slippery until some wear has developed because of use. It is sometimes useful to intentionally abrade new surfaces to provide better footing when the devices are in use.

Wooden step chocks are constructed with a 2- x 6-inch (50 mm x 150 mm) base approximately 30 inches (762 mm) in length. Centered on the base are progressively shorter lengths of 2- x 6-inch (50 mm x 150 mm) lumber stacked one upon the other. Each step is approximately 6 inches (150 mm) shorter than the one beneath **(Figure 4.35)**. The total number of steps is limited only by the length of the base. Experience has shown that it is better to construct wooden step chocks by laminating the pieces together with wood glue and screws, rather than with nails.

A step chock is installed by placing it on a firm, level surface and pushing the entire unit under the vehicle until the entire device is under the vehicle or one of the steps makes contact with the side of the vehicle. However, the chock should not be installed where it would interfere with the swing of the vehicle's doors. Any space between the highest step under the vehicle and the underside of the vehicle is then eliminated by driving a shim under the step chock.

Struts

Various equipment manufacturers now produce adjustable struts that can be used in a variety of materials and configurations **(Figure 4.36)**. Some consist of a square tube attached to a base plate to spread the load and provide more secure footing. The lower tube houses another tube that telescopes from the first one. Both tubes are perforated with a series of holes along both sides that allow a pin to be inserted to hold the tubes at the desired length **(Figure 4.37)**. Any space remaining between the top of the tube and the bottom of the vehicle can be taken up with a screw jack in the end of the tube. Some innovative rescue agencies have fabricated their own versions of these devices using wood and composite materials. These devices can be extremely effective

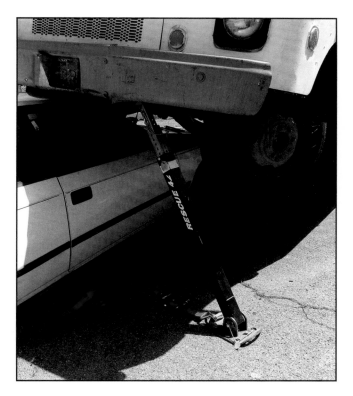

Figure 4.36 A rescue strut being used to stabilize a van.

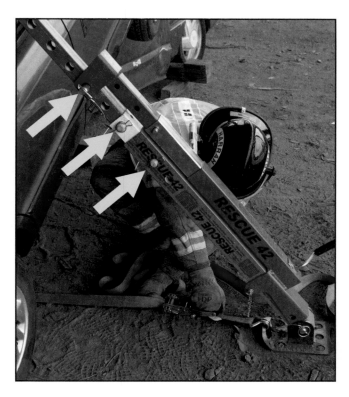

Figure 4.37 The arrows identify locking pin locations on a rescue strut.

when applied to the right situation. However, as with any other tool or device, there are conditions that do not lend themselves to their use and cribbing or step chocks may work better in these situations. Each individual extrication situation will dictate whether or not conditions are correct for using either cribbing or step chocks.

Shoring

The term "shoring" is used interchangeably for both the process and the materials and equipment. Shoring is used in the same way as cribbing and step chocks when the opening to be spanned is too large to make either cribbing or chocks a practical way to stabilize the vehicle. Shoring may consist of 4- x 4-inch (100 mm x 100 mm) or larger timbers of any length. For more information about shoring, rescuers should refer to IFSTA's **Technical Rescue for Structural Collapse**.

Rigging

Rigging is a general term for some of the other tools and equipment that are used to stabilize vehicles. Rigging includes using rope, chains, and webbing.

Rope. Rope is one of the most versatile and useful items carried on fire apparatus and rescue vehicles. It can be used for hoisting, lowering, rigging, crowd control, and securing and stabilizing vehicles.

The rope used must be of high quality to withstand the stresses exerted on it, but it does not have to be life safety rope unless it is used to suspend or support personnel. Rope rescue, including low-angle rescue, such as carrying an

Shoring — General term used for lengths of timber, screw jacks, hydraulic and pneumatic jacks, and other devices that can be used as temporary support for formwork or structural components or used to hold sheeting against trench walls. Individual supports are called shores, cross braces, and struts.

extrication patient up a slope in a basket litter, is beyond the scope of this manual. Therefore, the balance of this discussion will focus on the use of rope for securing and stabilizing vehicles.

Because non-life-safety rope is classified as "utility" rope, it may be made of manila fiber or any of the synthetics of which ropes are made. However, despite its great strength, nylon rope is not ideal for vehicle stabilization because it stretches under load. If a nylon rope must remain in place for an extended period, it may have to be retightened periodically. It is more efficient to use a different type of rope so that it can be applied and tensioned once and not have to be adjusted repeatedly during the operation.

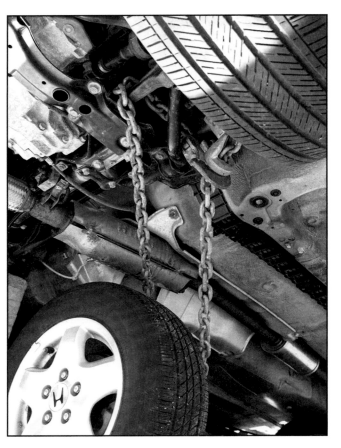

Figure 4.38 Chains can be used to "marry" two vehicles together to prevent them from shifting.

Chains. Only alloy steel chains should be used in vehicle extrication because they are strong and highly resistant to abrasion and chemical degradation **(Figure 4.38)**. Special alloys are available that are resistant to corrosive or hazardous atmospheres. The best chain for rescue work is Grade 80, also known as Grade 8 or Grade T. This chain can be identified by the 8 or T embossed on the links at regular intervals. Proof coil chain, also known as common or hardware chain, is not suitable for use in vehicle extrication operations. The minimum chain size generally used for extrication operations is 3/8-inch (10 mm). For any operation, it is important to match the rated strength of the chain to the tools being used and the job being done. Chain failures occur when the chain is abused or neglected in use or storage. Improper treatment of chain components leads to metal fatigue and chain failure. Chains should be inspected link by link for signs of wear or damage on a regular schedule. Remove defective chains from service.

Hooks and attachments should be made of the same alloy material as the rest of the chain. All chains should have an attached tag that has the safe load weight stamped or printed on it. Hooks and attachments should have at least the same strength rating, if not more, than the rest of the chain. In addition, the following safety rules should be observed when using chain:

- Do not drag a load with a chain under it.
- Do not cross, knot, or hammer a chain into position (for example, tying a knot in a chain to shorten it).
- Do not exceed the chain's listed safe working load.
- Do not use worn or damaged chains.
- Do not impact load a chain by lifting an object, dropping it, then suddenly stopping its fall. This increases the strain on the chain.
- Do not connect chain hooks to anything but the chain itself.
- Do not weld links in alloy chain or otherwise expose them to excessive heat.
- Do not use chain appliances (hooks, pins, links, etc.) that are not of at least equal strength to the load being handled.
- Do not attempt to splice a chain by placing a bolt through two links.
- Do not apply force to a kinked chain — make sure that all the links are straight.

With few exceptions, chains and webbing of the appropriate size and strength may be used interchangeably. From a safety standpoint, it is more important that rescuers know the capabilities and limitations of the chains and webbing available to them than which medium is used. Using chains and webbing beyond their limitations can result in their failure — perhaps catastrophically.

Webbing. Conventional webbing is made from the same materials used in synthetic ropes, so the same precautions and maintenance procedures apply. The size of webbing varies with the intended use, but most webbing used for lifting and pulling operations starts at about 2 inches (50 mm) in width. The strength requirements for webbing are the same as for chain used in the same situation. Disadvantages of webbing are that it is susceptible to ultraviolet light, abrasions, and chemical degradation which make it impractical for use in some extrication applications. If webbing must be used in a situation where it is susceptible to ultraviolet light for an extended period of time, abrasions, or chemical contamination, protect it with a salvage cover or similar material.

There are two main types of webbing construction: flat and tubular. Both are similar in appearance except when viewed cross-sectionally. Tubular webbing is woven in two ways: spiral and chain. Generally, the spiral weave is stronger and more resistant to abrasion than the chain weave.

Hand Tools

A wide variety of hand tools are used in vehicle and machinery extrication. Most of these tools are the same tools used for structural fire fighting and other emergency work. The sections that follow describe the wide variety of hand tools that rescuers will use including the following categories:

- Striking tools
- Prying tools
- Cutting tools
- Specialized hand tools
- Lifting tools
- Trench tools
- Mechanic's tools

NOTE: For a complete categorization of the various tools described in this section, refer to **Table 4.1, p. 151**.

Striking Tools

The most common and basic hand tools are striking tools. Most striking tools have a heavy metal head mounted on one end of a relatively long handle **(Figure 4.39)**. This category includes the following tools:

- Axes
- Battering rams
- Ram bars
- Punches
- Mallets
- Hammers
- Sledgehammers or mauls
- Picks.

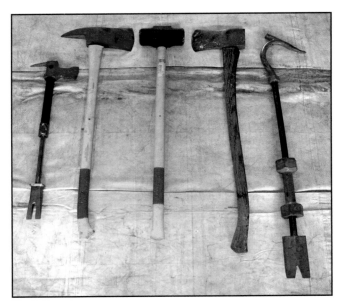

Figure 4.39 A selection of striking tools.

Striking tools can be dangerous and may cause serious crush or laceration injuries if used carelessly. High-velocity chips and splinters capable of piercing skin and eyes are sometimes produced when striking tools are used. In order to prevent injury, the following precautions should be taken:

- Wear proper protective clothing, helmet, and eyewear.
- Keep handles smooth.
- Ensure that all tool heads are well set.
- Keep the striking surface of the tool head free of chips and burrs.
- Keep axe blades clean and as sharp as their intended purpose and agency protocols dictate.
- Use striking tools with short, quick strokes. Long, sweeping strokes are more difficult to control and may strike anyone standing close by.

Prying Tools

Prying tools use leverage to provide a mechanical advantage. This means that using a prying tool properly can multiply the force applied. Prying tools are used to pry open doors, windows, hoods, and trunk lids of vehicles. These tools can even be used to lift vehicles or other heavy objects. The following tools are examples of hand prying tools:

- Pry-axe
- Crowbar
- Pry bar
- Spanner wrench
- Halligan (Hooligan) tool
- Claw tool
- Kelly tool
- Quic-Bar®

Crowbars and other prying tools are excellent for widening a small opening for larger power tools to fit into **(Figure 4.40, p. 152)**.

Table 4.1
Table 4.1 Hand Tools Listed by Categorization

	Striking	Prying	Cutting	Specialized	Lifting	Trench	Mechanic
Name of Specific Tool	Axes	Pry-axe	Chopping —Flat-head Axe —Pick-head Axe —Pry-Axe —Picks	Center Punch —Standard —Spring-Loaded	Screw Jacks —Bar Screw —Folding Screw	Short Handled Shovels	Sockets —Metric Set —Standard Set —Large Ratchet —Small Ratchet
	Battering Rams	Halligan	Snipping —Scissors —Shears —Tin Snips —Bolt Cutters —Wire Cutters	Glass Hammer	Rachet-Lever Jacks	Buckets —Collapsible Canvas —Metal	Wrenches —Metric Set —Standard Set —Adjustable —Open-end —Closed-end
	Ram Bars	Crowbar	Handsaws —Carpenter's Saw —Hacksaw —Coping Saw —Keyhole Saw —Windshield Cutters (Glass Saw)	Glass Saw			Pliers —Conventional —Channel-Lock® —Vise-Grip® —Wire Cutting
	Punches	Claw Tool	Knives —Pocket —Linoleum —Utility —V-Blade				Screwdrivers —Metric Set —Standard Set —Phillips head —Flat Head —Various Sizes
	Mallets	Pry Bar					Torx® Drivers (Star Drivers)
	Sledge-hammers	Kelly Tool					
	Mauls	Spanner Wrench					
	Picks	Quic-Bar®					

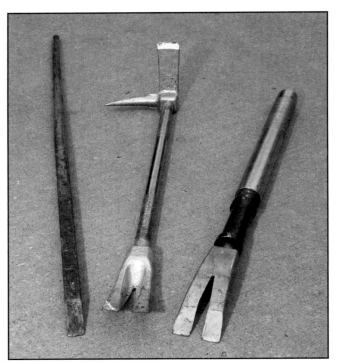

Figure 4.40 Three types of prying tools.

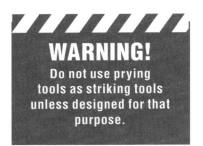

When used correctly, prying tools are safer than are striking tools because of the absence of ballistic movement. However, prying tools can be just as dangerous as other types of tools if used incorrectly. For example, it is unsafe to strike the handle of a pry bar with another tool or to use a makeshift extension (sometimes called a "cheater") on the tool handle. The most common type of cheater is a piece of pipe slipped over the end of a prying tool handle to lengthen it, thus providing additional leverage. Using a cheater can exert forces on the tool that are greater than the tool was designed to handle which can destroy the tool and perhaps cause serious injury to the operator or others. If a prying tool is inadequate for a particular application, an additional tool or a larger one should be used.

Cutting Tools

Cutting tools are the most diversified of the tool groups. Some cutting tools are designed to cut only specific types of materials. Misuse occurs when a tool is used to cut material that it was not designed to cut or to cut in a way for which the tool was not designed. Misuse can destroy the tool and endanger the operator. Manual cutting tools can be divided into the following four distinct groups:

- Chopping tools
- Snipping tools
- Saws
- Knives

Chopping Tools. These tools are characterized by a metal head with a cutting edge attached to one end of a relatively long handle. Chopping tools include the flat-head axe, pick-head axe, pry-axe, and various types of picks **(Figure 4.41)**. To ensure maximum cutting efficiency of these tools while preventing corrosion, the following precautions should be taken:

- Keep the cutting edge free of paint and covered with a thin coating of light-grade machine oil.
- Keep the blade sharp, but not so sharp that the cutting edge chips when the tool is used.
- Check tool handles regularly for looseness, cracks, splinters, or warping.
- Maintain cutting tools according to agency protocols.

Snipping Tools. These tools are used in situations where the material must be cut in a controlled fashion or where space does not allow larger tools to be used. They are most effective on relatively thin material that can easily fit within the jaws of the tool and are generally safer than other types of cutting devices when working close to a patient. Tools that fall into this category are various kinds of scissors or shears, tin snips, bolt cutters, and wire cutters **(Figure 4.42)**.

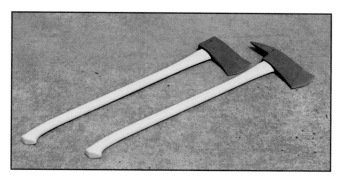

Figure 4.41 A flat head and a pick head axe.

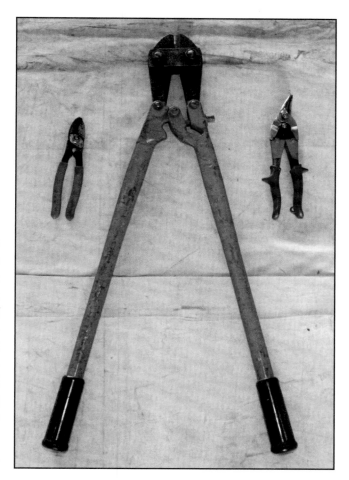

Figure 4.42 Three types of cutting tools.

The most common types of opposing-jaw metal cutters are bolt cutters and insulated wire cutters, sometimes called "hot wire" cutters. These tools are very similar in appearance, but they are not interchangeable. The most dangerous misuse is to use bolt cutters instead of insulated wire cutters; this misuse can result in electrocution. Only cutting tools approved by a recognized agency, such as Underwriters Laboratories (UL), Underwriters' Laboratories of Canada (ULC), or FM Global (formerly Factory Mutual), and maintained according to the manufacturer's recommendations should ever be used to cut energized electrical wire.

Saws. Handsaws are useful on objects that require a controlled cut but do not fit into the jaws of a manual, opposing-jaw cutter **(Figure 4.43, p. 154)**. Using handsaws is usually more time consuming than using powered saws or shears; however, handsaws are safer to use when working close to a patient or when working in a hazardous atmosphere. Handsaws commonly used for extrication include the following:

- Carpenter's saws
- Hacksaws
- Coping saws
- Keyhole saws
- Windshield cutters

The cutting efficiency of hacksaws can be increased by using two blades, installed in the same direction. However, this should only be done if the saw has an industrial quality frame. All saw blades should be kept sharp, clean, and lightly oiled. The cutting efficiency of any saw can be increased by periodically spraying the surface of the material being cut with bee's wax, a water based cutting fluid, or soapy water to reduce friction between the material and the saw blade.

The most specialized tool in this category is the windshield cutter or glass saw. This is a saw with a short, heavy blade composed of very coarse teeth. The windshield cutter is designed to quickly and efficiently remove a windshield from a vehicle. Glass saws consist of a glass cutting blade attached to a two-

> **WARNING!**
> Rescuers must follow their agency's protocols, but using insulated wire cutters to cut downed power lines to facilitate a vehicle rescue is NOT recommended.

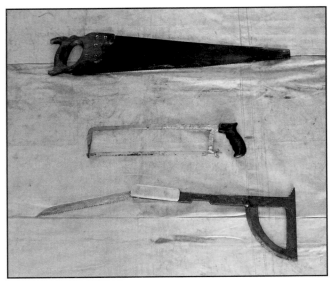

Figure 4.43 Examples of saws that might be used during an extrication operation.

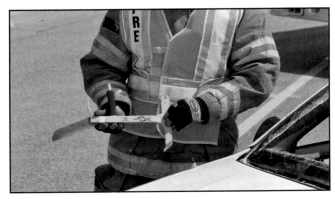

Figure 4.44 A glass saw is useful when cutting windshield glass.

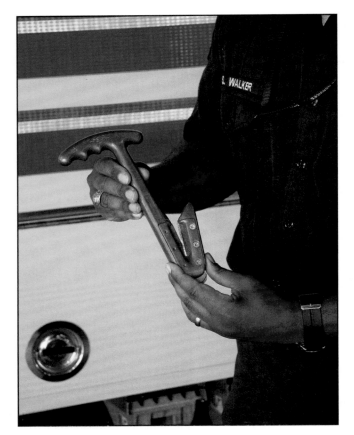

Figure 4.45 A V-blade knife can be used to cut seatbelts.

handed handle **(Figure 4.44)**. They are used to cut or saw through tempered safety glass. Some glass saws have a built-in spike or spring-loaded punch to help the user in creating the insertion point for the blade. When one of these devices is used, occupants in the front seat of the vehicle need to be protected from flying chips and splinters of glass.

Knives. Various types of knives may be useful in vehicle extrications. While a sharp pocket knife may be adequate in some situations, knives specially designed for vehicle rescue are usually more efficient. These specially designed knives include V-blade (seat belt) knives, linoleum knives, and utility knives **(Figure 4.45)**. Knife blades should be sharpened or replaced after each use to ensure that they are in optimum working condition for the next use.

Specialized Hand Tools

Some of the hand tools used in extrication are so specialized that they are almost never used for anything else. Examples of specialized hand tool are spring-loaded center punches and glass hammers.

Center Punches. There are two basic types of center punches: standard and spring-loaded. A standard center punch is similar to a small chisel but with a pointed end. A standard center punch can be used to break tempered glass, but it must be struck with another tool to provide the breaking force. A spring-loaded center punch looks very similar to a standard punch but provides its own breaking force when the tip is pressed against the glass.

Glass Hammers. Glass hammers consist of a pointed metal head attached to a plastic handle. They are used to break tempered glass by striking the glass with the point of the metal head. They are very effective at breaking glass, and some have a built-in seat belt cutter in the handle.

Lifting Tools

Except for pneumatic lifting bags, which are discussed later in this chapter, the primary lifting tools used in vehicle extrication are various forms of nonhydraulic jacks. The jacks most often used are various screw jacks and ratchet-lever jacks. Several types of nonhydraulic jacks are considered hand tools because they do not operate with hydraulic power. Although these tools are effective for their designed purposes, they do not have the same motive force as hydraulic jacks.

Screw Jacks. These are mechanical devices that can be elevated or depressed simply by turning a threaded shaft, making them among the easiest jacks to operate. Check screw jacks should be checked for wear after each use and kept clean and lightly lubricated, particularly the threaded shaft. The foot plates on which the jacks rest should also be checked for wear or damage. The two most common types of screw jacks used in vehicle extrication are the bar screw jack and the folding screw jack.

The bar screw jack is an excellent tool for stabilizing loads, but is considered impractical for lifting. The jack is extended or retracted by turning a threaded vertical shaft with a bar inserted into one of several holes in the jack's head.

The folding screw jack, also known as a scissor jack, consists of a top and bottom plate separated by levers that are drawn together or pushed apart by the action of a threaded shaft being turned. The main advantage of folding jacks is that when fully collapsed they fit into relatively small spaces (4- to 6-inch [100 mm to 150 mm] clearance). Folding jacks are not always stable under load and are therefore considered safe only for light loads.

Ratchet-Lever Jacks. Sometimes called Hi-Lift® or Handyman jacks, these jacks consist of a vertical metal shaft, with notches or gear cogs along one side that fits into a metal base plate **(Figure 4.46)**. A movable jacking carriage fits around the shaft and has two ratchets on the notched side. One ratchet holds the carriage in position while the other works with a lever to move the carriage up or down. The ratchet jack is a good medium-duty jack but is the least stable under load. This type of jack can be used for limited spreading and pulling operations in the absence of hydraulic rams.

Trench Tools

Due to space constraints in a trench, special scaled-down tools are sometimes needed to perform routine tasks such as removing dirt and debris. *Trenching tools* are short handled shovels with a blade that can be swiveled 90 degrees to form a hoe. Ideally, rescue units should carry picks and other tools equipped with short handles for working in trenches; the working ends of these tools may be scaled down as well.

Collapsible canvas buckets are used to remove dirt from trenches during rescue operations. Conventional metal buckets can also be used, but they increase the risk of injury to rescuers in the trench if a bucket is dropped from above. Ropes are attached to the bucket handles for hauling them up. Only buckets with secure handles should be used.

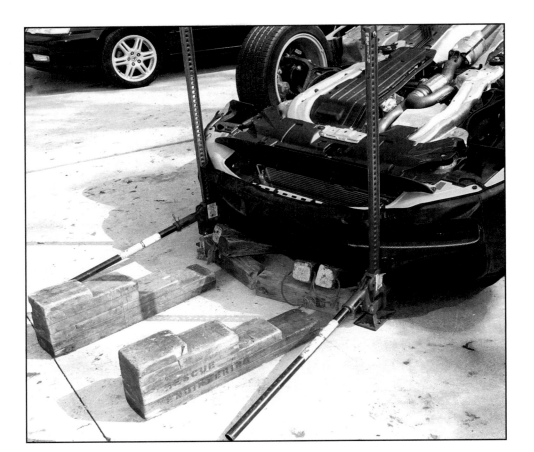

Figure 4.46 Ratchet jacks in use during an extrication training session.

Mechanic's Tools

In some cases, especially when working very close to a trapped patient, it is better to disassemble a part of the vehicle rather than use a power saw or similar tool to cut it. Disassembly eliminates the noise, vibration, and sparks that powered cutting tools produce. Rescue vehicles should carry a basic set of ordinary mechanic's tools — primarily sockets, wrenches, pliers, and drivers.

Sockets. Two sets of sockets — metric and standard — should be carried because vehicles manufactured outside the U.S. use nuts and bolts with metric dimensions, not standard (SAE). Each set should include deep sockets in a range of common sizes, 3/8-inch to 1¼-inch (8 mm to 28 mm), and at least one ratchet wrench or socket handle. Having two socket wrenches — one large and one small — is recommended. In addition to allowing more options in their use, if more than one wrench is available, more than one disassembly operation can be performed at the same time **(Figure 4.47)**.

Wrenches. Just as with socket sets, two sets of combination wrenches — metric and standard should be carried. Combination wrenches have an open head on one end and a closed head on the other end. Both sets of wrenches should include a range of common sizes. In addition to the combination wrenches, also adjustable wrenches of various sizes should be carried.

Pliers. A variety of types and sizes of pliers should be part of the tool inventory of any rescue vehicle **(Figure 4.48)**. Various sizes of the following types of pliers should be carried:

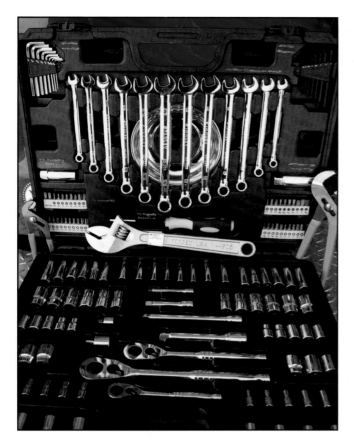

Figure 4.47 A mechanic's socket and wrench tool set. *Courtesy of Alan Braun, University of Missouri Fire and Rescue Training Institute.*

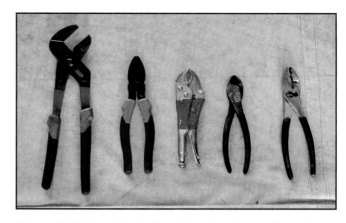

Figure 4.48 A variety of pliers that might be useful during extrication operations.

- Conventional pliers
- Channel-Lock® type pliers
- Vise-Grip® pliers
- Wire cutting pliers.

Drivers. The rescue vehicle's tool inventory should also include a variety of drivers — screw drivers and nut drivers. Include both Phillips head and flat screwdrivers in more than one size. Two sets of nut drivers — metric and standard — in a range of common sizes should be carried. Other drivers, such as Torx® drivers (sometimes called "star" drivers) should also be included.

Pneumatic (Air-Powered) Tools

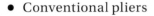

Pneumatic tools use the energy of compressed air for power. Air pressure can be supplied by vehicle-mounted air compressors, apparatus brake system compressors, SCBA tanks, or cascade system cylinders. The most commonly used pneumatic tools in extrication are pneumatic chisels/hammers and pneumatic wrenches.

Pneumatic Chisels/Hammers

Most pneumatic-powered chisels (also called air chisels, air hammers, or impact hammers) are designed to operate at air pressures between 90 and 150 psi (700 kPa and 1 050 kPa). Others operate up to 300 psi (2 100 kPa). Each tool

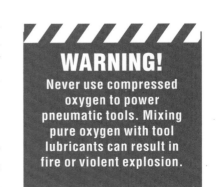

WARNING!
Never use compressed oxygen to power pneumatic tools. Mixing pure oxygen with tool lubricants can result in fire or violent explosion.

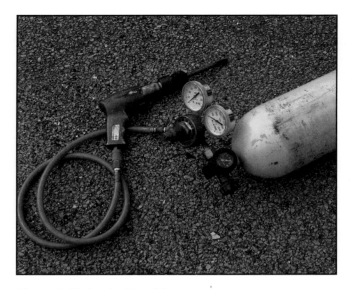

Figure 4.49 An air chisel kit.

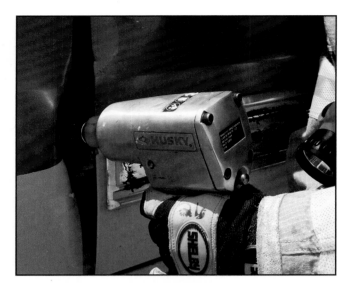

Figure 4.50 A pneumatic impact wrench being used to remove door hinge bolts. *Courtesy of Mark Stuckey, City of Owasso Fire Department.*

should be operated at the manufacturer's recommended operating pressure. In normal operation, they will use about 4 to 5 cubic feet (113 L to 142 L) of air per minute. Air chisels can be especially effective for auto extrication by cutting through the roof, roof support posts or doorjambs, seat bolts, and door lock assemblies. They are good for cutting medium- to heavy-gauge sheet metal and for popping rivets and bolts **(Figure 4.49)**. However, cutting heavier gauge steel or other metals requires larger air supplies and higher pressures.

A variety of air chisel bits are available to fit many vehicle extrication situations. In addition to cutting bits, special bits for operations such as breaking locks or driving in plugs are also available. All bits should be kept sharpened and free of defects at all times.

Pneumatic Wrenches

Air ratchets or "impact" wrenches are extremely useful for disassembling vehicle components. With an adequate air supply and the right size socket, these tools can remove nuts and bolts very rapidly **(Figure 4.50)**. Their chief disadvantage is that they are quite noisy in operation.

Pneumatic Saws

Pneumatic saws include both rotary and reciprocating saws that are effective for cutting a variety of materials. They are noisy and can produce sparks.

The pneumatic whizzer saw is an air-driven cutting device with several advantages over other types of power saws. At about 2 pounds (0.9 kg), the whizzer weighs about one-tenth as much as a circular saw, so it is much more maneuverable. Operating at 20,000 rpm, its 3-inch (75 mm) Carborundum blade cuts case-hardened locks and steel up to 3/4-inch (19 mm) in thickness. The tool has a clear Lexan® blade guard to protect the operator and the victim from flying debris. Driven by compressed air at 90 psi from an SCBA cylinder with a regulator, the whizzer operates much quieter than other power saws and will run for approximately three minutes from a full cylinder.

Pneumatic Lifting Bags

Pneumatic lifting bags devices allow rescuers to lift or displace objects that cannot be lifted with standard extrication equipment. Pneumatic lifting bags have a wide variety of applications in extrication operations. They can be inserted into openings that are too small for other lifting equipment, and they are relatively quick and easy to use. However, their use is not without some risks. To minimize these risks, operators should observe the following safety rules when using pneumatic lifting bags:

- Plan the operation before starting the work.

- Be thoroughly familiar with the equipment, its operating principles, capabilities, and limitations.

- Consult the appropriate operator's manuals and follow the recommendations for the specific system used.

- Keep all components in good operating condition and all safety seals in place.

- Have an adequate air supply and sufficient cribbing on hand before beginning operations.

- Position bags on or against a solid surface.

- Do not inflate bags against sharp objects — use a protective mat.

- Do not inflate bags fully unless they are under load.

- Inflate bags slowly and monitor them continuously for any shifting.

- Never work under a load supported only by lifting bags.

- Shore up the load with enough cribbing to support the load in case of bag failure.

- Interrupt the process frequently to increase shoring or cribbing — lift an inch, crib an inch.

- Make sure that the load is also supported by properly placed cribbing.

- Ensure that the top tier is solid when using box cribbing and that a protective mat is used.

- Avoid exposing bags to materials hotter than 220° F (104° C). Insulate the bags with a nonflammable material. Bags should be removed from service if any evidence of heat damage is seen.

- Do not stack more than two bags; center the bags with the smaller bag on top and inflate the bottom bag first (1/2 to 2/3 full), then inflate the top bag. If more height is needed, crib the object and deflate and reset the air bags.

 NOTE: Stacked bags can only lift the capacity of the lowest rated bag.

 There are three basic types of lifting bags: high pressure, medium pressure, and low pressure **(Figure 4.51)**.

 NOTE: A fourth type of bag is used for sealing leaks but has little or no application in extrication operations.

> **Pneumatic Lifting Bag —**
> Inflatable, envelope-type device that can be placed between the ground and an object and then inflated to lift the object. It can also be used to separate objects. Depending on the size of the bag, it may have lifting capabilities in excess of 75 tons (68 040 kg).

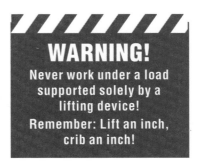

WARNING!
Never work under a load supported solely by a lifting device!
Remember: Lift an inch, crib an inch!

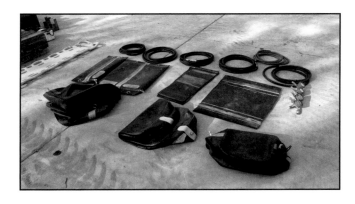

Figure 4.51 Examples of commonly used lifting bags, hoses, and protective mats.

High-Pressure Pneumatic Lifting Bags

High-pressure bags are constructed of neoprene rubber reinforced with either steel wire or Kevlar® aramid fiber and have a rough, pebble-grained, surface to improve purchase. Before inflation, the bags lie virtually flat and are about 1 inch (25 mm) thick. They come in various sizes that range from 6 x 6 inches (150 mm x 150 mm) to 36 x 36 inches (914 mm x 914 mm). The range of inflation pressure of the bags is about 116 - 145 psi (812 - 1 015 kPa). Depending on the size of the bags, they may inflate to a height of 20 inches (500 mm). The largest bags can lift approximately 75 tons (68 040 kg). An air bag's weight-lifting capacity decreases as the height of the lift increases and its maximum lift capacity is generally rated at one inch (50 mm) of lift. For example, a bag rated at 10 tons (9 072 kg) only lifts 5 tons (4 536 kg) to 8 inches (203 mm); one rated at 75 tons (67.5 t) only lifts 37 tons (33.3 t) to 20 inches (508 mm). To ensure the maximum, safe lift, cribbing or another suitable base should be used to position the bag as close as possible to the underside of the object to be lifted. Also remember to protect the bag from possible punctures by placing a protective mat or a piece of conveyor belt material between the bag and the object.

NOTE: The following formula will help rescuers determine the lift capacity of a high pressure bag: Length x Width x PSI divided by 2,000 = tons.

Low- and Medium- Pressure Pneumatic Lifting Bags

Low- and medium-pressure bags are considerably larger than high-pressure bags and are most commonly used to lift or temporarily stabilize large vehicles or objects. Their primary advantage over high-pressure air bags is that they have a much greater lifting range. Depending on the manufacturer and the model, these bags may be able to lift an object upwards of 6 feet (2 m). They are also safer than stacking high-pressure bags and they are easier to repair. The disadvantages of low- and medium-pressure lifting bags are as follows:

● Each bag is capable of lifting less weight than a high-pressure bag.

● They require twice as much space for insertion between the base and the object being lifted.

● They are more vulnerable to puncture than high-pressure bags.

Low and medium pressure bags do not operate the same as high pressure bags and can't lift a load straight up on their own; they must have a base or foundation point.

Depending on the manufacturer, a low- or medium-pressure lifting bag may be capable of lifting an object 6 feet (2 m) above its original position.

Low-pressure bags generally operate on 7 to 10 psi (49 kPa to 70 kPa), while medium-pressure bags use 12 to 15 psi (84 kPa to 105 kPa), depending on the manufacturer.

Electric Tools

In addition to the electrical lighting equipment discussed elsewhere in this chapter, a variety of electrically operated tools are used in vehicle extrication. These electric tools used can include spreaders, saws, cutters, and wrenches. Electrical saws are discussed along with other, power saws later in this chapter.

NOTE: These tools may be DC battery powered, 110-volt AC, or both.

Electric Spreaders and Cutters

Electrically powered spreaders and cutters are lighter and more portable than many of the hydraulic units. Like the hydraulic units, the electric spreader can be equipped with conventional spreaders for pushing and pulling, with optional shears, or with combination spreader/shears.

Electric Impact Wrenches

Electric wrenches are similar to the pneumatic impact wrenches discussed earlier in this chapter. They are used for the same purposes as the pneumatic versions. Depending upon the brand and model, they may or may not be as powerful as the pneumatic wrenches.

Electric Drills/Drivers

Improvements in the batteries used to power electric drills and drivers have made these tools extremely useful in vehicle extrication incidents. With replaceable battery packs and a variety of bits, these tools produce sufficient torque and rotational speed to be very effective for use in dismantling vehicle components **(Figure 4.52)**.

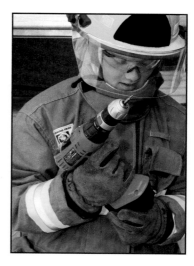

Figure 4.52 Rescuers now use a variety of battery powered tools such as this drill.

Hydraulic Tools

There are two categories of hydraulic tools used for vehicle extrication: powered and manual. While most agencies that deliver vehicle extrication services use powered hydraulic tools and equipment on most extrication incidents, there are still situations that require the use of manual hydraulic tools and equipment. The sections that follow describe both types of tools.

Manual Hydraulic Tools

Manual hydraulic tools operate on the same principles as powered hydraulic tools except that the hydraulic pump is manually powered by someone operating a pump lever. The primary disadvantage of manual hydraulic tools is that they operate slower than powered hydraulic tools and with more limited range of operation. Two manual hydraulic tools are used most frequently in vehicle extrication: the Porta-Power® system and the hydraulic jack.

Jack Safety

When using any kind of jack, hydraulic or otherwise, a good, solid base is the primary consideration, followed by adequate blocking and cribbing. The load must be blocked or cribbed as it is lifted to reduce the chances of it falling. The weight of the load being lifted is transmitted to the base of the jack. Therefore, to prevent the jack from sinking into the surface, place it on a weight-distributing base. This spreads the force placed on the jack. The base may be a wide board or steel plate; it should be solid, flat, and level. If it is not level, it should be shimmed level, making sure enough room remains to place the jack. Hydraulic jacks can only be operated within the orientation for which they were manufactured.

WARNING!
Never work under a load solely supported by a jack. Remember: lift an inch, crib an inch.

Porta-Power®. The Porta-Power® tool system is an auto body shop tool used for vehicle extrication. It operates by transmitting hydraulic pressure from a hand-operated pump through a hose to a tool assembly. A number of different tool accessories give the Porta-Power® a variety of applications.

The primary advantage of the Porta-Power® over the hydraulic jack is that the Porta-Power® has accessories that allow it to be operated in narrow places in which the jack will not fit or cannot be operated. The primary disadvantage of the Porta-Power® is that assembling complex combinations of accessories and the actual operation of the tool are time consuming.

Hydraulic Jacks. Hydraulic jacks are excellent devices for many heavy lifting situations and for shoring or stabilizing operations **(Figure 4.53)**. Hydraulic jacks operate on the principle that the pressure of liquids between two interconnected chambers of unequal size tends to equalize. A small chamber is used to pump fluid into a larger chamber. The energy applied is multiplied by the surface area differential to do more work in the large chamber. There is a check valve between the chambers that keeps the liquid from flowing back. Hydraulic jacks are available in capacities up to 20 tons (18 144 kg) or larger.

Power-Driven Hydraulic Tools

The development of power-driven hydraulic extrication tools has revolutionized the process of removing patients from various types of entrapments. The wide range of uses, the speed, and the superior power of these tools have made them the primary tools used in most extrication situations. These tools receive their power from hydraulic fluid under pressure supplied through special hoses from a pump, commonly referred to as the power unit. Hydraulic pumps can be powered by any of the following means:

- Compressed air
- Pressurized water
- Power-take-offs (PTOs)
- Electric motors
- Diesel or gasoline engines **(Figure 4.54)**

Any of these power units may be portable and carried with the tool, or they may be permanently mounted on a vehicle and connected to a hose reel. The tools powered by these units may be powered by manually operated pumps if the power unit fails. The following four basic types of powered hydraulic tools are used in vehicle extrication:

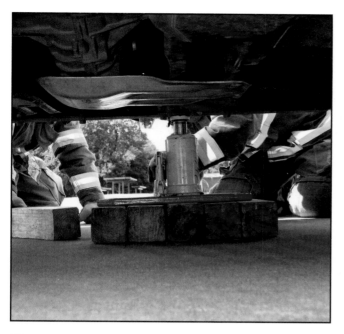

Figure 4.53 A hydraulic jack can be useful when lifting a vehicle.

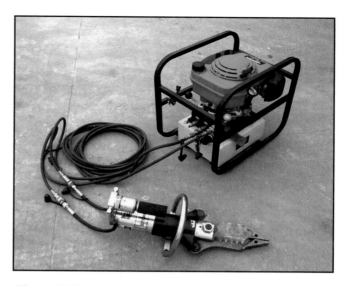

Figure 4.54 An example of a gasoline powered hydraulic unit with hoses and spreader/cutters.

- Spreaders
- Shears
- Combination spreader/shears
- Extension rams

Spreaders. Powered hydraulic spreaders were the first powered hydraulic tools to become available for vehicle extrication **(Figure 4.55, p. 164)**. They are useful for a variety of different operations involving either pushing or pulling. Depending on the brand and model, some tools can produce more than 49,000 psi (343 000 kPa) of force. The tips of some tools may spread apart as much as 41 inches (1 041 mm), although many smaller, lighter units are also in use.

Shears. Individual hydraulic shears are available for cutting roof support posts and other objects **(Figure 4.56, p. 164)**. These shears are capable of cutting almost any object (metal, plastic, wood) that will fit between their blades, although some models cannot cut case-hardened steel or high-strength low-alloy (HSLA) steel. Materials that shears cannot cut are often located at potential impact points and at the corners of the compartment, prime cutting locations for vehicle extrication operations. Shears are typically capable of developing up to 100,000 psi (700 000 kPa) of cutting force and have an opening spread of up to about 9 inches (229 mm).

Pedal cutters are shears that were originally designed for cutting reinforcing steel bars in construction. These powerful little devices cut accelerator, brake, and clutch pedal arms with ease. They can be used to cut virtually anything that will fit between the blade and the anvil. The blades don't actually cut hardened steel; they create compression fractures within the material.

> **CAUTION**
> Know the capabilities and limitations of the extrication tools and equipment available.

High-Strength Low-Alloy (HSLA) Steel — An alloy steel developed to provide better mechanical properties or greater resistance to corrosion than carbon steel. HSLA steels are different from other steels in that they are made to meet specific mechanical properties.

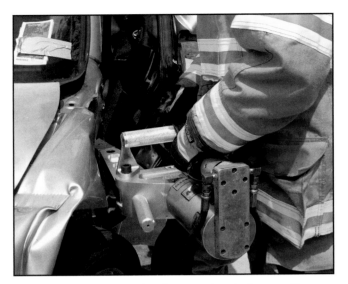

Figure 4.55 A set of hydraulic spreaders being used to pry open a door.

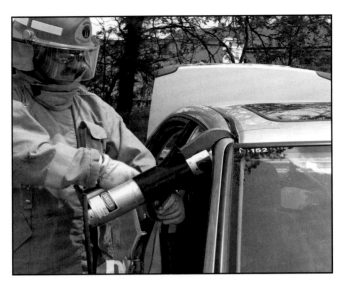

Figure 4.56 Hydraulic cutters or shears are useful when cutting vehicle components such as this door/window frame.

Combination Spreader/Shears. Several manufacturers of powered hydraulic extrication equipment offer a combination spreader/shears tool. This tool consists of two arms equipped with spreader tips that can be used for pulling or pushing. The insides of the arms contain cutting shears similar to those described in the previous section. These tools are excellent for use on small initial response vehicles or in areas where limited resources prevent the purchase of larger and more expensive individual spreader and cutting tools. The combination tool's spreading and cutting capabilities may be more or less than those of the individual units, although the spreading capability is usually less.

Extension Rams. Extension rams are designed primarily for straight pushing operations, although they are effective at pulling as well **(Figure 4.57)**. They are especially valuable when it is necessary to push objects further than the maximum opening distance of the hydraulic spreaders. The largest of these extension rams can extend from a closed length of 36 inches (914 mm) to an extended length of nearly 63 inches (1 600 mm). They open with a pushing force of more than 48,000 psi (336 000 kPa). The closing force is about one-half that of the opening force.

Telescoping extension rams are also available. From a retracted length of as little as 12 inches (300 mm), some telescoping rams will extend to 50 plus inches (1 250 mm). Unlike conventional hydraulic rams, telescoping rams cannot be used for pulling.

Power Saws

Power saws are available in various designs, depending upon the purpose for which they are intended. It is important that the operator know the limitations of each type of power saw. Used improperly, power saws can be very dangerous for both rescuers and trapped patients. However, following a few simple safety rules will prevent most injuries from power saws:

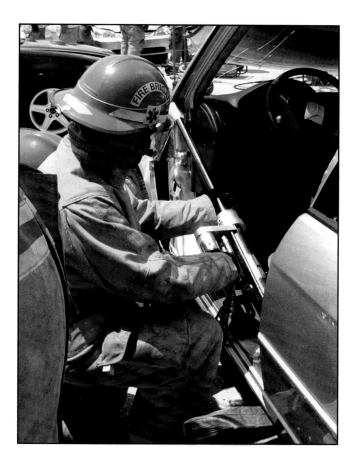

Figure 4.57 This rescuer is using a hydraulic ram to roll a dash forward.

- Match the saw to the task and the material to be cut. Never force a saw beyond its design limitations. Two things may occur: tool failure (including breakage) and/or injury to the operator.
- Use blankets or salvage covers to protect patients from the sparks, splinters, and debris chips created when using power saws.
- Wear appropriate protective equipment, including gloves, eye protection, and hearing protection because of the heat and noise generated by the cutting operation.
- Do not use any power saw when working in a flammable atmosphere or near flammable liquids.
- Keep unprotected and nonessential people out of the work area.
- Follow manufacturer's guidelines for proper saw operation.
- Keep blades and chains well sharpened. A dull saw is more likely to malfunction than a sharp one.

The saws described in the sections that follow may be powered by pressurized water, hydraulic pumps, gasoline, gas-oil mixtures, or electricity. Power saws can include the following types:

- Reciprocating
- Circular
- Rotary
- Chain

Electric Saws

The electric saws used in vehicle extrication, except for reciprocating saws, are simply electrically operated versions of the other power saws discussed in this section. There are electrically operated chain saws, reciprocating saws, and circular saws. Like all other tools, electrically operated tools have advantages and disadvantages. Among their advantages are that they are often lighter in weight and quieter in operation than gasoline-driven tools. However, their disadvantages may include being tethered to a power supply by a power cord, and unless they are designed to be intrinsically safe, they cannot be operated in potentially flammable atmospheres.

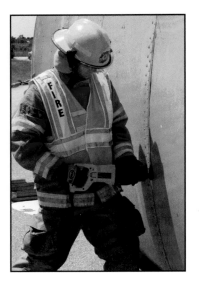

Figure 4.58 Reciprocating saws have become quite popular with extrication personnel.

Reciprocating Saws

These saws are easy to control and are well suited for cutting metal or wood because they produce far fewer sparks and airborne debris than does a rotary rescue saw **(Figure 4.58).** A reciprocating saw may be required when overhead cuts must be made or in areas where space is limited. This saw has a short, straight blade that moves forward and backward; an action similar to that of a handsaw. When equipped with metal cutting blades, reciprocating saws are also extremely effective on bus and automobile extrication incidents. Other than the frame, these saws can easily cut almost any portion of a bus or automobile body to provide access to patients. Reciprocating saws are also much easier to control and are safer to use than circular saws.

Reciprocating saws can also be powered by gasoline with certain disadvantages including the following:

- Heavier and more awkward than the pneumatic and electric models
- May not be used in confined or oxygen deficient spaces
- Produce carbon monoxide

Circular Saws

Unlike the gasoline-powered circular saws (rotary rescue saws) discussed later in this section, electrically operated circular saws used in vehicle extrication are usually the same as those used in construction. They are primarily designed for cutting wood and can be very useful when cutting shoring material on site. When equipped with a metal-cutting blade, they may also be used to make straight-line cuts. Other specialty metal-cutting saws and blades are available.

⚠️ **CAUTION**

The rotation of the blade of these saws creates significant torque that can cause the operator to lose control of the saw.

Rotary Saws

Also called "rotary rescue saws," these versatile tools may be used for cutting a variety of materials when equipped with the appropriate blade for the specific material being cut. In general, there are steel blades with carbide tips for cutting wood, and Carborundum® or other abrasive blades for cutting masonry and metals. There are diamond impregnated blades for virtually cutting anything. Because the abrasive blades can degrade when exposed to hydrocarbon vapors, these blades should not be stored in the same compartment with fuel containers.

Rescue saws must be used with extreme care to avoid injury to operators and trapped patients. Protect patients and rescue personnel in close proximity to the cutting operation from sparks when cutting metal and from chips and splinters when cutting wood. At least one charged hoseline should be standing by whenever metal is being cut. In addition to providing fire protection, water from the hoseline can be used to cool the saw blade by applying a fine mist to the blade while it is in operation. However, the cooling water must be started BEFORE cutting begins and continued throughout the cutting operation. Putting cold water on a hot blade may cause it to shatter and disintegrate. As with any other power tool, full protective clothing with face and eye protection should be worn when using circular saws.

Chain Saws

Both electric-, gasoline-, and hydraulically powered chain saws can be useful in some extrication situations. If chain saws are used, they should be powerful enough to penetrate dense material, yet lightweight enough to be easily handled in awkward positions. Chain saws equipped with carbide-tipped chains are capable of penetrating a large variety of materials, including light sheet metal. Although carbide-tipped chains cost almost four times as much as standard chains, but they last considerably longer.

While chain saws are capable of cutting the sheet metal and plastic parts of most vehicles, they often create more sparks, vibration, and noise than other saws. These characteristics can frighten trapped patients in close proximity to the cutting operation. Additionally, these patients are in danger of being struck by the cutting chain if it breaks during the cutting operation. Therefore, chain saws are sometimes used to cut windshields, but are primarily used to cut timbers for shoring and cribbing material, or for cutting trees and heavy brush to clear the scene.

Thermal Cutting Devices

To free trapped patients, it is sometimes necessary to cut through materials that are too dense to be cut with power saws. In these situations, a variety of thermal cutting tools can be used. Safety must remain a primary concern during any operation using thermal cutting devices. Cutting operations using thermal cutting devices are potentially dangerous. Observing the following safety rules will ensure that most malfunctions and injuries are avoided:

- Do not use cutting torches in any area in which the atmosphere may be flammable.

- Have charged handlines in place before beginning cutting torch operations. Handline personnel should wear appropriate personnel protective clothing and SCBA.

- Ensure that all cutting torch operators are experienced and efficient in using the tool in all situations.

- Train regularly in exercises that present a variety of cutting problems.

- Wear appropriate personnel protective clothing and eye protection when operating thermal cutting devices.

- Store and use acetylene cylinders in an upright position to prevent loss of acetone. When an acetylene cylinder is "empty" of acetylene, it still contains acetone. Never place empty cylinders on their sides.

- Handle cylinders carefully to prevent damage to the cylinder or the filler. A dent in the cylinder indicates that the filler may be damaged. If the filler is damaged, voids are created where free acetylene can pool and decompose, creating a potentially explosive condition. Dropping a cylinder may also cause the fuse plug to leak, creating a dangerous condition. Mark dented acetylene cylinders, and return them to the supplier.

- Avoid exposing cylinders to excessive heat. This means that an ambient air temperature exceeding 130°F (54°C) is undesirable for storing or using acetylene cylinders.

- Do not store acetylene cylinders on wet or damp surfaces. Cylinders rust at the bottom as protective paint is worn away.

- Store acetylene cylinders in an area physically separated from oxygen cylinders and other oxidizing gas cylinders. Segregate full acetylene cylinders from empty or partially full cylinders. Design storage areas to prevent acetylene cylinders from falling over.

- Perform a soap test (applying a solution of soap and water on fittings) to detect leaks after making regulator, torch, hose, and cylinder connections. Slow leaks in confined areas could permit acetylene to accumulate in concentrations above the lower flammability limit creating an explosive atmosphere. Acetylene has a wide flammability range: 2.5 percent to 81.0 percent by volume in air. Remove leaking cylinders to an open area immediately. Do not attempt to stop a fuse plug leak.

- Open acetylene cylinder valves no more than three-quarters of one turn. Do not use wrenches on cylinders that have handle valves. If the valve resists being turned, do not force it. Take the cylinder out of service immediately, and return it to the supplier for service.

- Do not use acetylene at pressures greater than 15 psi (103 kPa). Acetylene decomposes rapidly at high pressures and may explode as decomposition occurs.

- Do not exceed a withdrawal rate of one-seventh of the cylinder capacity per hour.

- Keep valves closed when not in use and when the cylinders are empty. After the valves are closed, bleed off the pressure in the regulator and in the torch assembly. Keep unconnected cylinders capped, whether they are full or empty, to prevent damage to fittings.

- Do not use grease or petroleum products on threads.

  The sections that follow describe the following varieties of thermal cutting tools:

- Exothermic cutting devices

- Cutting flares

- Plasma-arc cutters

- Oxyacetylene cutting torches

- Oxygasoline cutting torches

Exothermic Cutting Devices

Also known as *burning bars*, these devices are ultra-high-temperature burning tools that are capable of cutting through virtually any metallic, nonmetallic, or composite material. They cut through materials (such as concrete or brick) that cannot be cut with an oxyacetylene torch, and they cut through heavy gauge metals much faster. The device produces temperatures in excess of 8,000°F (4 154°C). The cutting bars or rods range in size from ¼- to ¾-inch (6 mm to 10 mm) in diameter and from 22 to 36 inches (550 mm to 900 mm) in length.

A similar exothermic cutting device is called an ARC-Aire®. This tool uses a hollow magnesium rod fitted into a handle that allows oxygen to flow through the rod. The rod is ignited by an electric striker and burns as the oxygen is increased. This tool produces temperatures from 6,000° to 10,000°F (3 298° to 5 520°C). The rods last between 15 and 30 seconds.

Cutting Flares

Also available for cutting metal and concrete are exothermic cutting flares. Approximately the size and shape of highway flares, cutting flares are also ignited in the same ways. Once ignited, these flares produce a 6,800°F (3 760°C) flame that will last from 15 seconds to two minutes depending upon the length and diameter of the flare. The obvious advantages of cutting flares compared to other exothermic cutters are the absence of a hose or power cord, and their light weight and portability.

Plasma-Arc Cutters

Like burning bars, plasma-arc cutters are also ultra-high-temperature metal-cutting devices, generating temperatures of up to 50,000°F (28 000°C). Plasma cutters work by sending an electric arc through a gas that is passing through a constricted opening. This high speed gas cuts through the molten metal. In operation, up to 200 amperes of electrical power is utilized. Air, nitrogen, and argon are just a few of the gases used. Air is the most common gas used for plasma cutters in the fire service. They work so fast that the heat traveling through the material being cut is minimal compared to other cutting devices. These tools don't work well in wet conditions, or poor conductive conditions.

Oxyacetylene Cutting Torches

Like the exothermic cutting device, the oxyacetylene cutting torch cuts by burning **(Figure 4.59, p. 170)**. It can be used for cutting heavy gauge metal that is resistant to more conventional extrication equipment. The torch preheats the metal to its ignition temperature, then burns a path in the metal with an extremely hot cone of flame caused by the introduction of pure oxygen into the flame. Like all other cutting devices that operate with a highly flammable gas and produce a flame, oxyacetylene cutting torches should be used with extreme caution.

Another hazard associated with cutting torches is the storage of oxygen and acetylene. Acetylene cylinders should always be kept in an upright position, whether they are in use or in storage. Acetylene is an unstable gas that is both pressure and shock sensitive. Acetylene storage cylinders, however, are designed to keep the gas stable and safe to use. The cylinders contain a porous filler of calcium silicate, which prevents accumulations of free acetylene within the cylinder.

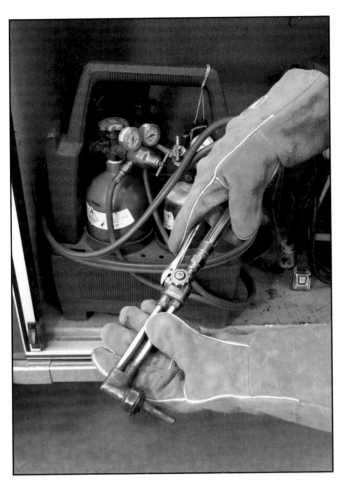

Figure 4.59 An example of an oxyacetylene cutting torch.

They also contain liquid acetone in which the acetylene is dissolved and stored in liquid form. When an acetylene cylinder's valve is opened, the gas leaves the mixture as it travels through the torch hose-line assembly.

Oxyacetylene cutting torches generate an extremely hot flame. For preheating metal, the flame temperature in air is approximately 4,200°F (2 316°C). When pure oxygen is added through the torch handle assembly, a flame of over 5,700°F (3 149°C) is created. This is hot enough to burn through iron and steel with relative ease.

Oxygasoline Cutting Torches

Petrogen® cutting torches, a relatively new cutting system, are fueled by a mixture of oxygen and gasoline, **(Figure 4.60)**. These systems use a conventional cutting torch and dual-hose configuration, but the fuel (gasoline) is delivered to the torch in liquid form. These systems produce a cutting flame in the range of 2,800° F (1 538°C). Oxygasoline cutting systems may be used underwater when special equipment is utilized.

In addition to the ready availability of gasoline and its relatively low cost compared to other fuels, the safety resulting from the fuel being delivered to the torch in liquid form is significant. Unlike systems that use gaseous fuels, in oxygasoline systems the flame cannot travel back through the supply hose.

Lifting/Pulling Tools

Often, rescue personnel have to lift or pull a vehicle or some of its components away from a patient. The vehicle or components may weigh several tons (or tonnes), and the lift or pull may range from only 1 or 2 inches (25 mm to 50 mm) to several feet (meters). A variety of extrication tools have been developed to assist in this task. These include winches, cranes, come-alongs, and block and tackles. (Because winches and cranes were discussed earlier in the chapter, they will not be discussed further here.) Durable leather or task associated gloves should be worn when working with wire rope or cables. Any broken strands are razor sharp and will cut anyone who handles them carelessly.

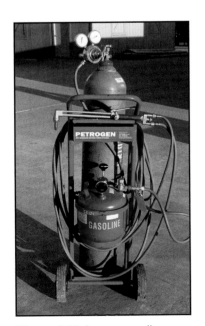

Figure 4.60 An oxygasoline cutting torch.

Come-Alongs

Another lifting or pulling tool often used is the come-along. The most common sizes or ratings of come-alongs are 1 to 10 tons (907 kg to 9 072 kg). This tool uses leverage and a ratchet/pulley mechanism to increase pulling capacity. The come-along has a drum that is rotated by a lever handle directly or through gear action. A cable or chain is attached to the drum which makes the effective pull of the come-along equal to the length of the cable. The come-along is anchored to a secure object, and the cable/ chain is run out to the load to be moved. Once both ends are attached, the lever handle is operated to pull the load toward the anchor point. The lever handles on some come-alongs are designed to bend before the chain or cable reaches the breaking point.

Block and Tackle

Because of their mechanical advantage in converting a given amount of pull to a working capacity greater than the pull, blocks and tackle are useful for lifting or pulling heavy loads. A block is a wooden or metal frame containing one or more pulleys called sheaves. Tackle is the assembly of ropes and blocks through which the line passes to multiply the pulling force (**Figure 4.61, p. 172**).

In vehicle extrication incidents, block and tackle may be very useful for stabilizing vehicles and similar applications. When using block and tackle, observe the following safety rules:

- Ensure that the rope is the right size for the weight being lifted and the blocks being used.

- Exert a steady, simultaneous pull on the fall line, and hold onto the gain.

- Ensure that the anchor to which the standing block is attached is strong enough to hold the load and the pull.

- Pull in a direct line with the sheaves.

- Pull downhill whenever possible.

- Allow no one to stand under or near the load in case the assembly fails.

- Lower suspended loads gradually, without jerking.

- "Mouse" open hooks to prevent slings or ropes from slipping off.

CAUTION

Do not use an extension handle with come-alongs. Only use the calibrated handle that came with the device.

CAUTION

Block and tackle is not considered to be sufficiently reliable for life safety applications.

Routine Operational Checks and Maintenance

To ensure operability and extend their functional lifetime, all rescue vehicles, tools, and equipment must undergo operational checks and maintenance on a routine basis. All personnel must be trained to perform these routine procedures for each type of apparatus, tool, and equipment the organization uses.

The organization's SOPs/SOGs should identify the frequencies and procedures to be followed for routine operational checks and maintenance on each type of equipment. The manufacturer's operations and maintenance manuals are excellent sources information on these topics.

A key part of any routine operational check and maintenance is to ensure that the proper fuels and lubricants are used during reservicing. The use of improper fuels and lubricants can severely damage emergency equipment and vehicles, causing them to fail at the most inopportune moment.

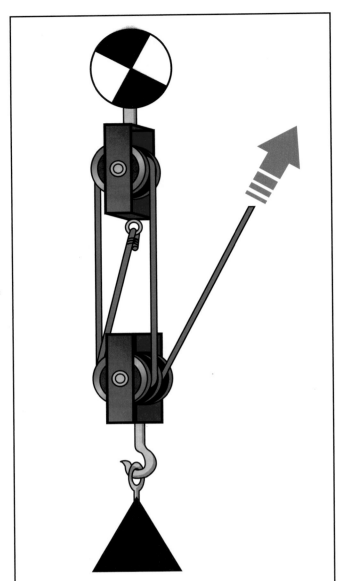

Figure 4.61 An example of a block and tackle system.

Summary

The tools and equipment required to perform safe and efficient vehicle extrication vary from the conventional manual and power tools carried on most fire apparatus to highly specialized and sophisticated devices. Likewise, the vehicles used by fire departments and other organizations that respond to vehicle extrication incidents also vary. Some are conventional municipal and wildland fire apparatus (engines and trucks); others are very specialized, dedicated rescue vehicles. To be most effective, rescue personnel must be thoroughly familiar with the tools and equipment available to them. The time spent training on each tool is very important. They must know the capabilities and limitations of extrication tools and equipment, and they must know how to operate them safely. Routine operational checks and maintenance are vitally for ensuring equipment operability and extended life.

Review Questions

1. What is the purpose of each type of personal protective equipment used by extrication personnel?

2. Discuss each type of rescue vehicle.

3. What are the advantages and disadvantages of the different types of rescue vehicle compartmentation?

4. What special equipment and accessories may be built into rescue vehicles?

5. What materials and equipment are used in stabilization efforts?

6. What are the advantages and disadvantages of each type of extrication tools and equipment?

7. What is the purpose of operational checks and maintenance?

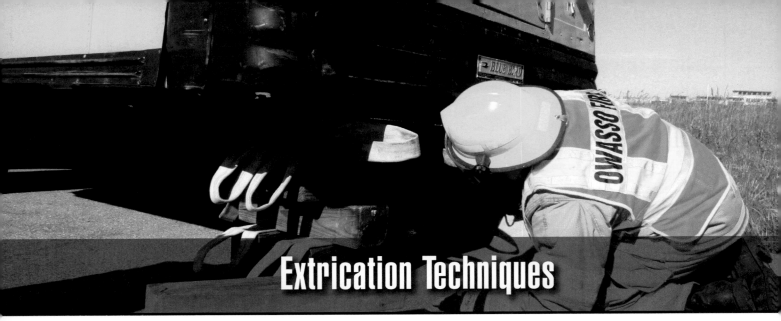

Extrication Techniques

Chapter Contents

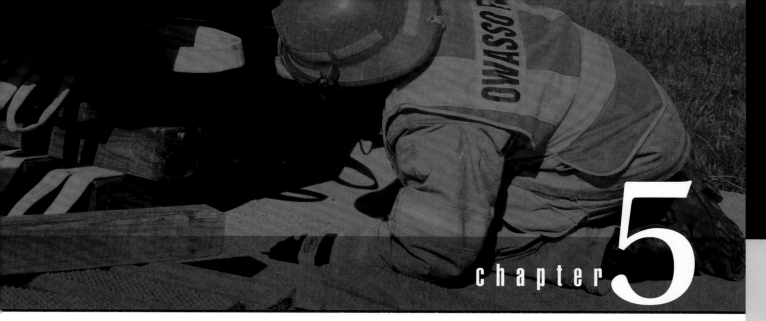

chapter 5

Key Terms

Job Performance Requirements

This chapter provides information that addresses the following job performance requirements (JPRs) of NFPA® 1001, *Standard for Fire Fighter Professional Qualifications* (2008), NFPA® 1006, *Standard for Technical Rescuer Professional Qualifications* (2008), NFPA® 1670, *Standard on Operations and Training for Technical Search and Rescue Incidents* (2009).

NFPA® 1001 JPRs

6.4.1

6.4.2

NFPA® 1006 JPRs

5.2.1	10.1	10.1.4	10.2	10.2.4
5.2.2	10.1.1	10.1.6	10.2.1	10.2.5
5.2.3	10.1.2	10.1.7	10.2.2	
5.5.1	10.1.3	10.1.8	10.2.3	

NFPA® 1670 JPRs

8.2.3	8.3.4
8.3.3	8.4.2

Extrication Techniques

Learning Objectives

1. Distinguish among the types of control zones established during extrication operations.

2. Describe the procedures for stabilizing vehicles found in different positions at extrication incidents.

3. Identify methods for lifting vehicles using a variety of equipment during extrication operations.

4. Identify procedures for removing vehicle glass.

5. Describe methods for displacing a vehicle's roof during extrication operations.

6. Explain the methods used for jacking or lifting steering columns and dashboards.

7. Describe the procedures for displacing or rolling a dashboard.

8. Identify the steps in performing a floor pan drop.

9. Describe the procedures for displacing and removing vehicle seats.

10. Identify methods used in cutting foot pedals during extrication operations.

11. Explain procedures used to enter a vehicle through the floor.

12. Describe methods to tunnel into vehicle passenger compartments.

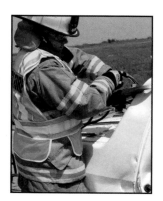

Chapter 5
Extrication Techniques

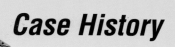

Case History

An early morning multivehicle accident with two patients heavily entrapped resulted in a large scale emergency response from several agencies. Following the establishment of incident command and size up, extrication personnel stabilized the vehicle containing the entrapped patients while medics began stabilizing several patients from other vehicles. With the vehicle stabilized, rescuers removed the driver's door and lifted the steering column from the driver's chest. Other rescuers removed the vehicle's roof, the driver's side B-post, and the back door. A hydraulic ram was used to roll the dash forward to free the driver's legs, and the driver's seat back was released to move the patient onto a backboard for removal. To free the passenger, the back seats were removed; the passenger seat back was lowered; and small hydraulic rams were used to roll the dash forward to free the passenger's legs.

Once emergency responders are at the scene of an extrication incident, they must first confirm that a patient has become trapped, and that there is a need for one or more patients to be extricated. If the initial size-up confirms the need for extrication, then a variety of tools and techniques can be used to safely and efficiently extricate the patient. How these tools and techniques are applied determine whether the operation is successful, and, in some cases, whether the patient survives.

When a patient is trapped and in danger, rescuers are justified in taking more forceful efforts to gain entry to the vehicle and reach the patient. In such situations, rescue personnel use extrication tools and techniques to remove doors and other vehicle components in order to gain access to the patient to stabilize their condition. These same tools and techniques can then be used to remove the vehicle from around the patient to safely extricate them from the vehicle. This chapter describes the techniques used to perform a variety of extrication procedures including the following:

- Glass removal
- Door and side panel removal
- Roof Removal
- Dashboard and steering column roll-up
- Vehicle seat displacement and removal
- Pedal displacement and removal
- Special entry techniques at unusual points of entry

Nonemergency and Emergency Entry

The approach rescue personnel take to entering a vehicle depends upon the situation. In a nonemergency situation where time and conditions are not life threatening, rescuers will make every effort to prevent damaging the vehicle. During emergency situations where a patient's life is in danger the vehicle can and will be sacrificed in an attempt to save the patient.

The question of priorities arises when a vehicle has not been structurally damaged to any great extent and it appears that the patient is not seriously injured. The patient may appear disoriented, as frequently happens with elderly people or small children may have been accidentally locked in a car. During an emergency, breaking a window to gain access is justifiable, but in a non-emergency situation less force is appropriate. Unlocking the car using an alternative method may prove effective, producing fewer hazards, such as glass fragments, with only a slight delay in time. A wire coat hanger or a locksmith's tool (an articulated piece of spring steel) can be inserted into the space between a window and its frame. From there it can be maneuvered to the door latch locking button to unlock the door.

On some vehicles, it is also possible to displace (pry) the side windows from the frame sufficiently to access the lock button. Using a thin screwdriver, a coat hanger that has been formed into a loop, or small saw blade to operate the lock button from outside the vehicle is often successful. It may also be possible to access the lock button by going through the crack between the door and the B-post. However, if the car has no visible lock button, this method cannot be used.

Unlocking doors has become more difficult due to industry modifications that keep doors from popping open on impact, antitheft devices, and child-proof door locks. The method of locking vehicle doors has changed from key operation to door locks operated digitally, electrically, or with vacuum power. The identification of the locking system on the vehicle is necessary before making attempts at unlocking the vehicle.

NOTE: Occasionally, the fire department or rescue unit may be called upon to assist a motorist who has simply locked his or her keys in the vehicle. In most areas, this is the responsibility of the police department. It is recommended that fire departments avoid this kind of activity because of liability concerns. Advise the person to call the police department or a locksmith for assistance.

Control Zones

As outlined in Chapter 2, *Extrication Incident Management,* control zones should be established around the incident scene. The *restricted (hot zone)* is the area immediately surrounding the vehicles involved. Only those directly involved in the extrication operation are allowed in this zone. Because of the amount of work to be accomplished and the limited time in which to accomplish it, this area should remain clear of unnecessary tools, equipment, and vehicle components. These items can create significant safety hazards to the extrication personnel and patients. The tools and equipment necessary for a given operation should be positioned in such a manner as to avoid creating fire, tripping, or other safety related hazards **(Figure 5.1)**. Vehicle components that have been removed should be moved a short distance away.

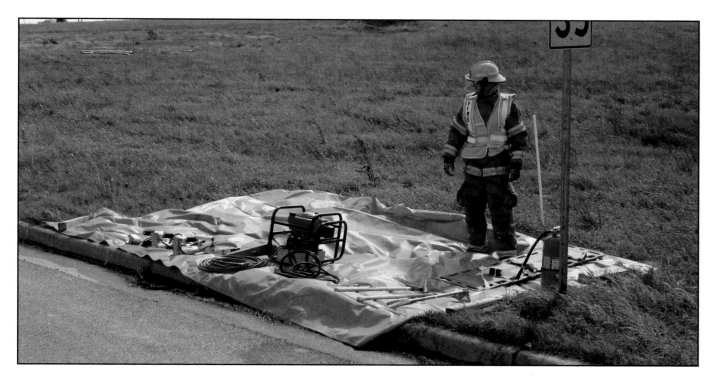

Figure 5.1 A rescuer setting up a tool and equipment cache.

The *limited access (warm or contamination) zone* can serve as a space where those in support of the extrication operation may function. Tool and equipment staging areas should be within this zone to allow the tools and equipment to be accessible but not in the way. This zone can also serve as a staging area for personnel.

The *support (cold) zone* is an ideal location for incident command and related functions to be conducted. The *crowd control line* around the outer edge of the cold/support zone creates a buffer between the public and the emergency operation. The incident public information officer may allow certain legitimate media representatives to cross the crowd control line if this is in accordance with local protocols.

"Safe the Vehicle" for Extrication

"Safe the vehicle" is the phrase which describes the list of procedures that need to be done to make the vehicle ready for extrication techniques of any kind include the following:

- Check and mitigate all hazards such as fluids or downed power lines.
- Check for number of patients and start triage.
- Stabilize the vehicle with cribbing and shoring.
- Make entry into the passenger compartment.
- Place the vehicle into park, set parking brake, pop hood, release trunk, unlock doors, roll down windows, move seats back and seatbacks backward, move electric pedal
- Disconnect the power supply(ies). When disconnecting the battery, disconnect the negative cable first, then the positive.

Vehicle Stabilization

Following scene assessment (refer to the information box for steps taken before stabilization), rescue personnel must stabilize each vehicle involved in the collision. This is necessary to prevent further injury to the patients, possible injuries to rescue personnel, and further degradation of the vehicle's structural integrity. Stabilization refers to the process of providing additional support at key points between the vehicle and the ground or other solid surface. The primary goal of stabilization is to maximize the area of contact between the vehicle and the ground to prevent any sudden or unexpected movement of the vehicle. Generally, a combination of cribbing, struts, ropes, webbing, and chains are used to accomplish these types of stabilization tasks. These techniques are discussed in the sections that follow. **Skill Sheet 5-1** describes several methods for stabilizing a vehicle.

Inexperienced rescuers may be tempted to test the stability of the vehicle as it is found — they must be trained to resist this temptation particularly if the vehicle is resting on its side, teetering on the edge of a cliff or embankment, or resting atop another vehicle. The slightest push in the wrong place may cause a vehicle to move significantly, perhaps compounding the patients' injuries.

In addition to being found upright, vehicles are found in positions such as on their side, upside down, or over an embankment. Under all circumstances, rescuers should use whatever means available to stabilize the vehicle. As always, the goal is to create as many points of contact between the vehicle and the ground as is reasonably possible given the resources available and the demands of the incident.

Vehicle Upright

Most vehicles involved in collisions remain upright. Even though all wheels are on the ground, some stabilization is required to ensure maximum stability for extrication operations. Vehicles should be stabilized to prevent movement in any direction.

The most common form of horizontal movement involves the vehicle rolling forward or backward on its wheels. This movement can be prevented by chocking the wheels with conventional wheel chocks, pieces of cribbing, or other suitable objects. If the vehicle is on flat ground, the wheels should be chocked fore and aft. If it is on a slope, the wheels should be chocked on the downhill side **(Figure 5.2)**. The vehicle's mechanical systems, such as parking brake and transmission, can also be used to help prevent horizontal movement. Automatic transmissions should be placed in "park." Depending upon the relationship of the vehicle to the slope, manual transmissions should be placed in reverse gear to prevent forward movement or placed in the lowest forward gear to prevent backward movement. The vehicle's parking brake should also be set.

The standard operating procedure (SOP) in some departments is to deflate all four tires to stabilize an upright vehicle. Removing the valve core, snipping off the valve stems with wire cutters, or pulling the stems out with pliers will quickly and safely accomplish deflation. However, this action also allows the vehicle to move as it settles onto its rims and thus could impart negative energy (potentially harmful movement) into the passenger compartment, so not all

CAUTION

Do not rely on mechanical systems – even if they are operable – as the sole means of stabilization.

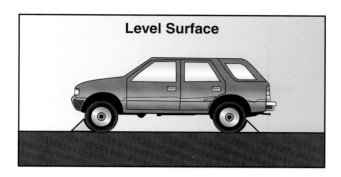

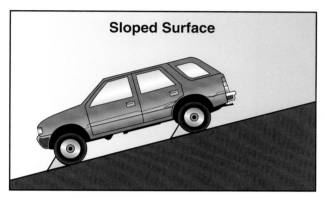

Figure 5.2 Methods for chocking a vehicle on a flat surface and on a slope.

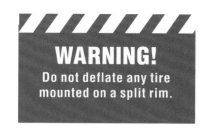

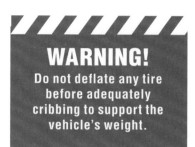

departments advocate this practice. Again, local agency protocols must be followed.

Deflating the tires does prevent the vehicle from rising as it gets lighter when the roof and other components are removed. However, if the tires are to be deflated, it should only be done after cribbing has been installed to support the weight of the vehicle.

There are numerous ways to prevent a vehicle from moving vertically — that is, to prevent it from settling or suddenly dropping. Step chocks, cribbing, jacks, and pneumatic lifting bags are most often used for this purpose.

Both wooden and plastic step chocks can be used when vehicles are upright. They are effective and quick and easy to install. At least four step chocks are needed to provide adequate stabilization. The situation will dictate the best method to use in any particular incident.

Cribbing, especially when used with wooden or plastic wedges, is relatively easy to install. However, installing cribbing usually takes longer than using step chocks. Cribbing is most often installed in a box formation until enough cribbing is installed to support the vehicle **(Figure 5.3, p. 182)**.

Different types of hydraulic and mechanical jacks can be used to support the frame of the vehicle. Their primary advantage is that they can be adjusted to the required height without the need for wedges. Their disadvantages are that they can be time-consuming to install, have limited range of motion, and are not as reliable as some other forms of stabilization.

Although they are designed primarily for lifting, pneumatic lifting bags can also be used for temporary support — if no other means is available. Usually, two or more bags are needed and may be installed along one side, in opposing positions on both sides, or under the front and rear of the vehicle. Lifting bags take time to deploy, and they do allow some vehicle movement even when the bags are fully inflated. Therefore, pneumatic lifting bags should only be used in conjunction with appropriate cribbing.

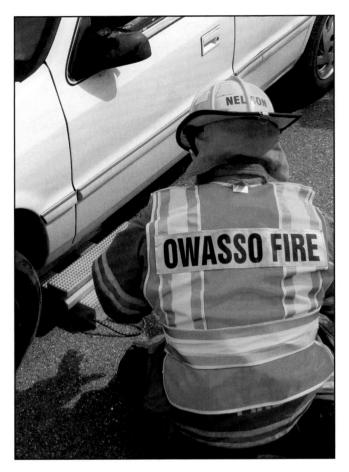

Figure 5.3 Extrication personnel creating a box crib.

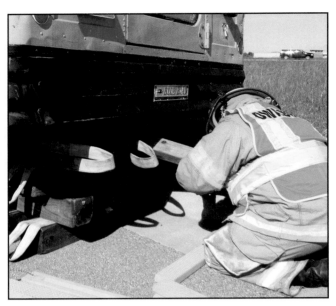

Figure 5.4 Rescuers should not place their hands between a vehicle and the crib being constructed.

When using any of these stabilization methods, rescue personnel must be careful to avoid placing their heads, hands, or any other part of their bodies under the vehicle while installing the stabilizing device. There is always the possibility of the vehicle dropping suddenly and unexpectedly, injuring or even killing anyone beneath it. To prevent any crushing hand injuries should a sudden drop occur, each piece of cribbing should be grasped from the sides, set outside of the vertical plane of the vehicle, and pushed into position under the vehicle with a tool or another piece of cribbing **(Figure 5.4)**.

As in all extrication operations, the simpler the stabilization operation the better, as long as the technique used is safe and effective. Experience has shown that for stabilization most vehicles require support at a minimum of four points and perhaps six **(Figure 5.5)**. Obviously, it takes less time to install support at four points than six, but the situation will dictate how much support is needed and where it should be installed. The following two options are the most common cribbing techniques rescuers use:

1. *Four-Point Support* — Although commonly called a "four-point crib," the means employed may involve the use of cribbing or any of the other equipment described in this chapter. Regardless of what equipment is used to support the vehicle, in a four-point crib the support is placed aft of the front wheel well and at the equivalent point forward of the rear wheel well on both sides of the vehicle.

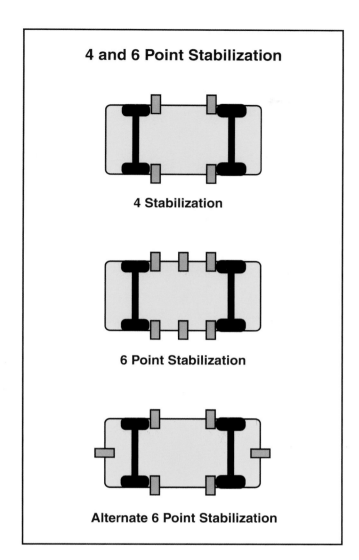

4 and 6 Point Stabilization

4 Stabilization

6 Point Stabilization

Alternate 6 Point Stabilization

Figure 5.5 Examples of 4- and 6-point stabilization.

2. *Six-Point Support* — A six-point crib is most often needed to support a vehicle that is in danger of collapsing in the middle such as when the doors are opened or removed or when the roof is removed from a unibody vehicle. Cribbing should be installed under the middle of both sides of the vehicle. However, it is possible that additional support may also be needed under the front and rear of the vehicle.

Vehicle on Side

When a vehicle has come to rest on its side, establishing fire protection is a high priority because gravity causes fuel, oil, and other fluids to flow into areas where they do not belong **(Figures 5.6, p. 184)**. These fluids may come into contact with hot exhaust system components or electrical components that can serve as sources of ignition. At least one 1½-inch (38 mm) or larger hoseline should be charged and ready **(Figure 5.7, p. 184)**. If fuel has been spilled, Class B foam should be applied to suppress the production of flammable vapors.

The exposed doors on the top side and rear may or may not be operable. If they are, occupants can escape through the door/window openings. If the vehicle is not on fire and rescue personnel are going to assist occupants through these

CAUTION
Fire in the area of loaded bumpers or damage to loaded bumpers may cause the bumpers to discharge, hurling the bumpers at high speed.

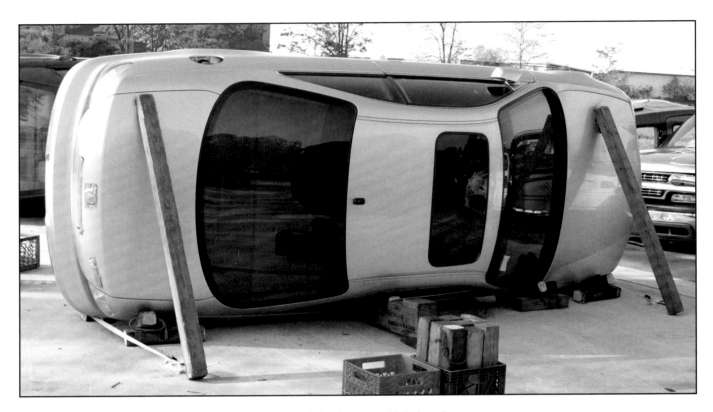

Figure 5.6 Vehicles on their sides require cribbing and shoring at multiple locations.

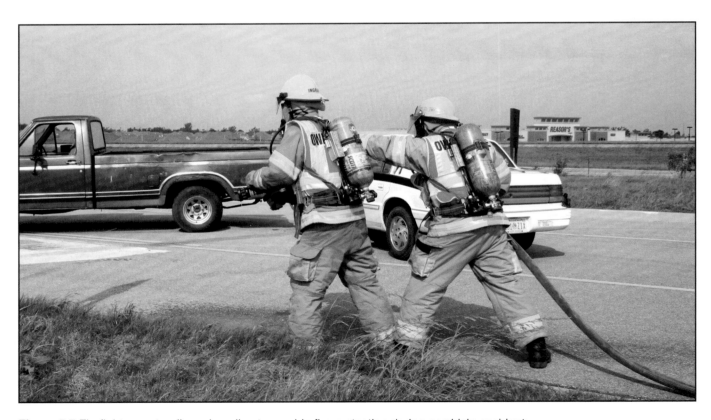

Figure 5.7 Firefighters extending a hoseline to provide fire protection during a vehicle accident.

openings, they should first stabilize the vehicle. A four-point crib with step chocks and wedges may be sufficient. Again, depending upon the situation, rescue personnel should use the best means available to quickly and safely prevent the vehicle from moving in any direction. This may involve the use of cribbing and/or step chocks as previously described, but it may also involve the use of webbing and rope.

When a vehicle has come to rest on a sloping, sandy, or other unstable surface, webbing/rope may be needed to stabilize the vehicle. The webbing/rope may be used alone or in combination with shoring or step chocks. Webbing, ropes, and/or chains can be attached to the vehicle and to a secure anchor point. Rope and webbing should be protected from chafing and/or contact with chemicals (such as battery acid) that may reduce their strength and cause them to fail. The need for redundancy must be weighed against other factors in the situation when deciding whether to back up rope or webbing with a second system.

Vehicle on Its Roof

When a vehicle has come to rest upside down, the same fire potential exists as with the vehicle on its side, so the same fire protection should be prepared. The vehicle's roof posts may be supporting the chassis more or less intact, or they may have collapsed. If the posts have collapsed, the normal window openings may have been reduced to narrow slits, too small to serve as access openings. If the A- and B-posts have collapsed but the vehicle has a rear door, it may still be operable and can be used to access the occupants, or the rear window can be removed. The occupants are likely to be hanging upside down, being held in place by their seat belts. They cannot survive long in this position, so they must be extricated as quickly and safely possible. After establishing fire protection, stabilizing the vehicle is critical.

Because the roofs of most vehicles are rounded above the door openings, and their surfaces have a smooth, painted finish, there is less purchase for cribbing or step chocks in contact with the roof surface than with other parts of the vehicle. Because of the rounded contours of vehicle roofs, it may also be necessary to support the vehicle front and rear with cribbing and/or Hi-Lift® jacks **(Figure 5.8)**.

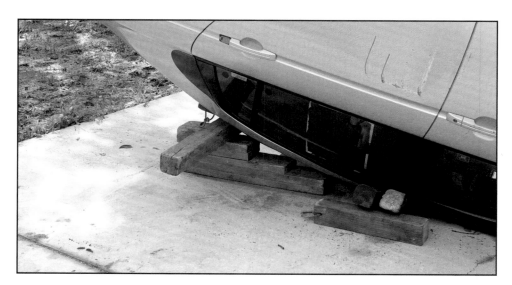

Figure 5.8 Upside down vehicles present unique cribbing situations.

Vehicles in Other Positions

Because of the dynamic forces involved in collisions, vehicles can come to rest in a variety of positions other than those already described. For example, a vehicle may be found at a steep angle resting against a tree, an embankment, other solid object or partially atop another vehicle. Just as with spinal immobilization of an injured patient, the challenge in stabilizing a vehicle in an unusual position is to stabilize as it is found — without moving it. This may involve the use of box cribbing or wooden or pneumatic shores to span the distance between the vehicle and a stable surface. It may also involve the use of tow trucks.

One technique used to stabilize vehicles in these situations is "marrying" or binding the vehicles together. This technique is used when two or more vehicles and/or objects are in contact with each other. Due to the changing conditions sometimes caused by operations, these vehicles and/or objects must be made safe throughout the rescue process by securing them to each other.

The "marrying" of vehicles together may be the only stabilization process available in extreme situations. "Marrying" is the process of providing additional support at key points between the vehicle(s) and the ground or other solid surfaces or anchors. The primary goal of "marrying" is to maximize the area of contact between the vehicle and the ground to prevent any sudden or unexpected movement of the vehicle.

Generally, a combination of cribbing, struts, ropes, ratchet straps, come-alongs, and chains are used to accomplish this type of stabilization task **(Figure 5.9)**. Only equipment with the manufactured approved working load limits should be used. **Skill Sheet 5-2** describes this process.

Sometimes it may also be necessary to use wreckers, cranes, and other large equipment to assist with stabilizing and "marrying" vehicles together, especially when large buses, trucks, or other heavy duty vehicles are involved. When patient removal has been accomplished additional equipment may be needed, such as; wreckers, cranes, fork lifts, etc. to safely retrieve stabilization equipment.

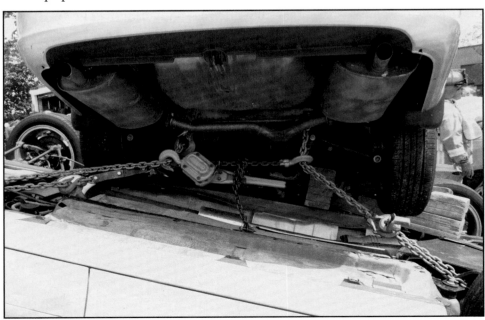

Figure 5.9 An example of two vehicles "married" together with chains and cribbing.

!!! caution "CAUTION"
    Loads and center of gravity may shift during extrication processes.

Use of Recovery Vehicles (Tow Trucks and Cranes)

If a tow truck or rescue crane is already on the scene, it may be a very valuable resource for stabilizing vehicles. In some cases, depending upon the situation and the other resources available, it may be prudent to wait for a tow truck or rescue crane to arrive before attempting to stabilize a vehicle. For example, if the vehicle is teetering on the edge of a high cliff or a bridge and the rescue units on scene do not have the necessary equipment to secure the vehicle, it may be safer for both the trapped occupants and rescue personnel to wait for a tow truck or rescue crane that is already en route. Attaching the cable from a tow truck or rescue crane winch to an unstabilized vehicle can provide the initial stability needed for rescue personnel to safely access the trapped patients.

NOTE: The Incident Commander (IC) or rescue personnel should maintain control of the scene while using tow trucks, rescue cranes, or other resources to assure a safe operation. Freelancing should not be allowed even by other agencies. The scene is under the control of rescuers until all extrication and rescue operations are complete.

Lifting

In order to stabilize a vehicle, it is sometimes necessary to remove other objects involved in the incident away from or off of the vehicle being stabilized. For example, if the vehicle struck a tree, power pole, or a building, the struck object may have collapsed onto the vehicle, trapping the occupants inside. The challenge in these situations is for rescue personnel to be able to lift the collapsed object from the vehicle while limiting the amount of vehicle movement.

Depending upon the situation and the resources available on scene, lifting objects from crashed vehicles may involve the use of pneumatic lifting bags, jacks, levers, or even booms or cranes. The most critical point in these operations is the security of the attachment of the lifting mechanism to the object being lifted. If the attachment should fail during the lift and allow the object to drop back onto the vehicle, the time and effort will have been wasted and it may have done more harm than good.

In some cases, the object resting on the vehicle may be too massive to be lifted intact. This situation may require the object to be divided into pieces that can be lifted. If the object is a tree or wooden power pole, it can be cut into smaller, more manageable pieces with a chain saw. The point of the operation is to free the underlying vehicle while making as few cuts as possible. Also, to the extent possible, the crushed vehicle must be stabilized to reduce the amount of reaction movement when the overlying burden is lifted. The same is true if the overlying object is made of metal and will be cut with a power saw, oxyacetylene cutting torch, or other thermal cutting device. If the overlying object is a wood frame wall, it can be cut into sections with a chain saw or rotary saw. If it is a masonry wall, it can be cut into smaller pieces with a rotary saw — or if necessary, broken apart using an electric concrete breaker (jack hammer).

In cases of this type where the IC is convinced that the operation is not a rescue but a body recovery, one other option remains — removing the vehicle from the object. This option involves supporting the overlying object so that it will not settle any further and lowering the vehicle enough that it can be pulled from beneath the object. If the vehicle's tires are still inflated, the valve cores can be removed or the valve stems cut off to allow the tires to deflate. If this creates the necessary clearance, the vehicle can then be pulled out with a tow truck's winch. If deflating the tires does not create the needed clearance, it may be necessary to use shovels to dig out beneath the vehicle's wheels.

Lifting can also be done to accomplish the following:

● Help position the vehicle for better stabilization (very common!)

● Lift one vehicle off another to gain access into the lower vehicle

● Lift a vehicle off of a trapped patient

The sections that follow discuss various vehicle lifting methods using a variety of equipment.

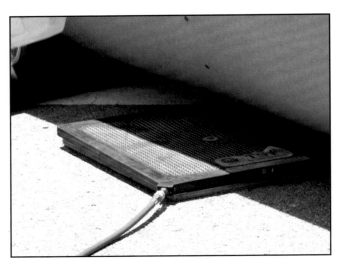

Figure 5.10 Air lifting bags should have a piece of plywood or mat material placed under them to protect them from damage.

Using Air Bags

Vehicles can be lifted using low, medium, or high pressure air bags designed for lifting heavy objects. The procedures for using air bags to lift a vehicle are found in **Skill Sheets 5-3**. When using air bags to lift a vehicle, rescuers should protect the bags from being damaged by using solid pieces of plywood or heavy duty mat material as large as or larger than the air bag being used. Place one piece of the plywood or mat or industrial belt material below the air bag. This will protect the air bag from glass and sharp edges **(Figure 5.10)**.

NOTE: Never exceed the manufacturer's recommendations for the amount to be lifted or the number of bags to be stacked on top of one another. When stacking air bags, the load to be lifted should never exceed the rating of the lowest rated bag.

Using Low and Medium Pressure Air Bags

The following actions should be performed when using low pressure air bags during extrication operations:

● Check hazards, patients, continuous vehicle stabilization, determine patient location.

● Crib the vehicle in a way to allow the insertion of the air bag ⅔ of the way under the object to be lifted.

● Protect the bag from punctures.

● Lift an inch, crib an inch.

● Ensure the pivot side (opposite of the lift side) of the object is well cribbed, to avoid crushing the patient(s).

● Reminder: it is only necessary to lift the object enough to remove the patient properly.

Using High Pressure Air Bags

The following actions should be performed when using high pressure air bags during extrication operations:

- Check hazards, patients, continuous vehicle stabilization, determine patient location.

- Assess the load to be lifted.

- Crib the vehicle in a way to allow the insertion of the air bag 2/3 of the way under the object to be lifted.

- Protect the bag from punctures .

- Lift an inch, crib an inch.

- Use the proper lifting bag for the weight to be moved or displaced.

- Put the largest airbag on the bottom.

- Stack only two airbags at a time.

- Insert the air bags under the object for a straight lift upward.

- Inflate the lower bag according to the manufacturer's instructions to the desired lift.

- Inflate the top bag according to the manufacturer's instructions, if lift is not achieved. If the lift is still not achieved, crib the object, and deflate the bags.

- Adjust the lifting platform higher.

- Repeat the above steps until desired lift is met.

- Do not inflate either bag fully.

- Inflate or deflate an inch, crib an inch. Never use the bags as your only means of cribbing.

- Follow the bag movement with cribbing to prevent sudden drop of lifting devices in case of failure.

- Use simple commands like "up on red," "hold on red," or "down on red" to perform these maneuvers to control the operation. The control operator should concentrate on commands given to him by the air bag rescue operator and carefully monitor the air bag lifting evolution. If the operator sees something fail, the operator can take corrective action. The operator can also see how much to lift or lower a load and see that the equipment is functioning correctly.

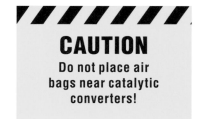

CAUTION
Do not place air bags near catalytic converters!

Using Jacks

The following guidelines should be followed when using jacks during extrication operations:

- Crib the opposite side or end of the object to be raised.

- Establish a firm base to set the tool against so that the tool being used will not be pushed into the ground. Cribbing or platform can be used to provide a good base.

- Install the equipment as to insure good footing on the ground and the lifting object so the distribution of weight is spread over more area.

- Lift an inch, crib an inch.

NOTE: Never allow the object that is being moved to come back into the area it is being moved away from. It is important to prevent re-impingment of the object onto the patient. It is only necessary to move the material being lifted or moved the amount needed to extricate the patient. **Skill Sheet 5-4** describes the procedures for lifting a vehicle using a jack.

Using Levers

The lever is the simplest of all devices: it is a rigid bar, either straight or bent, that is free to move on a fixed point called a *fulcrum*. The lever works by transferring a force from one place to another while at the same time changing the direction of the force. The detailed procedures for lifting a vehicle or part of a vehicle using a lever are found in **Skill Sheet 5-5**.

Fulcrum — Support or point of support on which a lever turns in raising or moving something.

The potential mechanical advantage of a lever can be calculated by measuring the distance between the load and the fulcrum and the fulcrum and where the force is applied. The potential mechanical advantage of a lever can be calculated by measuring the distance between:

1. the load and the fulcrum and

2. the fulcrum and where the force is applied.

If the length of the lever is three times as long on the force side of the fulcrum as on the load side, the lever has a 3-to-1 mechanical advantage. Thus, if you have a 300-pound load to lift and a 3:1 lever, it will take 100 pounds of force to lift the load. There are three classifications of levers; these are determined by the location of the fulcrum as it relates to both the load and the force.

Class I Lever

The Class I lever is the most efficient to use to move objects vertically. A load is applied at one end of the lever and the lifting force is applied at the other end, with a fulcrum located between the two. Crowbars, pry bars, and most fire service forcible entry tools are examples of Class I levers **(Figure 5.11)**. A seesaw is another example of a Class I lever.

When using a Class I lever, it is very important to consider the stability and strength of the surface upon which the fulcrum rests. Both the fulcrum and the foundation on which it rests must be capable of holding twice the weight of the load to be lifted. If the load is 100 pounds, it will take 100 pounds of force to lift it. That means that the fulcrum must be capable of holding 200 pounds.

Class II Lever

A Class II lever is the next most useful and efficient lever. Class II levers are used to move objects horizontally. It consists of a fulcrum at one end, a load in the middle, and a force on the other end. Wheelbarrows, furniture dollies, and pulleys are types of Class II levers **(Figure 5.12)**.

Class III Lever

A Class III lever is used when force may be sacrificed for distance. It places a load on one end, the fulcrum on the opposite end, and the force in the middle. Shovels and brooms are types of Class III levers **(Figure 5.13)**. This class of lever is the *least* efficient method of lifting. As a mechanical *disadvantage*, it depends upon the rescuer's strength to move the load, not the multiplication of the force.

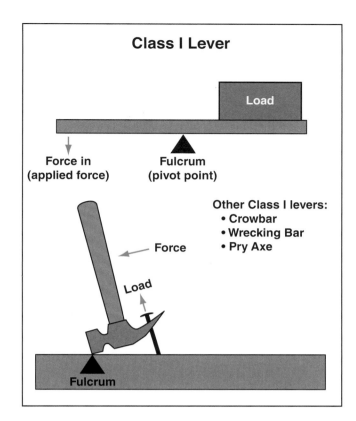

Figure 5.11 This illustration shows how a Class I lever works.

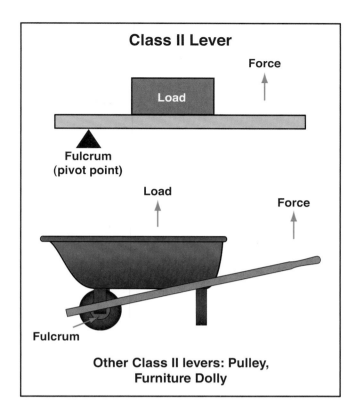

Figure 5.12 An example of how Class II levers work.

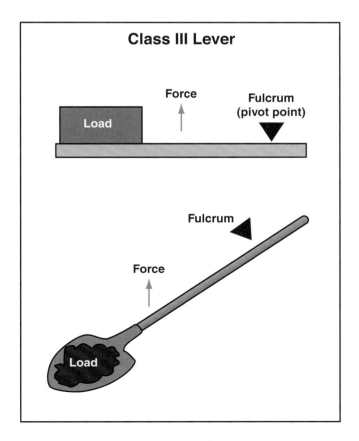

Figure 5.13 This is an example of a Class III lever.

Using Chains, Wire Rope, Synthetic Slings, and Hitches

A *sling* is an assembly that connects the load to the crane. Slings are used to stabilize, lift, pull, or move objects. The procedures for using slings to lift a vehicle are described in **Skill Sheet 5-6**. There are three commonly used materials for the manufacture of slings: chain, wire rope, and synthetic fibers.

Chains

Rescue chain can be used to help move wreckage away from a patient and to tie down unstable objects. Chain slings can be used for rugged applications in harsh environments where flexibility, abrasion resistance, and long life are required. Rescue chain can be used to help move wreckage away from a patient and for tying down unstable objects.

In selecting chain, it is best to use a Grade 8 or 10, also called Grade 80 or Grade 100, alloy steel chain. When using Grade 8 or 80 chain, it is also important to use hooks that have an equal or greater rating. This grade can absorb shock loads better than other grades of chain rated at the same strength. The use of chain for slings is limited due to its weight.

There are several other precautions to be aware of when using chain including the following:

- Do not exceed the listed safe working load of the chain. All chain should have an attached tag that has the safe load weight stamped or printed on it.

- Remember that links can break without warning.

- Place padding between the chain and the load to create a better gripping surface and to protect the chain from damage.

- Use padding, such as planks or heavy fabric, around sharp corners on the load to protect links from being cut.

- Do not expose chain to cold temperatures for long periods of time.

- Do not permit chain to become kinked or twisted while under stress.

- Make sure that the load is seated in the hook.

- Do not attach chain hooks to the loads. Attach hooks only to the chain.

- Avoid sudden jerks in lifting and lowering the load. Do not shock load the chain.

- Remember that chains may create a sparking hazard.

- Do not tie a knot in a chain.

- Chain can be very slippery when lifting steel. Watch for shifting loads.

- Use a chain gauge to check chain regularly for fatigue and stretching.

- Destroy damaged or worn-out chains.

- Do not reweld broken links on alloy chain.

Chain should be inspected regularly because failures can occur if the chain has been abused or neglected during use or storage. Improper treatment of chain components can lead to metal fatigue and chain failure. Chain should be regularly inspected link by link for signs of cracks, nicks, gouges, bent links, corrosion, elongation, or any other defects. Defective chain should be removed from service.

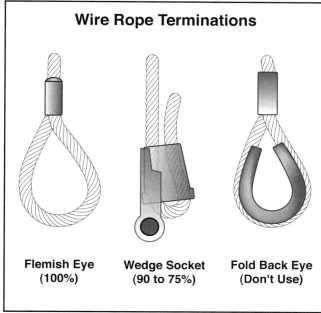

Figure 5.14 Examples of wire rope fittings and terminations.

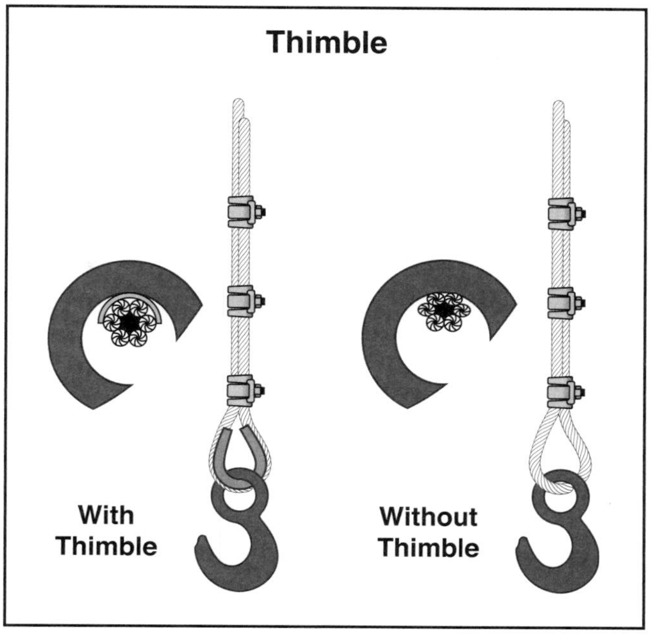

Figure 5.15 This illustration shows how a wire thimble can be used to protect wire rope.

Wire Rope

Wire, such as plow steel cable, is the strongest type of material used for slings. It may be constructed in one of the following forms:

- *Braided wire rope* — a wire rope formed by plaiting component wire ropes.
- *Cable laid rope* — a wire rope composed of six wire ropes wrapped around a fiber or wire rope core.
- *Strand laid rope* — a wire rope made with strands (usually six or eight) wrapped around a fiber core, wire strand core, or independent wire rope core.

Wire rope fittings and terminations are available in a number of designs **(Figure 5.14)**. The Flemish eye is the most reliable and efficient termination and must be done in a shop. The Flemish eye does not reduce capacity. The Wedge socket is the next most reliable type of termination. If it is properly manufactured and installed, it will only reduce capacity by 10-20 percent. The Fold-back eye termination is the least reliable and should not be used.

It may be necessary during an incident to construct wire rope terminations using cable clips. These clips reduce capacity by about 20 percent, so it is vital that rescuers become familiar with how to position and tighten these very useful devices. The clips are installed in succession and torqued (tightened) according to manufacturer's specifications. If the wire rope needs to be attached to a hang point that would cause the cable to bend sharply, it is important to use a *thimble* **(Figure 5.15)**. The thimble guides the cable into a natural curve shape and helps to protect the wire rope.

Some important points about wire rope are as follows:

- Keep from kinking to avoid damage and loss of integrity
- Will be damaged by sharp bends or edges

- Must not be tied in a knot (either cable or wire rope). This places severe stress on the strands, causing them to break

- Remember that kinetic energy is stored in the cable during hauling. In the event of cable failure, it can whip around violently, resulting in severe injury hazard

- Requires edge protection or softeners to protect wire rope from damage due to sharp edges

- Should be destroyed when a wire rope sling is deemed out of service due to wear or damage

Wire rope inspection should be done on a regular basis. The following conditions are unsafe and are signals that the wire rope must be discarded:

- Broken wires – depends on location

- Crushed strands

- Kinks, birdcages (outer strands displace from the core forming a cage), and protruding core

- Stretch, diameter reduction

- Abrasion and corrosion

- Fatigue and electric arc

Synthetic Slings

Synthetic round slings and web slings are frequently used in rescue work for quickly setting up anchors and attachments for lifting, stabilizing, pulling, and moving operations. Synthetic slings have the following characteristics:

- Tend to mold around the load, adding additional holding power **(Figure 5.16)**

- Do not rust and are non-sparking

- Are lightweight, making them easier and safer to rig

- Have no sharp edges, thereby reducing injury potential

- Are more elastic than chain or wire rope and can absorb shock loading better

- Are not affected by moisture and are resistant to many chemicals

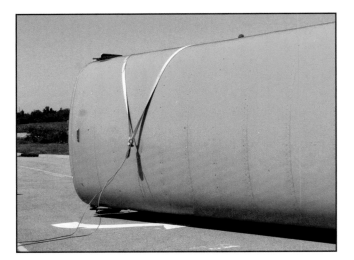

Figure 5.16 A synthetic sling material molds itself to the shape of this bus.

- Are damaged more easily than cable slings. Must be protected from sharp edges in a rescue situation
- Neither Nylon nor polyester are very resistant to temperatures greater than 200°F (93°C)

Whenever any sling is used, the following practices must be observed:

- Destroy any slings that are damaged or defective.
- Do not shorten slings with knots, bolts, or other makeshift devices.
- Make sure that sling legs are not kinked or twisted.
- Do not load slings in excess of their rated capacity.
- Make sure that slings used in a basket hitch have the loads balanced to prevent slippage.
- Make sure that slings are securely attached to their loads.
- Protect or pad slings from the sharp edges of their loads.
- Be sure that suspended loads are kept clear of all obstructions.
- Keep all personnel clear of loads about to be lifted and of suspended loads.
- Do not EVER place hands or fingers between the sling and its load while the sling is being tightened around the load.
- Avoid shock loading. Jerking the load could overload the sling, causing failure.
- Do not pull a sling from under a load when the load is resting on the sling. Lumber can be used to allow space to remove the sling and prevent shifting of the load and damage to the sling.
- Do not drag slings on the ground or floor.

Despite the inherent toughness of synthetic slings, they can be cut by repeated use or from failure to provide proper barrier protection. Edge guards, movable sleeves, and coatings are available to increase the life of the sling. Synthetic slings should be inspected every 30 days and after each incident on both sides, in good light as follows:

- Pay particular attention to the stitching and ends for wear
- Check the body of the sling for cuts, tensile damage, abrasion, punctures, snags, chemical damage, and heat damage
- Remove any sling that shows excessive wear or damage from service.

Round Slings. A round sling, also known as an endless sling, is a synthetic sling – usually polyester fibers twisted into yarn bundles -- made from a continuous loop of yarn and covered with a jacket. The yarn bundles are twisted into multiple, but separate continuous strands. These strands form the load-bearing members of the sling, and the number of strands in the sling determine its strength. Continuous load-bearing strands are covered with a polyester jacket that is primarily a protective covering that reduces the potential of mechanical and physical damage to interior strands. Round slings may be used for vertical, choker, basket, or bridle slings.

Web Slings. Web slings are commonly available as endless, standard eye, and twisted eye. The endless sling has both ends of one piece of webbing lapped and sewn together to form a continuous piece. They can be used for vertical, bridle, choker, and basket hitches. The standard eye and eye sling is a single

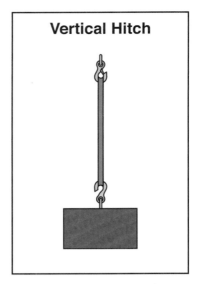

Figure 5.17 An example of a vertical hitch.

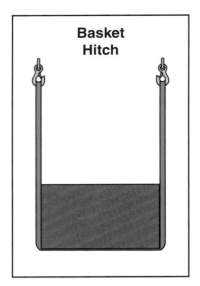

Figure 5.18 An illustration showing a basket hitch.

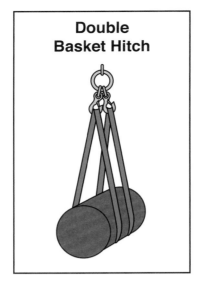

Figure 5.19 Double basket hitches are more stable than single basket hitches.

piece of webbing sewn with an eye at either end in the same plane as the sling body. The twisted eye sling is a single piece of webbing with the eye at either end sewn at 90 degrees to the plane (tapered or full width) of the sling. The twisting allows for better rigging of chocker slings.

Hitches

When a sling, regardless of type, is attached to a load, it is termed a hitch. A hitch is a sling configuration whereby the sling is fastened to an object or load, either directly to it or around it. Common hitches are described in the sections that follow.

Vertical hitch. A vertical hitch is a method of supporting a load by using a single leg of rope, chain, or webbing. The full load is carried by a single leg, which is one straight piece of chain, rope, or webbing **(Figure 5.17)**. This hitch should not be used in the following cases:

- Load is hard to balance.
- Center of gravity is hard to establish.
- Load is loose.
- Load extends past the point of attachment.

Basket hitch. A basket hitch is a sling configuration whereby the sling is passed under the load and has both ends on the hook or a master link **(Figure 5.18)**. This hitch supports the load by having one end of the sling attached to a hook. The sling is then wrapped around the load, and both "eyes" of the sling are attached to the hook. A basket hitch is not designed to keep a load balanced or stabilized.

Double Basket Hitch. A double basket hitch is more stable than a single basket hitch. The double basket hitch uses two single slings wrapped at separate locations in the same manner **(Figure 5.19)**. This hitch allows for locating the center attachment hook over the estimated center of gravity, and permits

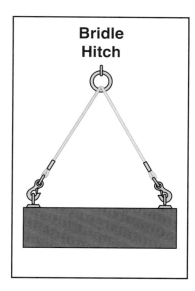

Bridle Hitch

Figure 5.20 Bridle hitch slings have 2 or 3 "legs" that attach to the load to be lifted.

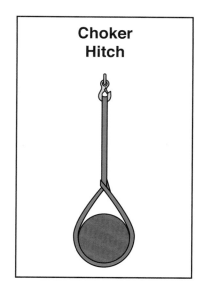

Choker Hitch

Figure 5.21 Choker hitches create a vise-like grip on the load being lifted.

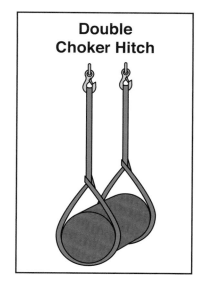

Double Choker Hitch

Figure 5.22 An example of a double choker hitch.

the wrapping of the slings to either side of the center of gravity. It is possible to use a "double wrap" basket hitch that makes contact all the way around the load surface for increased securing of the load, which is especially good for cylindrical loads.

Bridle hitch. A bridle hitch is a sling configuration consisting of 2 or 3 "legs" attached to the load. The slings are secured to a single point, which is usually in line between the center of gravity and the anchor (lifting point) **(Figure 5.20)**. The bridle hitch can provide very stable lifting, stabilizing, moving, and pulling due to distribution of the load onto the multiple slings.

Choker hitch. A choker hitch is a sling configuration with one end of the sling passing under the load and through the other end of the sling. This sling is secured back onto itself and creates a vise-like grip on the load **(Figure 5.21)**. A potential problem with the choker hitch is one of stability of the load.

Double choker hitch. A double choker hitch has two single slings spread apart around the load. This hitch does not make full contact with the load surface, but it can be double wrapped to help control or hold the load. When using straps in pairs, hooks should be arranged on the straps so that they will pull from the opposite sides to create a better gripping action **(Figure 5.22)**.

Using Rigging

Rigging is defined as a length of rope/chain/webbing attached to a load for the purpose of stabilizing, lifting, pulling, or moving objects. Basic components are hooks and shackles/eyes for termination points so that connections can be more easily made to the load. The heavy equipment company may supply the rigging; if so, employees of the company will be responsible for the care, maintenance, selection, and attachment of the rigging to the load and to the crane. Rescue personnel may be asked to assist with attaching the rigging to the load or manning guidelines. The sections that follow described various equipment associated with rigging.

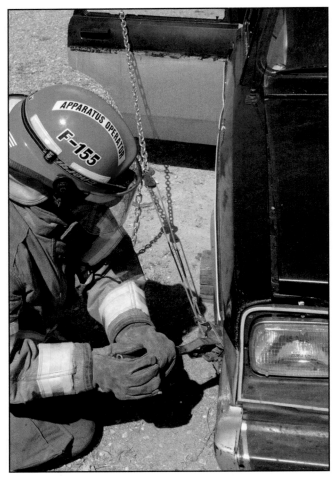

Figure 5.23 A rescuer using a cable winch come-along to pry a car door out of the way.

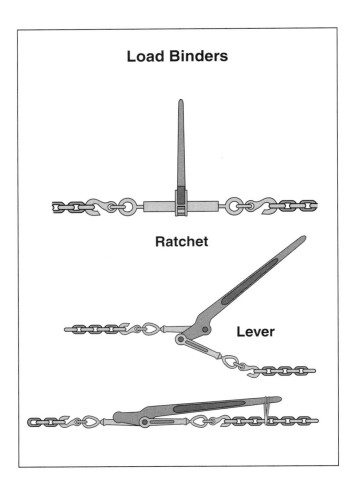

Figure 5.24 Ratchet and lever type load binders.

Clevis hook — A type of hook attached at the end of a rope, web sling, or chain engineered for rapid connection; commonly used during vehicle extrication and rescue incidents.

Tighteners

A number of different types of tighteners can be used for adjusting rigging. These include wire rope tighteners, cable winches, load binders, chain hoists, and turnbuckles.

Wire Rope Tighteners. Wire rope tighteners can be used for lifting light loads as well as tightening cable tiebacks and other rigging. Care needs to be taken not to overload them.

Cable Winch (come-along). Cable winches are 2 to 3 feet (.75 m to 1 m) long, so their use may be limited in confined spaces. When using a cable winch, the length of the handle and the strength of one person provide the overload limit. If care is not taken, cable can foul during rewinding **(Figure 5.23)**.

Load Binder. Load binders are most commonly used with chain assemblies. The ratchet type is more reliable, and it is important to wire tie the handle for safety. They have a 50:1 ratchet action, but only an 8-inch (200 mm) take-up **(Figure 5.24)**.

Chain Hoist. A chain hoist can lift up to 6 tons with 100 lbs. of pull. It is critical that rescuers not overpull by using more than one person. These tighteners have a large take-up (up to 10 feet [3.1 m]), and some only require a 12-inch (300 mm) clearance **(Figure 5.25)**.

Turnbuckles. Turnbuckles are a commonly used tightening device that can be used to do the final tightening of tiebacks, freeing a cable winch to do other jobs. The maximum take-up can vary from 8 to 24 inches (200 mm to 600 mm), depending on what type is used. The hook ends of turnbuckles are only ⅔ as strong as the eye or jaw ends **(Figure 5.26)**.

Rigging Fittings

The basic components of rigging fittings are hooks, shackles, and eyes. Hooks and shackles provide a way to lift loads without directly tying to the load. They can be attached to wire or fiber rope, blocks, or chains. The Clevis and eye-types are engineered to enable rescuers to make rapid chain-to-hook connections. Hooks should have a latch or mouse closing device to keep slings or traps from slipping off the hook. Hooks can be moused by using rope yarn, seizing wire, or shackles **(Figure 5.27)** Shackles should be used when loads are too heavy for hooks to handle safely. Ring, hook, and shackle components of slings should be made from forged alloy steel. The pins used in each shackle are *not* interchangeable with other shackles. The pin should be screwed in all the way and backed off one-quarter turn before loading.

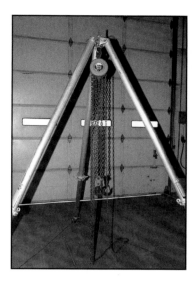

Figure 5.25 One type of chain hoist system.

Mouse — To tightly wrap or cover the open end of a hook with a material to prevent an object from slipping off the hook.

Shackle — A U-shaped metal device that is secured with a pin or bolt across the device's opening. Another type of shackle is a hinged metal loop that is secured with a quick-release locking pin mechanism.

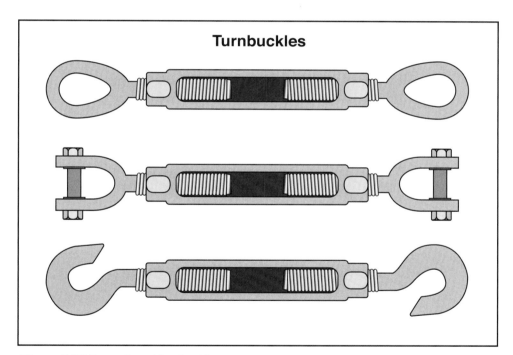

Figure 5.26 Examples of turnbuckles.

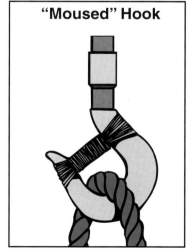

Figure 5.27 A hook that has been wrapped or "moused" to prevent slings or traps from slipping off the hook.

Glass Removal

One of the fastest and easiest ways of gaining access to the interior of a vehicle is by removing glass from the vehicle. Removing the glass may be necessary if the doors are inoperable, the doors are operable but locked, or the roof needs to be removed or flapped. There are multiple types of glass used in vehicles: laminated safety glass, tempered glass, polycarbonates, Lexan®, ballistic, and enhanced protective glass (EPG). Rescuers should continuously monitor new developments in automotive glass.

Removing Laminated Safety Glass

Removing windshields and laminated rear windows is somewhat more complicated and time-consuming than removing tempered side or rear windows. This is mainly because of the difference in glass types. **Skill Sheet 5-7** describes the methods and procedures for removing windshields and other laminated glass.

Windshields and rear windows constructed of laminated safety glass do not disintegrate and fall out like tempered glass windows. Because more laminates are being added to windshields, it may not be as easy to chop through the windshields of newer vehicles. Rescuers should protect vehicle occupants from glass dust and chips that may be produce during the removal process. To protect themselves, rescue personnel should wear full PPE to include eye protection. The following hand tools can be used to remove or cut laminated glass:

- Commercial windshield removal tool
- Reciprocating saw
- Handsaw with a coarse blade such as those used in commercially produced rescue tools
- Air chisel
- Baling hook

In most modern vehicles, the windshield, the two A-posts, and the forward edge of the roof are part of the structural integrity of the vehicle body and should remain in place unless they hinder rescue and extrication efforts. If windshield removal is necessary, remove the glass while leaving the A-posts and roof edge intact to maintain a minimum of structural integrity. If the windshield or rear window must be removed, the glass may have to be cut on all four sides. Sometimes a patient impacts the windshield and the windshield must be removed from around the patient. **Skill Sheet 5-8** describes two methods for removing a windshield from around a patient.

Removing Tempered Glass

If it is necessary to break a window to access a patient, choose a window as far away from the patient as possible, and protect the patient from glass dust and chips. To protect themselves, rescue personnel should wear full PPE including eye protection.

Removing side and rear windows made of tempered glass is a relatively simple operation. These windows can easily be broken by being struck with a sharp, pointed object such as a glass hammer or a windshield wiper arm. They may also be broken by a spring-loaded center punch being pressed against the glass. These tools are usually applied at a lower corner of the glass but they may work at any point on the glass surface. When using a spring-loaded center punch, the hand holding the tool should be braced with the other hand to increase control of the tool. Having control prevents the rescuer from sticking a hand into the glass when it breaks. It also prevents the center punch from being pushed through the window opening and possibly striking a vehicle occupant who may be near the window **(Figure 5.28)**. A standard center punch or Phillips® screwdriver can also be used. Both of these tools must be driven into the glass with a hammer or other striking tool. The pick end of a pick-head axe or Halligan tool will also work if nothing else is available.

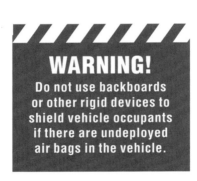

WARNING!
Do not use backboards or other rigid devices to shield vehicle occupants if there are undeployed air bags in the vehicle.

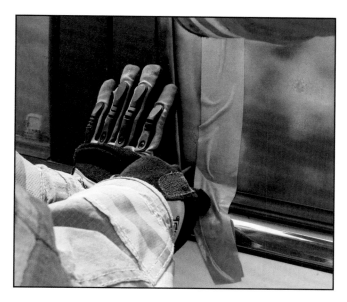

Figure 5.28 A rescuer demonstrating the proper hand positions for using a center punch.

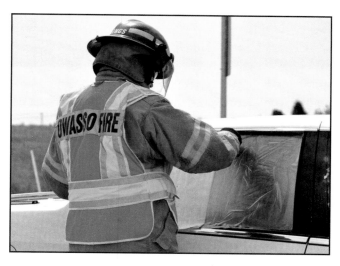

Figure 5.29 Contact paper can be used to control glass fragments when removing vehicle glass. *Courtesy of Sonrise Photography.*

One method of controlling the glass fragments is to apply a sheet of self-adhering contact paper to the surface of the glass **(Figure 5.29)**. Once broken, the glass adheres to the contact paper. Another method of controlling breaking glass is to place duct tape on the windows and then spray the glass surface with an aerosol adhesive that forms a coating on the glass. This coating sets up in seconds and allows the glass to be broken and retained in a sheet. Then the glass can be removed in sheets instead of tiny pieces **(Figures 5.30a and b)**.

As mentioned earlier, some rear windows are tempered glass and some are laminated. If a window does not respond to removal techniques for tempered glass, it is probably laminated glass and must be removed in the same way as a windshield. If the glass resists all attempts to remove it, it is probably the newer 1/3 inch (9 mm) glass that is virtually unbreakable. This glass can be left intact while doors and other vehicle components are removed. **Skill Sheet 5-9** describes the procedures for removing tempered glass.

Removing Other Types of Glass

Rescuers should also be trained to remove other types of glass such as enhanced performance glass, polycarbonates, Lexan®, and ballistic glass. The following sections described the procedures for removing these types of glass.

Enhanced Performance Glass (EPG)

- Cut the lower part of the window horizontal.
- Pry out the lower section of the glass
- Pull the glass out and downward

Removing Other Types of Glass (continued)

Polycarbonates and Lexan®:

- Normal tools do not work.
- Doors must be removed or a purchase point must be made into the glass using a saws-all, rotary, or circular saw.
- After removal or creating a purchase point, use the saw to complete the cut.
- An alternate method is to use CO_2 to freeze Lexan® glass followed by breaking the glass with a sharp object.

To date, these styles of glass are only to be used in the tops and rear glass behind the passenger according to NHTSA in the United States.

Ballistic Glass:

- Removal of this glass will mean removal of the doors.
- Some door such as up armored military vehicles, armored vehicles, or security vehicles may need the use of a cutting device to cut open the doors by the hinges if possible.
- Take special care as to not allow the door to come down on any tools or body parts.

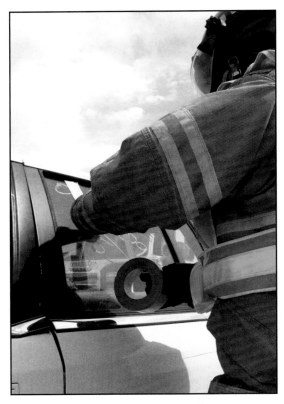

Figure 5.30a Duct tape can be applied to create handles for rescuers to use to lift out a window.

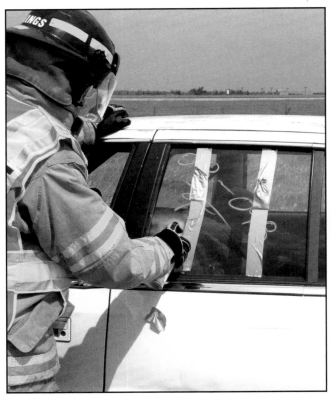

Figure 5.30b Spray adhesive can then be applied to bind the window's glass fragments prior to breaking the glass.

Door/Side Panel Removal

When removing the glass from a crashed vehicle does not allow sufficient access to those inside the vehicle, other means must be used. The most obvious means is by simply opening the vehicle's doors. If the doors will not open because they are locked, the interior door lock release can be reached through the window opening. If unlocking the doors does not allow them to open when both the inside and outside latches are used simultaneously, the doors must either be forced open or removed from the vehicle entirely. On two-door vehicles, it is sometimes advantageous to also remove the side panel between the door opening and the rear wheel well.

Prior to conducting any door or side panel removal operation, rescuers should peel away any trim or plastic components on the vehicle's interior around the area being removed. This helps the rescuers identify the location of any seat belt pretensioners, air bag gas cylinders, or other safety devices. It also helps prevent the trim and plastic pieces from breaking loose and striking patients or rescuers during extrication operations.

Creating Purchase Points

When removing a door from a vehicle, you must first determine which side of the door the rescuers are going to start with (hinge side or latch side). There are several opinions and schools of thought on this subject. Local policies/procedures and the conditions found at an incident will dictate which side rescuers start on first.

Whichever side rescue personnel plan to start with, they must first gain a purchase point to use the tools selected to open the door. This can be done in a wide variety of ways with a wide variety of tools. We will discuss the techniques involved with several tools.

Using a Halligan (Hooligan) Bar

Place the adz end of the Halligan either between the door and the fender for the hinge side or the door and the post for the latch side. Then hit the tool into the space with a flat-head axe or a sledgehammer and rotate the tool up and down to create an opening for the tool to be used to open the door **(Figure 5.31)**.

CAUTION
Avoid rocking the patients when using hand tools to make purchase points.

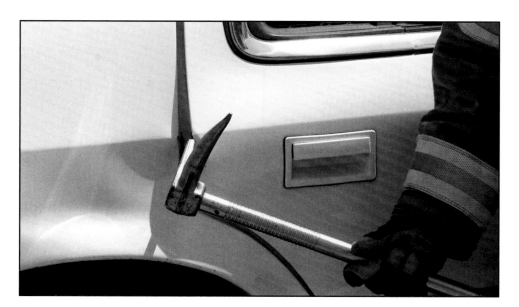

Figure 5.31 A halligan bar can be used to create purchase points into which hydraulic spreader tips can be inserted.

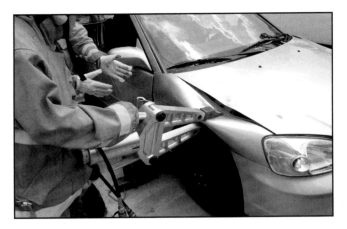

Figure 5.32 A fender crush procedure can create a purchase point by pulling the fender away from the door edge.

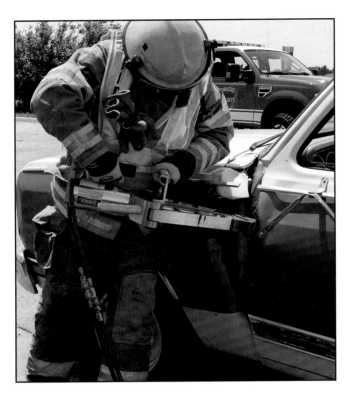

Figure 5.33 Hydraulic spreaders being used to pry open a vehicle door from the hinge side. *Courtesy of Mark Stuckey, City of Owasso Fire Department.*

Using a Pry Bar

Place the pry bar in the same spot as described previously and knock it into place with a striking tool. Then pry from side to side instead of up and down. It will be necessary to move the pry bar up and down the slot to achieve enough of an opening for the door opening tool to fit in.

Using a Hydra Ram/Rabbit Tool

These manually operated hydraulic spreaders can also be used to create purchase points. Agencies use these tools often for forcible entry on residential and commercial doors, but they are also very good for gaining purchase points on doors, hoods, and trunks. To use this tool, simply place the spreader tips into the space between the door and the fender and/or post and manually pump the handle until the opening is of the appropriate size.

Using Hydraulic Spreaders

The majority of the time, hydraulic spreaders can be used to gain a purchase point. Use a fender crush technique to gain an opening between the fender and the door **(Figure 5.32)**. This allows the rescuers to spread the fender out of the way and cut or spread the hinges to remove the door **(Figure 5.33)**. This method also allows rescue personnel to only have to bring a spreader and the cutter to the vehicle.

To use this technique, a rescuer should open the spreaders and place one arm in the wheel well on the front fender. The other arm of the spreaders is placed on top of the fender and close the spreaders. Closing the spreaders will crush the fender and create an opening between the door and the fender.

This method must be practiced before using it during an actual extrication. When trying this for the first time, the spreader often slides off the top of the fender before it crushes it. When this happens it is often difficult to make a second attempt at the same location, so it will be necessary to move to another spot on the fender and attempt to crush it again.

To avoid this error, the spreader tip edge can be fit into the space between the fender and the hood. If this can be done, the spreader arms will not slide off the hood and instead will bite down onto the fender and crush. Raising the back end of the spreader slightly above a 90 degree angle this will help prevent the tool from slipping.

Using a spreader in the window opening to spread the upper and lower parts of the door away from the roof rail and pillars is another method for using hydraulic spreaders. Many leading rescue technicians recommend using a vertical crush to create purchase points and pop open doors. This method forces the door away from the patient and often pops open a door without repositioning the spreader and without the use of any other tools, thus making it quicker to extricate the patients. Safety is always a concern when performing extrication, and even more so with the latest technology. Caution must always be exercised when operating around air bags.

Door Forcing/Removal

If the doors cannot be opened, they will have to be forced or removed. Even if a door is ultimately removed from the vehicle, having the door open makes removal easier. As is true of most evolutions in emergency rescue, there is more than one way to open or remove a jammed door.

NOTE: Frontal air bags, side-impact air bags, head protection systems, and seat belt pretensioners can be unintentionally deployed when doors are being forcibly opened or removed.

Rescue personnel should always maintain control over a door they are attempting to open or remove to prevent injury to patients and rescuers alike. This can be accomplished by attaching webbing, straps, rope, chains, or other materials to door and maintaining tension on the material and door to prevent it from striking personnel **(Figure 5.34, p. 206)**.

If the vehicle door contains an air bag, a cable (possibly yellow) will be exposed between the door and the A-post when the door is removed. If the wires between the door and the A-post must be cut, after the battery has been disconnected and the reserve power dissipated, the wires should be separated and cut one at a time with handheld cutters — never with power shears. Cutting the yellow wire in these situations deploys any undeployed airbag systems and should be avoided.

A Hi-Lift® jack can be used to open a door by crushing or weakening the door's collision bar. Once this has occurred the jack is repositioned over the Nader pin to roll door down and off of the Nader pin. **Skill Sheet 5-10** describes the procedures for using a Hi-Lift® jack to open a door. Caution should be used when using Hi-Lift® jacks. If not deployed properly, they can slip easily and be very dangerous.

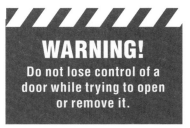

WARNING!
Make sure that rescuers, patients, and loose objects (including seat belt buckles) are out of the deployment path of any air bags, head protection systems, or seat belt pretensioners.

WARNING!
Do not lose control of a door while trying to open or remove it.

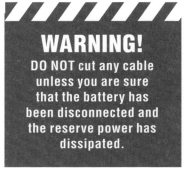

WARNING!
DO NOT cut any cable unless you are sure that the battery has been disconnected and the reserve power has dissipated.

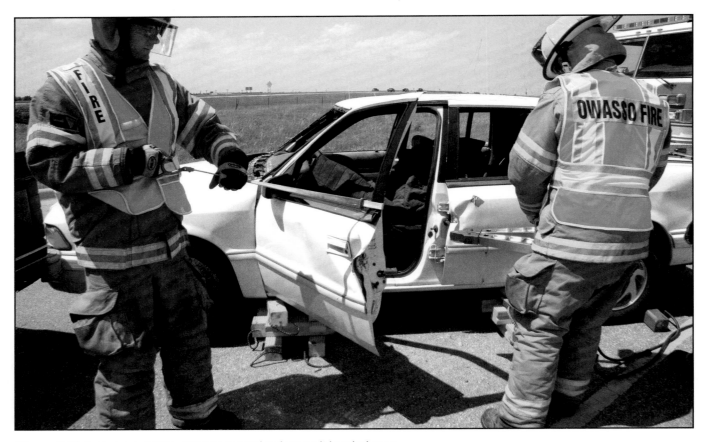

Figure 5.34 A rescuer using a strap to control a door as it is pried open.

Nader pin — The bolt on a vehicle's door frame that the door latches on to in order to close the door.

Another method uses power ratchets, power impact wrenches, or manual socket sets to remove the bolts on the door's hinges. Rescuers must gain access to the hinges through the door's exterior then either loosen and remove the hinge bolts or over-tighten the bolt heads to shear them off **(Figure 5.35)**. If the door latch mechanism works the door can be removed. If the latch mechanism does not work, the door can be bent towards the back of the vehicle using the Nader pin as a hinge. The door hinges may also be cut with variety of tools. With the hinges disconnected, the rescuers can operate the door latch mechanism to unhook the door from the Nader pin and remove the door from the vehicle. This method works very well for removing doors on vehicles equipped with air bags in the doors. This procedure is addressed in **Skill Sheet 5-11**.

Perhaps the fastest and most commonly used method of forcing or removing a jammed door is with hydraulic or electric spreaders. After protecting those inside the vehicle, a safety strap is looped loosely around the B-post and the door frame. The tips of the spreader are inserted into the seam between the door and the B-post above the door lock. The spreader is then opened in a downward and outward direction **(Figure 5.36)**. This motion allows the door latch to roll off the Nader pin and open the door. **Skill Sheet 5-12** describes the procedures for using hydraulic or electric spreaders to open or remove a door.

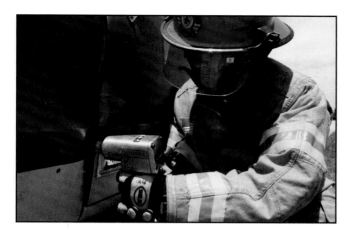

Figure 5.35 Pneumatic impact wrenches can be used to remove hinge bolts. *Courtesy of Mark Stuckey, City of Owasso Fire Department.*

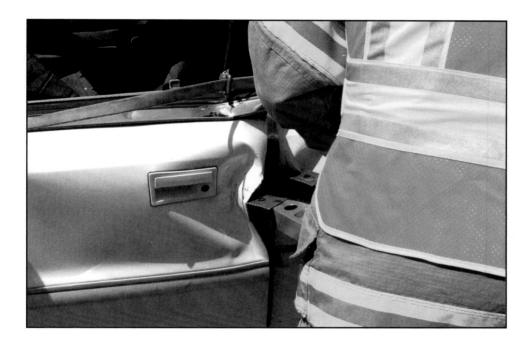

Figure 5.36 Hydraulic spreaders are useful in opening or removing jammed vehicle doors. *Courtesy of Sonrise Photography.*

Factory Third/Fourth Doors

Some automobiles and light trucks are available from the factory with a third (and sometimes fourth) door that is smaller than the regular door. On automobiles and light trucks, the third door is located directly aft of the driver's door **(Figure 5.37, p. 208)**. Some light trucks now have this type of door on both sides of the vehicle. Regardless of how many of these doors a vehicle has, there is no B-post between the front door and the third/fourth door. Since there is no B-post, the front door latches to the leading edge of the third/fourth door. Therefore, the third/fourth doors cannot be opened unless the adjacent front doors are opened first.

Factory third/fourth doors latch at the top and bottom, and even though some of them have inside door handles, they can normally be opened only when the front door is open. On some light trucks (but not all), the third/fourth door hinges are slightly exposed behind the trailing edge of the door. This exposure allows access to these hinges, and they can be cut from outside the vehicle with power shears. All factory third/fourth doors have a window

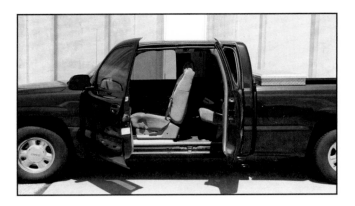

Figure 5.37 A pickup equipped with a factory built third door.

with tempered glass. However, since the inside door handle (if so equipped) will not work with the front door closed, there is no advantage to breaking this window in an attempt to gain access into the vehicle.

Total Sidewall Removal

Another method for gaining access to patients is total sidewall removal or the removal of both doors and the B-post along one side of the vehicle. An advantage to this method is that it provides a wide access way to the patient to perform extrication and disentanglement as well as provides wide access for patient removal. This method starts with releasing the rear door latch from the Nader pin. Next the B-post is cut away from the roof and spreaders are used to disengage the B-post from the rocker panel. Finally, the whole assembly (rear door, B-post, and front door) are swung towards the front of the vehicle pivoting on the front door/A-post hinges **(Figure 5.38). Skill Sheet 5-13** describes the procedures for performing a total sidewall removal.

Third Door Conversion

The term *third door conversion* refers to the technique that is sometimes used to create a wider door opening on two-door vehicles. Because rear seat passengers in two-door vehicles are virtually trapped as long as the front seats are intact and in place, it is sometimes necessary to remove the wall of the vehicle to allow the passengers to escape or to allow rescuers to gain access to them for medical evaluation and stabilization **(Figure 5.39)**. Reciprocating saws and spreaders are two useful tools in performing third door conversions. **Skill Sheet 5-14** describes the procedures for performing a third door conversion.

Kick Panel Removal

When a vehicle driver's feet and legs are pinned by the brake and/or clutch pedal, it is often necessary to move the kick panel out of the way to allow access to the patient's feet. One of several ways to create this access is to perform a kick panel roll-up. To make a kick panel roll-up, the door is removed as described earlier. The kick panel roll-up is easier to complete if the front fender is removed. In either case, shears are used to cut through the A-post at its base and make a relief cut in the A-post at the dashboard level. If the fender has not been removed, an air chisel or reciprocating saw is used to cut the skin of the kick panel from the base of the A-post forward to the wheel well and vertically to the level of the top door hinge. This cut should allow the skin of

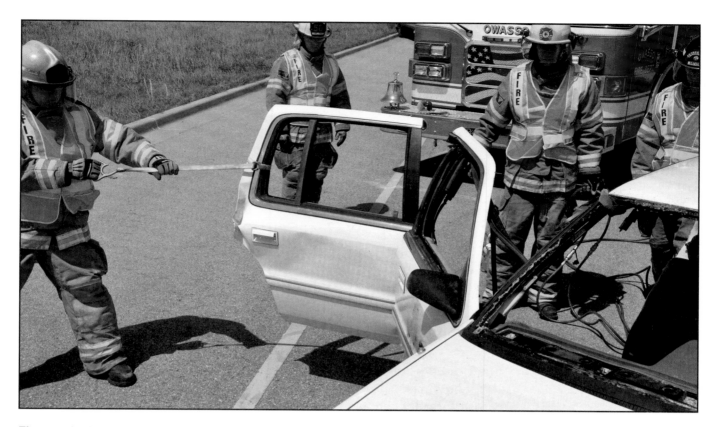

Figure 5.38 A total sidewall removal provides rescuers with better access to patients inside a vehicle. *Courtesy of Sonrise Photography.*

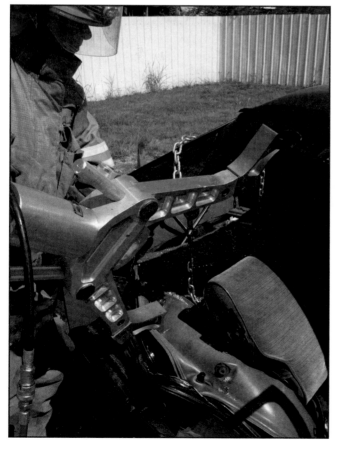

Figure 5.39 A rescuer creating a third door conversion.

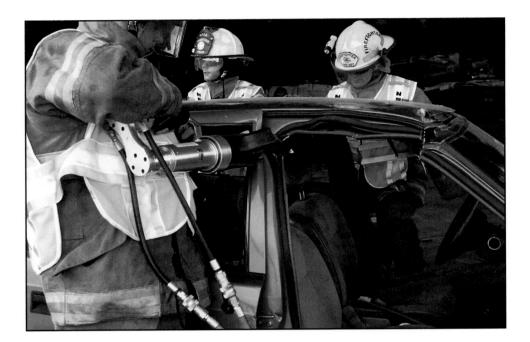

Figure 5.40 Rescuers can help protect the vehicle's structural integrity by leaving the windshield and A-posts intact, cutting the remaining B- and C-posts, and removing the roof.

the kick panel to be pulled outward and upward to expose the substructure. After the substructure has been cut away with an air chisel or reciprocating saw, a spreader can be used to fold the kick panel upward exposing the foot well area.

Roof Displacement and Removal

Gaining access to trapped patients by removing part, or all, of a vehicle's roof is a common and frequently performed evolution. Flapping or removing the roof also eliminates the possibility of Side Impact Protection Systems (SIPS) or inflatable window curtains deploying.

Roof Removal

Because unibody vehicles are designed to function as a unit, removing the doors and roof can seriously compromise the vehicle's structural integrity. Therefore, a step chock or other support should be placed under the B-post of unibody vehicles before removing the roof. Because the windshields, A-posts, and forward edge of the roof on modern cars are part of the structural integrity of the vehicle body, they should remain intact and the roof should be cut just behind the A-posts. The roof can then be removed by cutting the remaining door posts and lifting the entire roof off as a unit **(Figure 5.40)**. These cuts should be made just below the roof level to avoid cutting into the seat belt pretensioners (commonly found in the B-posts) or side airbag gas cylinders (commonly found in the C-posts) **(Figure 5.41a and b)**. **Skill Sheet 5-15 Methods 1 and 2** describe two approaches to removing a roof from an upright vehicle.

Flapping a Roof

Historically, it was SOP in some agencies not to remove the roof but merely to fold it back onto the trunk or forward onto the hood **(Figure 5.42)**. These procedures were sometimes called *making a roof flap* or simply *flapping the roof*.

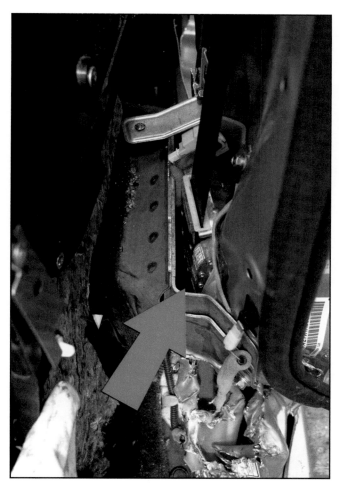

Figure 5.41a A seatbelt pretensioner inside the lower portion of a B-post.

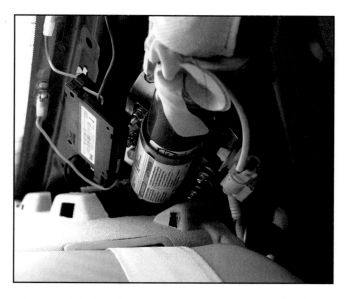

Figure 5.41b An airbag compressed gas cylinder inside the lower portion of a C-post.

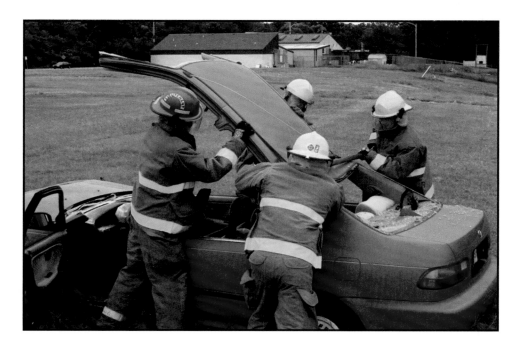

Figure 5.42 Extrication personnel flapping an upright vehicle's roof.

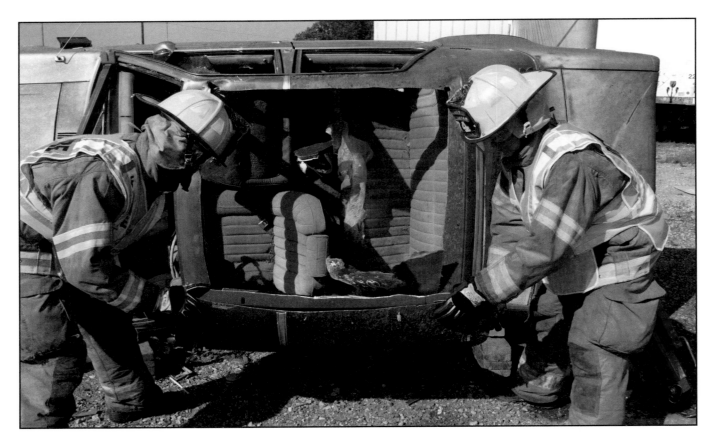

Figure 5.43 Rescuers flapping the roof of a vehicle that is on its side.

Flapping a roof forward did eliminate the need for removing the windshield. However, flapping a roof takes as long as removing it and may not serve as well. In addition, the materials used in the construction of some newer vehicles may prevent the roof from being folded, so removing the entire roof is the only option. **Skill Sheet 5-15 Method 3** describes the procedures for removing a roof from an upright vehicle.

Entry through the Roof with Vehicle on Its Side

Gaining access through the roof of a vehicle on its side can be very effective. Using an air chisel or reciprocating saw, a vertical cut is made in the roof panel about 6 inches (150 mm) away from the edge of windshield down to a point near the ground. A similar vertical cut is then made about 6 inches (150 mm) away from the edge of the rear window. A horizontal cut is then made connecting the top ends of the two vertical cuts. The roof panel can then be flapped down, exposing the headliner **(Figure 5.43)**. The headliner support struts can be cut with shears or bolt cutters. If necessary, the headliner can be cut out with a knife in the same pattern as the roof panel. **Skill Sheet 5-16** describes the procedures for flapping a roof when the vehicle is on its side.

Jacking or Lifting a Steering Column and Dashboard

Jacking or lifting a steering column and dashboard should not be confused with pulling or rolling a steering column and wheel. Jacking or lifting is intended to "lift" the steering column and dashboard straight up and off a patient to

> **CAUTION**
> Do not wrap a rescue hook or chain through a steering wheel.

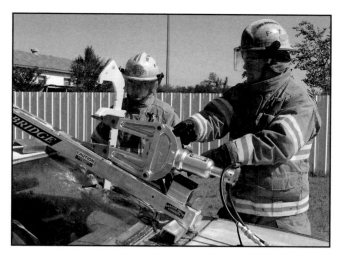

Figure 5.44 A rescue hook, bridge, and hydraulic spreaders in position to lift a steering column.

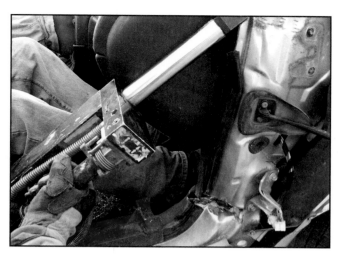

Figure 5.45 A hydraulic ram being used to roll a dashboard. *Courtesy of Alan Braun, University of Missouri Fire and Rescue Training Institute.*

relieve respiratory compromise. Rescuers pierce the windshield with a hook or other tool, then a rescue hook or chain is hooked or wrapped around the steering column. The hook or chain is placed under the steering column and as close to the dash as possible thus preventing the steering wheel from flying into the patient.

Once in place, a bridge is placed across the windshield extending from the firewall to the top of the roof. Next, hydraulic spreaders, a ram, or other lifting device is placed on the bridge in-line with the steering column and dash. The hook or chain is placed above the chosen lifting tool, if a chain is used, the chains hook should be connected to the chain after it is wrapped around the steering column and bridge. Now the lifting process can begin **(Figure 5.44)**. This process can relieve respiratory compromise safely and in much less time than other methods. The procedures for jacking or lifting a steering column and dash are described in **Skill Sheet 5-17**.

Displacing or Rolling a Dashboard

After a front-end collision, patients are often pinned under the steering wheel and/or wedged under the dashboard. To free the patient(s), rescuers should displace or roll the entire dashboard away from those in the front seat.

Displacing or rolling a dashboard can be accomplished in several ways. Each depends upon the vehicle's condition, the available tools, and the local policies and procedures **(Figure 5.45)**. Cribbing or other suitable spacers should be inserted under the base of the A-post on unibody vehicles, or between the frame and the body on full-frame vehicles, to prevent the dashboard from returning to its original position. The extension ram can be retracted and removed. The procedures for displacing are described in **Skill Sheet 5-18 Method 1** and those for rolling a dash are found in **Skill Sheet 5-18 Method 2**.

NOTE: This procedure can often be accomplished without removing the windshield, without removing or flapping a roof, and often by removing only one door. Remember *TIME IS IMPORTANT!*

CAUTION

When applying the dash displacement or rolling techniques, rescuers must protect themselves and the entrapped patients from any undeployed front-impact or knee-bolster air bags.

Floor Pan Drop

The floor pan drop may be used to disentangle the patient's feet from entrapment. Instead of raising the dash, the floor pan drop moves the floor pan down and away from the patient's feet. This method is particularly effective in incidents of front and side impact collisions.

This process involves making cuts that greatly resemble a dashboard lift but with no cuts made to the upper A-post or fender rail. Cuts are made in the lower A-post and rocker channel to allow the floor pan to be lowered. **Skill Sheet 5-19** describes the procedures for performing the Floor Pan Drop.

Vehicle power cables (hybrid vehicles), brake lines, fuel lines, and other cables that extend along the inner side of the rocker channel under the vehicle should be identified before beginning this technique to avoid increasing the risks to the rescuers and patients. A charged 1½-inch (38 mm) hoseline should be positioned for use in case of fire.

Seats: Displacement and Removal

A vehicle's seats are designed to allow the occupants to sit in relative comfort for long periods of time. To accomplish this end, the driver's seat and front passenger's seat are usually adjustable to a greater or lesser extent. The range of adjustments vary from a simple mechanical system for moving the seat forward or backward or adjusting the angle of the seatback, to electrically operated systems with 8-way movement and adjustable lumbar support. The seats in some newer automobiles also contain the side-impact air bags. These features designed to increase passenger comfort and safety can sometimes cause injuries to passengers and rescuers alike.

To be adjustable forward and back, vehicle seats slide in tracks mounted on the floor of the vehicle. Small metal teeth hold the seats in the desired position in the tracks. However, the inertial forces generated by a high speed impact often break the teeth of these mechanisms allowing the seats to move rapidly forward carrying the seat occupants with them. If the vehicle is not equipped with front-impact and knee-bolster air bags, the driver may "submarine" under the dashboard — that is, become wedged under the dashboard and/or entangled in the steering wheel and brake pedal. In these cases, it may be necessary to move the seats to access the patients.

The seats of many newer automobiles contain side-impact air bags. In most vehicles so equipped, the air bags can be disabled by cutting the cable between the sensor and the air bag. This cable is usually in a corrugated black plastic sheath inside the outer edge of the seatback near the bottom.

The seatbacks on bucket seats in many vehicles can be reclined several degrees. On bucket seats that do not recline, it will be necessary to cut the seat frame on both sides in order to lower the seatback. If there are SIPS in the seats, the seat frame must not be cut, as this can deploy the air bags.

Seat Displacement

Before a seat is moved, any patients must be properly packaged as dictated by their injuries and closely monitored during the seat movement. If a patient cannot be packaged without moving the seat, the seat must be left in position and the vehicle removed from around the patient. In general, it is better to move

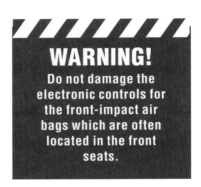

WARNING!
Do not damage the electronic controls for the front-impact air bags which are often located in the front seats.

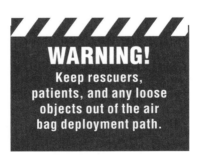

WARNING!
Keep rescuers, patients, and any loose objects out of the air bag deployment path.

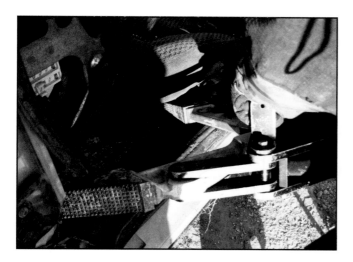

Figure 5.46 Hydraulic spreaders can be used to displace a seat. *Courtesy of Alan Braun, University of Missouri Fire and Rescue Training Institute.*

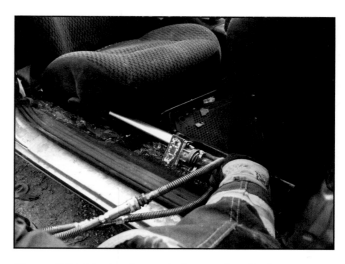

Figure 5.47 A hydraulic ram being used to displace a seat. *Courtesy of Alan Braun, University of Missouri Fire and Rescue Training Institute.*

the vehicle from around the patient by displacing or rolling a dashboard than to move the seat. If the patient can be properly packaged and monitored, the seat can be moved to facilitate removing the patient from the vehicle.

One method for displacing the front seat involves the use of a hydraulic or electric spreader. Rescuers should position the spreader with one tip on the seat's lower frame directly above the seat runner. Then they should place the other tip against the A-post at a point higher than the seat frame. A piece of cribbing may be placed between the spreader tip and the post to prevent the post from buckling. Next, they should open the spreader arms to move the seat towards the rear of the vehicle **(Figure 5.46)**.

Another method uses hydraulic rams to displace the front seat. With this method, rescue personnel position the ram between the corner of the seat's lower frame, directly above the seat runner and the firewall or A-post. A piece of cribbing can be positioned between the firewall and the heel of the ram to prevent it from pushing through the firewall. Next the ram is extended to move the seat towards the rear of the vehicle **(Figure 5.47)**.

NOTE: This method is more effective if two rams are used at the same time, one on each side of the seat.

Seatback Displacement/Removal

If it is necessary to lay the seat back to a horizontal position, the seat frame must be cut at its base on both sides of the seat. To make this cut easier and more controlled, the upholstery covering the seat frame should be stripped away. Then, rescuers can use cutters or shears to cut both sides of the seat frame at its base **(Figure 5.48)**. Once this has been accomplished, the rescuers can carefully lay the seat back horizontal or remove it, if necessary.

Front Seat Removal

It is sometimes necessary to remove a front seat entirely — such as to provide room to work on a rear seat passenger. In this case, the seat mounts at the point of attachment to the tracks can be cut with shears. Or, they can be broken

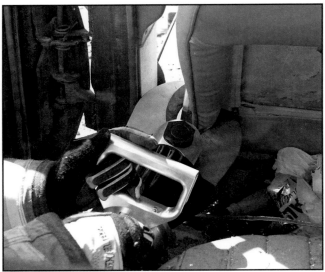

Figure 5.48 Extrication personnel can cut the frame of the back of a seat in order to allow the seat to be reclined.

away by inserting the tips of a spreader between the rocker panel and the bottom of the seat frame. Once the attachments on the door side are loose, the tool can be inserted between the seat and the transmission hump to separate it from the track on the inside.

NOTE: Depending on the situation, it may be easier to simply unbolt the seat mounts from the brackets.

Pedals

It is not uncommon for the brake pedal to pin a vehicle driver's right foot to transmission housing or driveshaft tunnel. If the vehicle has a standard transmission, the clutch pedal may also pin the other foot. In either case, the pedal must either be moved away from the patient's foot or removed entirely. Once access to the pedal area has been accomplished — either through the door opening or after a kick panel roll-up — the pedals can either be cut or moved out of the way.

Cutting Pedals

If available, a hydraulic pedal cutter can be used to quickly cut the pedal arms and free the patient's feet. Extrication personnel should exercise caution when operating hydraulic pedal cutters around a patient's legs and feet to avoid causing injury to the patient. To prevent a pedal from twisting and pinching the patient's leg or foot, a web strap should be wrapped around the pedal and tension should be placed on the strap to pull the pedal away from the patient's extremities. To cut the pedals, rescuers should cut high on the pedal arm with the cutting tool and then remove the pedal from the area around the patient's leg or foot.

Displacing Pedals

If space allows, a hydraulic spreader may be used to bend the pedals out of the way. If not, the pedals can be moved by securely attaching a chain, web strap, or rope around the pedal arm near the foot pad and pulling laterally. The pull can be applied by a number of rescue personnel physically pulling on the attachment **(Figure 5.49)**. It can also be applied by forming the attachment into a short loop and slipping one end of the loop over a spreader tip. The other tip is placed against the rocker panel near the A-post. When the tips are spread apart, the attachment pulls the pedal clear of the patient's feet.

Other methods include the following:

- If the doors are still attached, the pedal can be moved by strapping it to the frame of a partially opened door. Opening the door fully will move the pedal **(Figure 5.50)**.

- The pedal can also be bent upwards by strapping it to the steering wheel and then turning the wheel.

- Rescue personnel can also use the same tools used in jacking or lifting the steering column and dashboard to move the pedals away from a patient's feet.

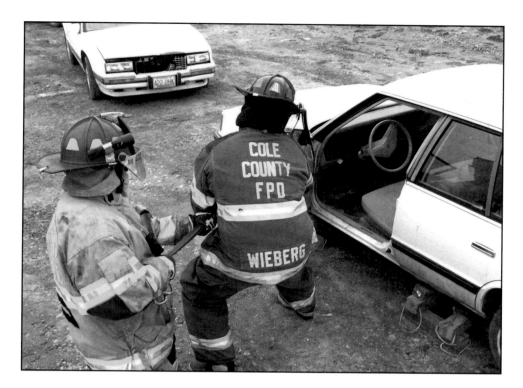

Figure 5.49 Rescuers can use webbing to pull vehicle foot pedals away from a patient's feet. *Courtesy of Alan Braun, University of Missouri Fire and Rescue Training Institute.*

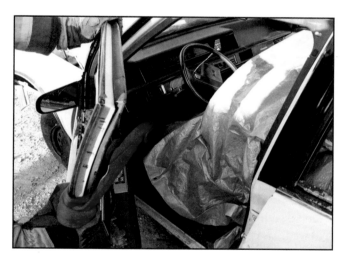

Figure 5.50 The webbing can be attached to a door and the door used to provide leverage to move the foot pedals. *Courtesy of Alan Braun, University of Missouri Fire and Rescue Training Institute.*

Entry Through the Floor

Gaining access through the floor of a vehicle may be necessary if the vehicle has come to rest upside down and there is limited access to the windows. In any such case, entry through the sides of the vehicle is difficult if not impossible. A far easier technique is to enter the vehicle through the floor.

Prior to cutting, rescuers must identify the locations of any fuel and hydraulic lines. On hybrid cars, rescuers should look for high voltage cables that run from the high voltage batteries (usually in the rear of the vehicle) forward to the engine compartment. Firefighters should be in position with charged hoselines, 1½ -inch (38 mm) or larger, and fire extinguishers to provide fire protection for both the patients and the rescuers. Rescuers should check the interior of the vehicle before cutting to ensure that patients are not in contact

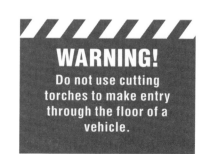

WARNING!
Do not use cutting torches to make entry through the floor of a vehicle.

with the portion of the floor that is about to be cut. If it is not possible to determine the location of patients through conventional openings, the drain plugs in the bottom of the floor pan should be removed. The patients may be visible through the resulting holes. Cutting torches should not be used to gain entry because of the fire hazard presented by floor covering materials and any fuel that may have spilled if the vehicle is overturned.

There are two ways to enter a vehicle through its floor. The choice of which way is best is determined by the type of vehicle, the number of trapped occupants, their locations within the vehicle, and their conditions. One way is to mark an area approximately 2 feet x 2 feet (0.6 m x 0.6 m) over the rear foot well area between the rocker panel on unibody vehicles (or the inside of the frame on frame vehicles) and the centerline of the vehicle. If little is known about the occupants, cutting in this area is least likely to cause additional injury to those inside the vehicle. Cutting through the sheet metal floor pan is best done with a medium- to heavy-duty air chisel, reciprocating saw, or keyhole saw. Using one of these tools, three sides of the square are cut — one parallel to the rocker panel or frame and two more from the ends of the first cut toward the centerline. Once the metal has been cut away, pull or cut away any remaining floor coverings on the interior of the vehicle. The flap thus created can then be bent upward and toward the centerline allowing a rescuer to enter the vehicle to assess the condition of those inside.

NOTE: The floor coverings may be used as guards over the jagged edges of the entry.

The other way to gain access to the vehicle's interior through its floor can be used only on unibody vehicles and if the front passenger seat is unoccupied. Using a spreader, the bottom of the passenger door is pried away from the rocker panel at least far enough to allow the blade of an open shear to be inserted into the opening — farther if possible. The rocker panel is then cut through at a point near the base of the A-post and at a point near the B-post. A reciprocating or rotary saw can then be used to extend these cuts toward the centerline of the vehicle. The flap of floor board, with the passenger seat attached, can then be lifted and folded toward the centerline of the vehicle. It may be necessary to cut the seatback from the passenger seat as it is being rotated out of the vehicle.

Tunneling

Due to the position and condition of the vehicle, it may be necessary to tunnel under the vehicle to gain access to the passenger compartment as follows:

- Safe the vehicle
- Determine access and egress points
- Check the vehicle's integrity from the outside ground surface to the upper roof rail to prevent roof collapse if load is compressing downward and entry is being made through the side of the vehicle

CAUTION
Trunks or other vehicle compartments may contain a variety of hazards.

- Remove trunk lid, rear deck, and seat back to gain entry into the passenger compartment through the trunk if necessary
- Remove patients located in the rear of the vehicle first prior to accessing patients in the front of the vehicle
- Recline seats back, mechanically force/spread or cut the seat backs out of the way for front patient access and removal

Summary

Rescuers should choose the easiest route available to gain access into a vehicle. They should first try to open the doors normally, but if they are jammed, the windows would be the next logical choice. Once a suitable opening has been created, at least one medically qualified rescuer should be placed inside the vehicle to begin stabilizing the patient and to protect the patient while disentanglement procedures are in progress. Initial medical assessment and treatment must follow local EMS protocols.

Once the patient's injuries have been assessed, treatment and preparation for removal from the vehicle can be performed simultaneously. It is important to remember that in most cases the vehicle is removed from the patient and not the reverse. Various parts of the vehicle, such as the steering wheel, seat, pedals, and dashboard, may trap the occupant. Their own and the patient's safety should be foremost in the rescuers' minds when selecting and applying the method of extrication.

Review Questions

1. What is the purpose of each control zone established at a vehicle extrication incident?

2. What tools, equipment, and techniques are used to stabilize a vehicle if it is found upright?

3. Which tools and equipment are useful in lifting a vehicle?

4. What safety precautions should rescuers follow when removing vehicle glass?

5. Which techniques are used to gain access into a vehicle passenger compartment through the side of the vehicle?

6. What is the difference between flapping a roof and roof removal?

7. What tools and equipment are useful in jacking or lifting a steering column or dashboard?

8. Why may it be necessary for rescuers to cut foot pedals during vehicle extrication operations?

REMINDER: Not all agencies advocate the following procedures and practices. Local agency procedures and protocols must be followed.

For example: Some agencies advocate deflating vehicle tires during extrication operations while others do not. The concern here is whether a sudden release of air pressure could result in the transmission of negative energy into the passenger compartment.

Another example would be removing lifting devices (such as rams, jacks, and air bags) once the object has been lifted and properly cribbed. A device might be left in place in case additional lifting is required or removed if needed in another location or to provide additional space for working around the vehicle/equipment. This depends upon the amount of equipment the responding agency has and its procedures.

The following skill sheets present a snapshot of various procedures utilized during extrication operations. As always, local agency procedures and protocols must be followed.

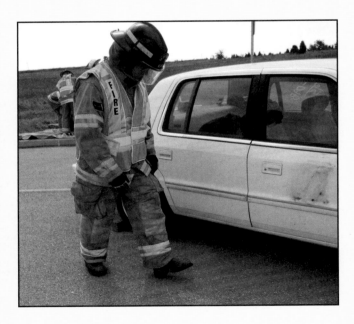

Method 1 - Vehicle/Equipment Stabilization Using Step Chocks

Step 1: Determine vehicle's orientation (upright, on side, upside down) and determine the need for stabilization. (Is the vehicle occupied? Is the vehicle in danger of causing damage or injury to life or property if it should move?)

Step 2: Determine vehicle's construction, condition, and integrity.

Step 3: Determine whether to use a four-point or six-point support.

Step 4: Identify support locations on the vehicle. Stabilization devices should be positioned at locations that will provide maximum stabilization and support to the vehicle without obstructing vehicle doors and windows.

Step 5: Determine whether the ground under these support locations will support the vehicle's/equipment's weight.

CAUTION: When installing any type of stabilization or lifting device (step chocks, cribbing, wedges, struts, or air bags) under a vehicle/equipment, extrication personnel shall not place any other part of their bodies under the vehicle/equipment. The vehicle may drop or move suddenly causing injury or death. To prevent hand injuries should a sudden drop occur, each piece of cribbing should be grasped from the sides, set outside of the vertical plane of the vehicle, and pushed into position under the vehicle with a tool or another piece of cribbing.

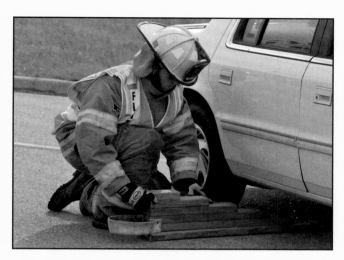

Method 1a - Vehicle/Equipment Stabilization Using Step Chocks (No Lifting)

a. Position step chocks at support locations.

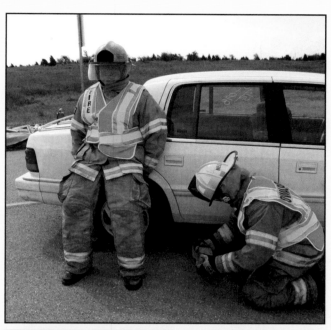

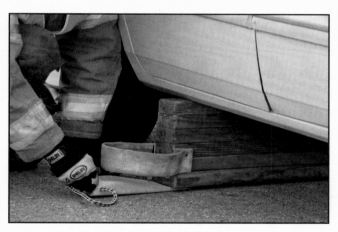

b. If the step chock is not high enough to provide support, it may be necessary to first construct a box crib to rest the step chock on or use a wedge to raise the step chock.

c. Slide the step chock into position under vehicle until it makes solid contact with the vehicle's support point. To remove the tension off the suspension system, it may be necessary to use wedges and/or shims under the step chock to provide the maximum amount of contact between the crib and the vehicle.

d. Repeat the process until at least four step chocks are supporting the vehicle.

e. The vehicle's tires can be left inflated or deflated depending on local policy.

f. Evaluate and maintain the integrity of the step chocks.

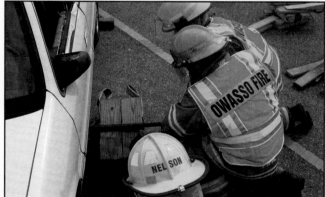

Method 1b - Vehicle/Equipment Stabilization Using Step Chocks (Lifting)

a. Position step chocks at support locations.

b. If the step chock is not high enough to provide support, it may be necessary to first construct a box crib to rest the step chock on.

c. Slide the step chock into position under vehicle until it makes solid contact with the vehicle's support point. A wedge should be positioned under each step chock to allow the chocks to be further tightened during the operation. To remove the tension off the suspension system, it may be necessary to lift the vehicle slightly to get the step chock into position. This must be accomplished without imparting any negative energy to the patient(s).

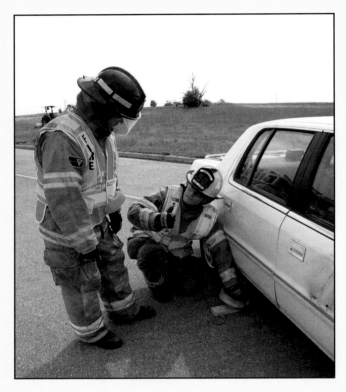

d. Repeat the process until at least four step chocks are supporting the vehicle.

e. The vehicle's tires can be left inflated or deflated depending on local policy.

f. Evaluate and maintain the integrity of the step chocks.

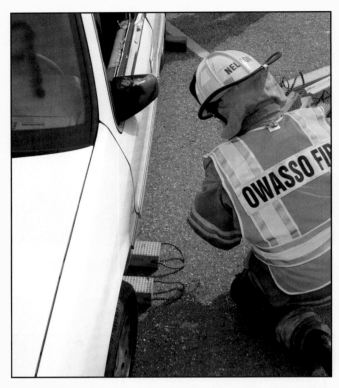

Method 2 - Vehicle Stabilization Using Cribbing, Wedges, and Shims

a. Position sufficient cribbing material at each support location.

b. Construct a crib base.

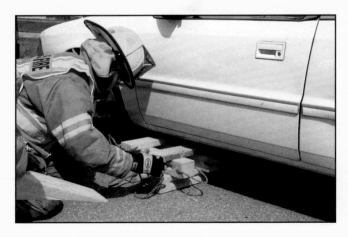

c. Add the next layer of cribbing allowing the ends of the cribbing pieces to extend 3 or 4 inches (75 mm to 100 mm) beyond the individual pieces of the base.

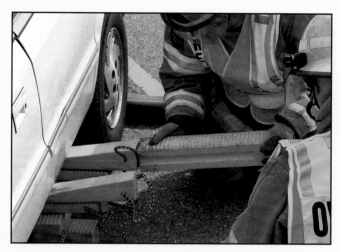

d. Add additional layers as needed, overlapping the crib corners as described above.

e. Use wedges and shims to provide the maximum amount of contact between the crib and the vehicle.

f. Repeat the process until at least four cribs are supporting the vehicle.

g. Evaluate and maintain the integrity of the cribbing.

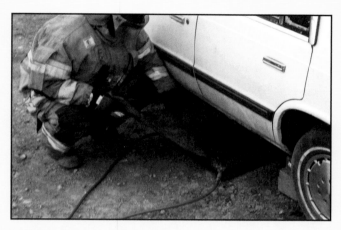

NOTE: Use a solid crib instead of a box crib when building a base for the air bag.

CAUTION: Placing plywood on each side of a high pressure bag may result in slippage as the bag contour rounds out

b. Connect air bags according to manufacturer's recommendations.

c. Position the air bags at the support locations.

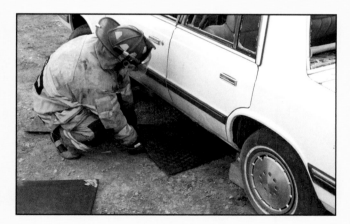

Method 3 - Vehicle/Equipment Stabilization Using Air Bags

NOTE: In this usage, the air bag is used to provide supplemental stabilization not lift.

a. Place one piece of the plywood or mat material below the air bag. Use solid pieces of plywood or heavy duty mat material as large as or larger than the air bag being used. This will protect the air bag from glass and sharp edges and give the bags a solid base for maximum safe lifting, if needed.

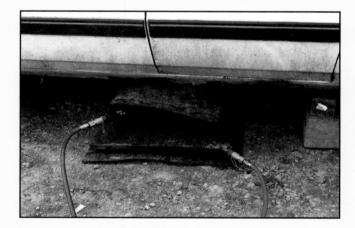

d. Pressurize bags slowly and evenly until they come in contact with the vehicle.

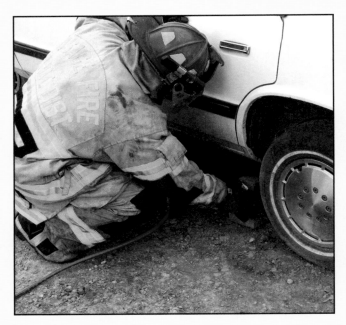

e. Install cribbing under the vehicle to ensure the vehicle does not fall or shift should a bag fail.

f. All airbags should be used in accordance with manufacturer's design and capacity.

g. Evaluate and maintain the integrity of the cribbing.

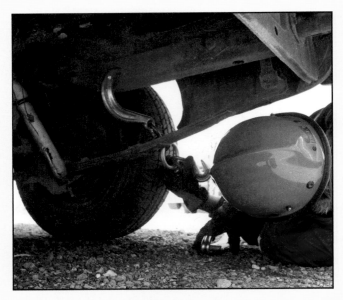

Method 4 - Vehicle Stabilization Using Webbing, Ropes, and Chains

a. Attach webbing, ropes, or chains to anchor points on the vehicle.

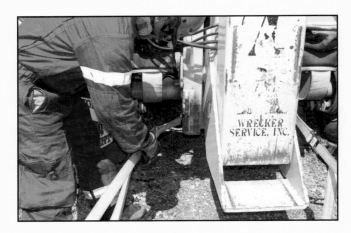

b. Secure the webbing, ropes, or chains to anchor points on the ground vehicles, large trees, intact utility poles, bombproof anchors, adequate sign posts, bridge parts or apparatus that have had the keys removed and wheels chocked. Careful thought must be given when selecting ropes, chains, or webbing to make sure the device selected is fit for the task in condition and ability.

NOTE: Any webbing, rope, chain, or cable must be rated for the load for which it is intended.

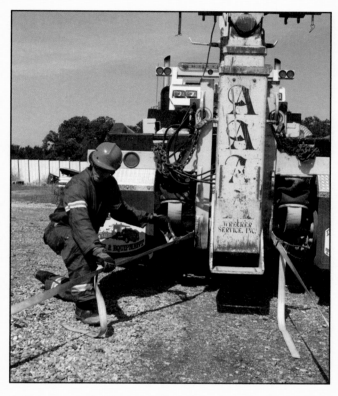

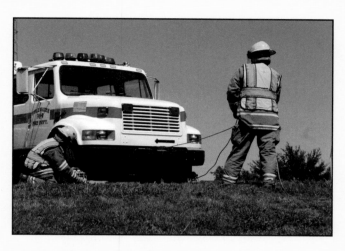

Method 5 - Vehicle Stabilization Using a Recovery Vehicle with a Winch or Rescue Crane

a. Ensure the recovery vehicle is on stable ground, emergency brake is set, and wheels are chocked to prevent the vehicle from moving.

c. Remove slack from the webbing, ropes, or chains.

d. Evaluate and maintain the tension of the stabilization equipment used.

NOTE: The more redundant the number of anchor points and devices, the more stable the vehicle will be.

CAUTION: Do not over tighten the first several straps as this may cause the load to shift.

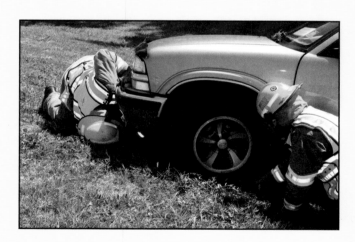

b. Attach tow cable or arm to vehicle to be stabilized.

c. Remove slack from tow cable or arm to stabilize the vehicle.

d. Many agencies employ heavy winches and cranes for removal and stabilization of vehicles during extrications.

CAUTION: Placing personnel in the path of a loaded winch cable may result in injury or death if the cable in event of cable failure.

CAUTION: Do not over tighten the cable as this may cause the load to shift.

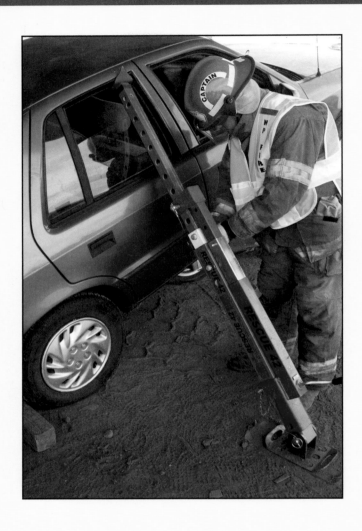

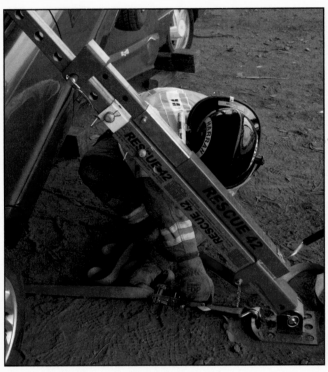

Step 1. Stabilize the vehicle or object that poses the greatest potential for movement.

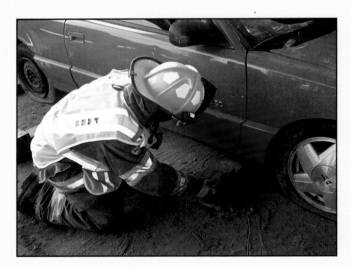

Step 2. Stabilize the vehicle or object that poses the next greatest potential for movement.

Step 3. Select from the available equipment those tools and equipment for the attachment.

Step 4. Fill the voids between the vehicles/objects using appropriate stabilization equipment.

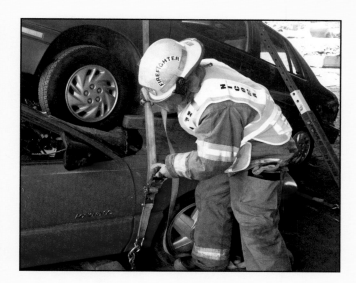

Step 5. "Marry" or attach the vehicles/objects together to minimize movement.

NOTE: Placement of stabilization equipment should not interfere with patient access or egress. When "marrying" vehicles together, avoid anchoring to movable parts of the vehicle, such as; wheels, and steering or suspension components. The process of "marrying" the vehicles/objects together should not cause one vehicle/object to crush or cause additional structural damage or injury. The amount of tension used to secure the vehicles/objects should be sufficient to minimize movement without causing undue damage.

Step 6. Assess the potential for movement of all vehicles and/or objects throughout the extrication operation by evaluating and maintaining the integrity of the cribbing.

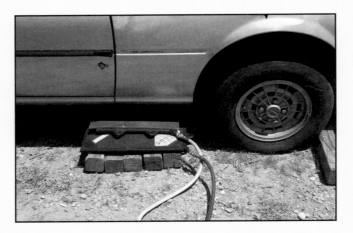

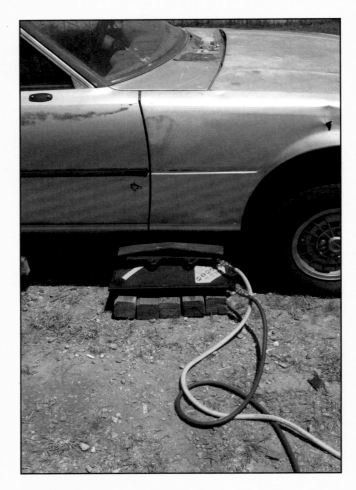

Step 1: Place one piece of the plywood or mat material below the air bag, if needed. Use solid pieces of plywood or heavy duty mat material as large as or larger than the air bag being used. This will protect the air bag from glass and sharp edges.

Step 2: Position the air bags.

NOTE: For maximum lifting ability, place the bags on the ground directly beneath the lowest, solid portion of the vehicle frame. If the manufacturer recommends it, stack two bags on top of each other. Be sure to place the larger bag on the bottom. They can then be inflated one at a time to double the amount of lifting height. Inflate the bottom bag first. Remember that your system is limited to the lowest rated bag you use and that after 2 inches (50 mm) of lift, the bag is out of its maximum lift capacity. If it is necessary to use a crib for the lift, use a solid crib instead of a box crib when building a base for the air bag.

WARNING: If positioning is faulty, one of the bags or pieces of cribbing can be violently thrown out, resulting in serious injury or death to emergency personnel. Consult the manufacturer of your air lifting bags to determine whether they can be used in this manner.

Step 3: Start to inflate the bags slowly. As the vehicle starts to lift, construct box cribs at each end of the vehicle. This is done as a precaution in case the air bag fails.

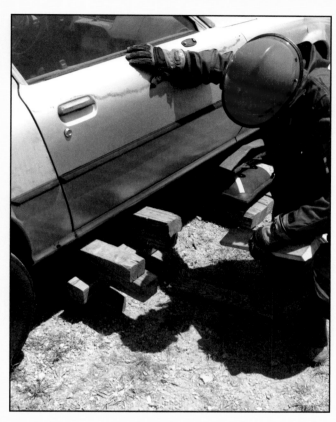

Step 4: Once the desired height is achieved, deflate the air bag slightly until the vehicle is resting firmly on the cribbing.

Step 5: Evaluate and maintain the integrity of the cribbing.

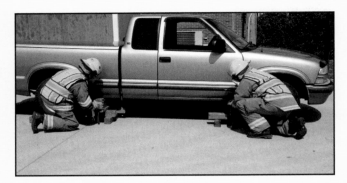

Step 1: The opposite side or end of the object to be lifted should be resting on cribbing. This will GREATLY reduce the chances of the object moving and becoming more dangerous.

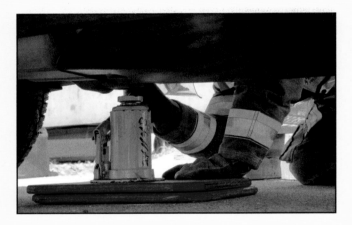

Step 2: Select the lifting device to be used (jack or air bag).

Step 3: Position the jack so it is directly beneath a solid portion of the vehicle frame, yet can be operated without rescuers needing to lie beneath the vehicle.

NOTE: To get the maximum lift from the jack, stack cribbing beneath the fully retracted jack until the pushing end of the jack is nearly in contact with the vehicle frame. This will allow the vehicle to be lifted the full height of the jack travel distance.

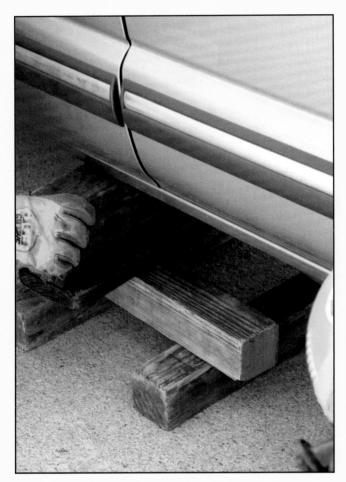

Step 4: As the vehicle starts to lift, construct at least one box crib or insert at least one step chock in the area of the lifting. If possible, construct box cribs at each end of the vehicle for added stability. Cribs are placed as a precaution in case the jack fails.

Step 5: Once the jack has reached its maximum travel distance and sufficient cribbing is in place, lower the jack until the vehicle is resting firmly on the cribbing.

Step 6: Retract the jack and add additional cribbing beneath it to raise the vehicle further, if necessary. Again, it is very important to continue to keep building box cribs as the vehicle/equipment is raised.

Step 7: Evaluate and maintain the integrity of the cribbing.

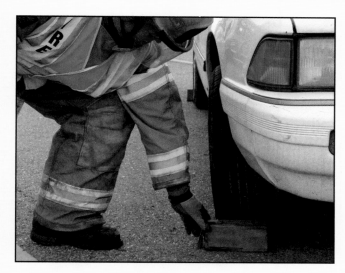

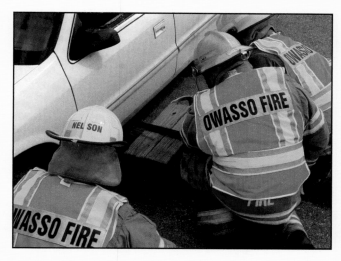

Step 1: Secure all items needed such as lever, fulcrum, cribbing, and chocks.

Step 2: Chock and stabilize vehicle to be lifted.

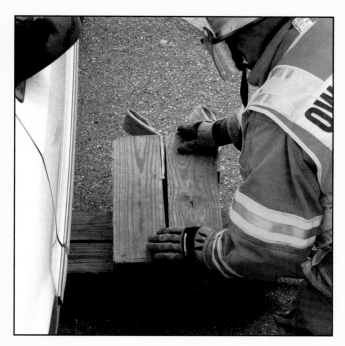

Step 3: Position prepared fulcrum or build a crib bed to act as a fulcrum.

Step 4: Make sure the area of the vehicle to be lifted is strong enough to be lifted and that access to the patient will not be impeded before placing fulcrum (block, cribbing, or whatever the lever will teeter on). Also the surface that the fulcrum is placed on must be stable and able to support it.

Step 5: Place the pry bar or other lever in position.

NOTE: The lever must be of good length and strong enough to support the loads placed on each of its two ends. The closer the fulcrum is to the object and the farther towards the upper end of the lever the weight or pull is applied the more capable the system is.

Step 6: Slowly add downward pressure to the end of the pry bar until the vehicle begins to move.

Step 7: Additional personnel will be needed to place cribbing and/or to apply force to the lever.

Step 8: Capture the vertical progress of the vehicle lift by installing cribbing.

Step 9: Evaluate and maintain the integrity of the cribbing.

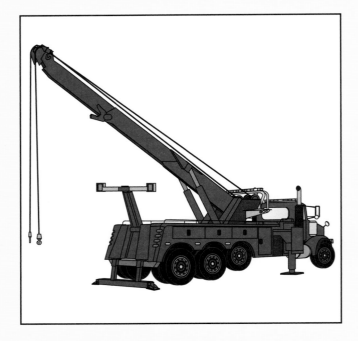

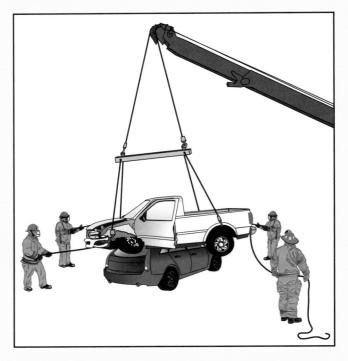

NOTE: If the lifting vehicle has outriggers, ensure they are extended and secured. Also, ground support may need to be placed such as steel squares.

Step 1: Make sure the lifting mechanism is capable of the job that is being asked of it and that it has the reach needed. Operators experience should be considered here as well.

Step 2: Stabilize the vehicle as much as possible before operating around the vehicle that is to be lifted.

NOTE: Careful consideration should be given to the amount of weight to be moved or lifted. Selecting the right sling make-up whether it be a chain, webbing, cable or rope, is vitally important.

Step 3: When applying the sling the operator must be able to predict the movements that will take place. Anchoring systems may be needed to limit or stop the movement of a particular type. In addition tag lines may be used to control expected and unexpected movements.

Step 4: All moving forces applied to the sling should be activated slowly and only when personnel are in safe positions.

NOTE: When lifting a vehicle/equipment with a crane and sling, cribbing will depend on where the vehicle/equipment is being lifted from and to, as well as a variety of other factors.

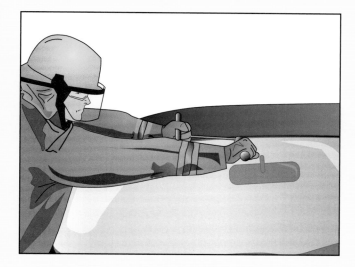

Step 1: Cover patients with a blanket, tarp, or fire resistant material to protect them from glass fragments.

Step 2: Identify the method to be used to remove the windshield based upon windshield type, windshield condition, and equipment available.

Method 1 - Removing a Windshield by Removing the Seal

NOTE: This technique works on most vehicles where the windshield is either: 1) secured by glue from the top or outside of the window seal or 2) inserted and floats within the seal. On other vehicles, the windshield may be glued from the bottom rendering this technique ineffective.

a: Place the blade of a commercial windshield removal tool under the windshield seal. The starting point is not a factor.

b: Hold and stabilize the seal removal tool with one hand, place the other hand on the attached cable and handle and begin to pull towards oneself, ensuring that the blade of the tool remains against the windshield and under the seal at all times.

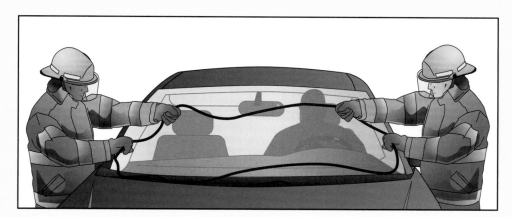

c: Continue until the entire seal has been cut. Upon completion, remove the outer portion of the seal from the windshield.

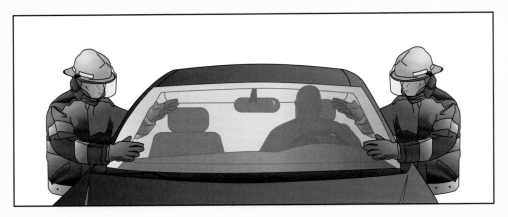

d: Push the windshield outward from the interior of the vehicle. An alternate option of removal is to place duct tape handles or suction cups onto the outer portion of the windshield and remove.

e: Upon removal of the windshield, position it away from the rescue scene to ensure safety of personnel.

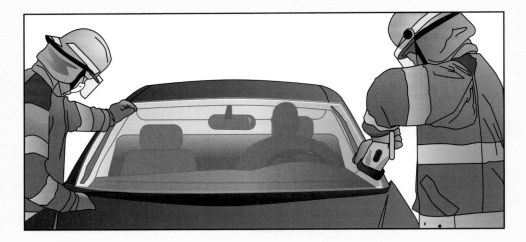

Method 2 - Cutting a Windshield

NOTE: Glass removal methods that produce glass fragments and dust require that rescue personnel should be in full PPE and wearing eye and respiratory protection. Patients should also wear eye and respiratory protection during such procedures.

a: Saw operator cuts two slits in the glass to be removed using reciprocating saw, handsaw, air chisel, or other tool.

 — Cut one side of the window.

 — Cut the other side of the window.

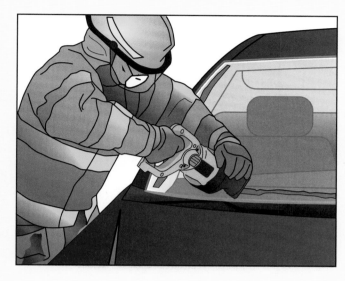

b: Cut the lower portion of the window connecting each side cut near the bottom of window.

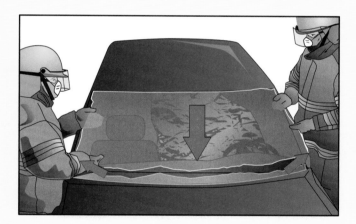

c: Saw operator and other glass-removal team member position themselves on opposite sides of the window.

d: Each team member grasps the glass near bottom cut.

e: Raise the glass moving bottom outward, using care not to break the glass.

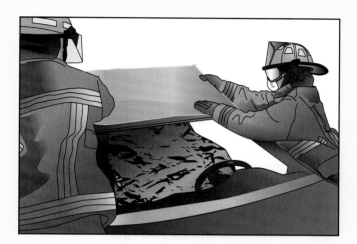

f: Remove the glass, pulling down to dislodge from frame and folding back over roof.

g: Place the glass out of the way of operations per local protocol.

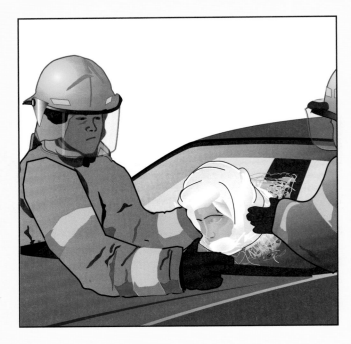

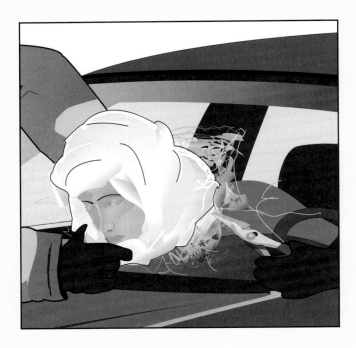

METHOD 1 - Pulling Glass

Step 1: After stabilizing the vehicle, protect the patient from further injury by padding the protruding body part and having someone hold it to stabilize it. Work a towel, blanket, or sheet between the body part and the windshield.

NOTE: It is imperative to stabilize the weight of the patient's body as well as the protruding body part. For example, the body weight may need to be supported from inside the vehicle as well as supporting the head or protruding part from the outside.

Step 2: Start pulling glass from around the body part using pliers or another type of suitable tool. It may also be necessary to cut the plastic laminated sheet away using tin snips or shears.

Step 3: When enough glass has been moved away, carefully move the body part back through the windshield under the coordination of EMS personnel.

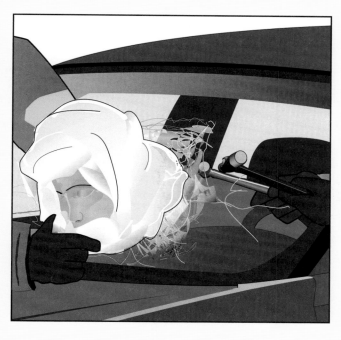

METHOD 2 - Pulverizing Glass

NOTE: An alternative to "pulling" or picking glass away from the protruding part involves pulverizing the glass and then peeling away the plastic laminate. To pulverize the glass:

Step 1: Place the face of a ball peen hammer on the inside of the windshield adjacent to the impaled body part.

Step 2: Gently tap the glass on the outside (opposite of the hammer face on the inside) with the peen. This will effectively turn the glass to dust on both sides of the windshield.

Step 3: Carefully remove the plastic laminate.

Step 4: Create a large enough space between the body part and the windshield, pad adjacent sharp edges and slowly remove the impaled part under the coordination of EMS personnel.

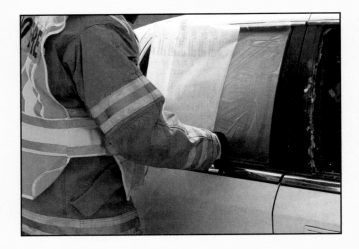

NOTE: Glass removal methods that produce glass fragments and dust require that rescue personnel should be in full PPE and wearing eye and respiratory protection. Patients should also wear eye and respiratory protection during such procedures.

NOTE: Some agencies apply a sheet of self-adhering contact paper or adhesive spray to the window, if available. Apply 2 vertical strips of duct tape to form handles on contact paper, if using it.

Step 1: Select the tool that you are going to use to break the glass.

Step 2: Ensure patients are protected from glass fragments.

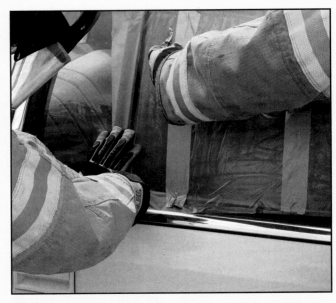

Step 3: Place a center punch or other tool in the lower corner of the window.

Step 4: Brace the hand holding the center punch with the opposite hand to prevent the rescue from pushing the hand with the punch through the broken glass.

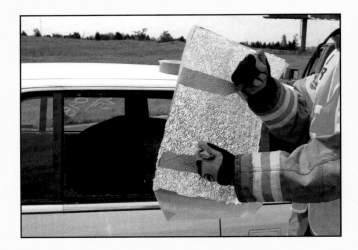

Step 5: Break the window with the punch or other tool.

NOTE: When using a striking tool, take precaution to use pillars to block/stop tool swing.

Step 6: Clear the remaining glass from the window opening.

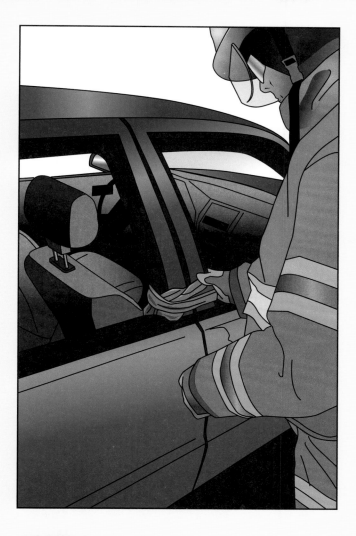

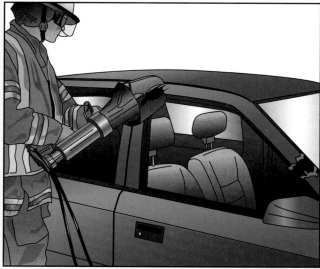

NOTE: Hi-Lift® jacks carried on emergency apparatus should be dedicated to extrication tasks only. Steel jack base foot pieces should be modified by the application of a raised expanded metal gripping surface and a ball release pin and chain installed to allow for easy attachment/removal of the base plate. The standard factory-issue Cast Top-Clamp Clevis is not suitable for extrication operations. Purpose built devices such as Jackmates™ should be used instead. Personnel should ensure that all jack components are capable of performing extrication operations.

Step 1: Deploy cribbing to control and manage the force of the door opening or lash the door to the adjacent post. This cribbing should be placed to restrict the door from opening in a violent dynamic action and creating a dropping and/or shearing action onto the rescuers feet. This cribbing should not interfere with the personnel operating the jack.

Step 2: If the window is framed with a solid frame attached to the door, separate from the roof line, cut or remove it.

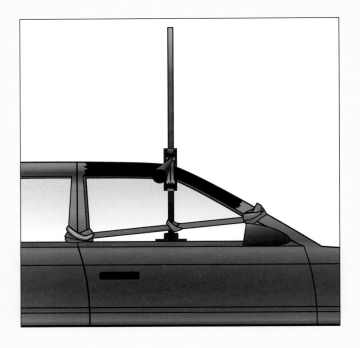

NOTE: The jack's operating lever should be placed in the raised position prior to positioning the jack.

Step 3: Position the base of the jack towards the middle of the door in order to attack the doors internal collision bar. Position the base of the jack in order for it to "grab" the inner panel/skin of the door.

Step 4: Secure the main bar of the jack towards the base plate with 1 inch (25 mm) tubular rescue quality webbing. In a passenger vehicle, secure one end of the webbing around the posts on either side of the door. Personnel need to be assigned to monitor each end of the webbing.

NOTE: A balance needs to be achieved between tension on the jack to hold it in place and excessive tension that might prevent the jack from operating.

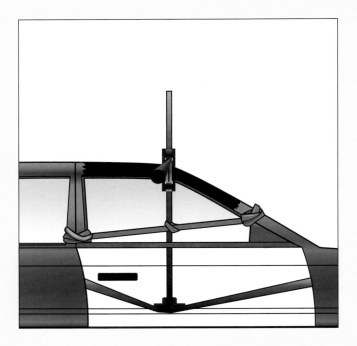

Step 5: Place the working end to the jack on the upper section of the door frame.

NOTE: Personnel assigned to the rear post side of the webbing need to assist the tool operator by keeping the tool operator out of the door and tool potential strike zone.

Step 6: Operate the tool in order to crush or weaken the door's collision bar.

NOTE: Change out personnel operating the tool to avoid fatigue.

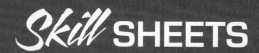
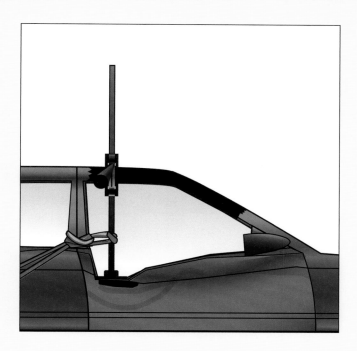

Step 7: Once the collision bar has been weakened, move the base of the jack to a position over the Nader pin. Place the base of the jack in order for it to "grab" the inner panel/skin of the door. Operate the Jack in a fashion to "roll" the door "down" and off of the Nader Pin.

NOTE: It may be necessary to reposition the jack closer to the Nader pin during the operation to effectively roll the door off the Nader pin. Personnel should look for opportunities to cut the Nader pin or latching mechanism during this operation.

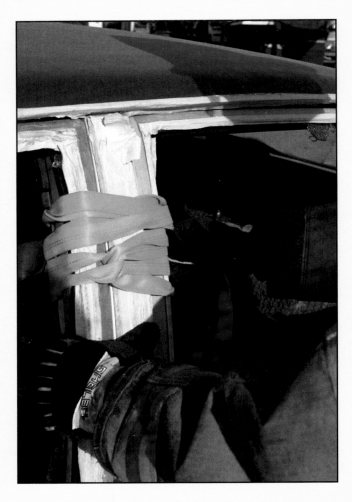

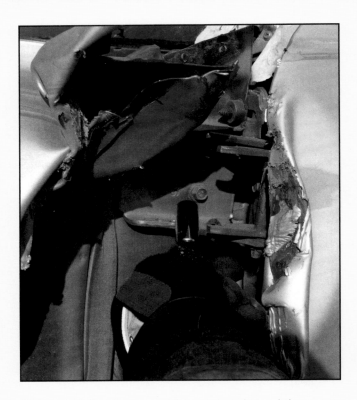

Step 5: Select the appropriate socket size and the appropriate type of socket for power ratchet, power impact wrench, or manual socket set.

Step 1: Gain access to hinge side of the door.

Step 2: Determine how door hinges are bolted onto or attached to the post.

Step 3: If the hinge is bolted to the post, determine the bolt head size.

Step 4: Deploy cribbing to control and manage the force of the door opening or lash the door to the B-post. This cribbing should be placed to restrict the door from opening in a violent dynamic action and creating a dropping and/or shearing action onto the rescuers feet.

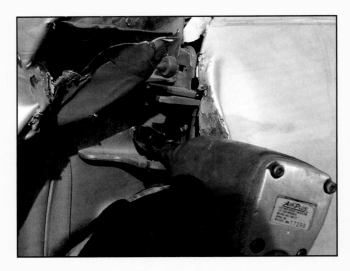

Step 6: Attempt to unscrew the bolt to release the hinge from the post. If bolts will, loosen then remove them.

Step 7: If Step 6 is unsuccessful, attempt to snap the bolts off by over tightening them.

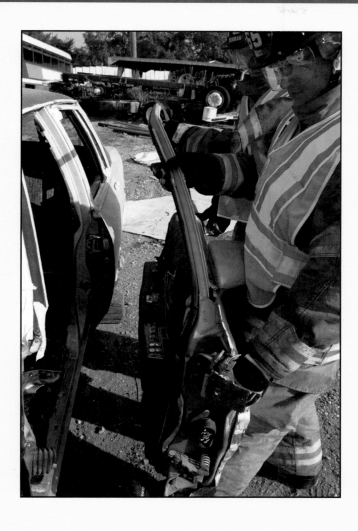

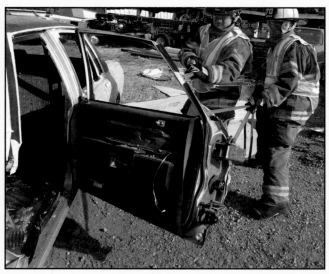

Step 8: Once hinges have been released, attempt to open the door latch mechanism to release the door from the Nader pin. If the door latch mechanism works, simply remove a door.

If the door does not release from the Nader pin it may be necessary to bend the door back away from the patient using the Nader pin as a hinge.

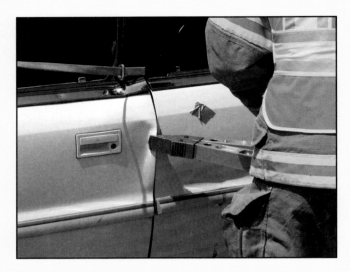

Note: Peel interior trim and plastic prior to any spreading or cutting operations. This will allow rescuers to locate any pretensioners, gas cylinders, or other safety devices.

Step 1: Create a purchase point using any of the various methods used in your area.

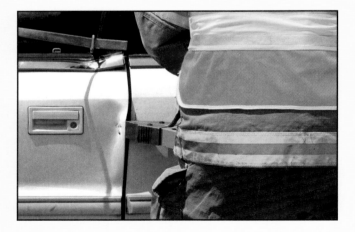

Step 2: Insert the tips of the spreader slightly above the door lock, at a downward angle. Place the tips in such a position that they push the door outward and toward the ground.

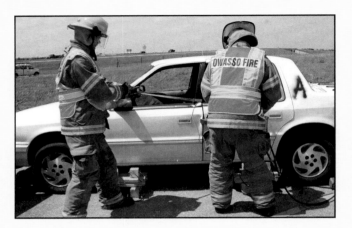

Step 3: One person should maintain control of the door using a strap to prevent the door from striking anyone. Never use personnel and the door butt method to maintain control in close proximity when prying the door. A rope, chain, strap, or tubular webbing should be used to tether the door.

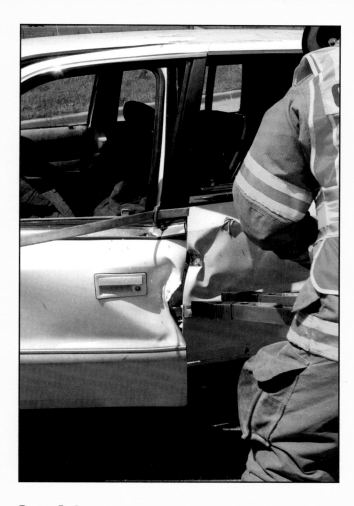

Step 4: Open the spreader arms until the door opens.

NOTE: Freeing a door from a Nader pin is not always this easy and may require repositioning the tool or the angle of the tool several times to get the best purchase to overcome the Nader pin or other latching mechanism. Parts of the door may tear away without releasing the door from the retaining point.

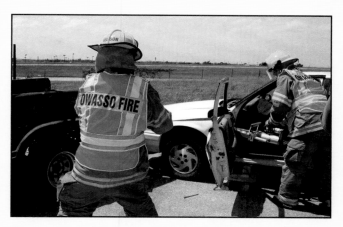

Step 5: (Front and Back Doors) - Force the door down and away from patients and rescue personnel. Never use personnel and the door butt method to maintain control in close proximity when prying the door. A rope, chain, strap, or tubular webbing should be used to tether the door. Peel interior trim and plastic prior to any spreading or cutting operations. Insert the spreader slightly above the first hinge. It is important to aim the tips of the spreader so the door is being pushed down and away from the vehicle.

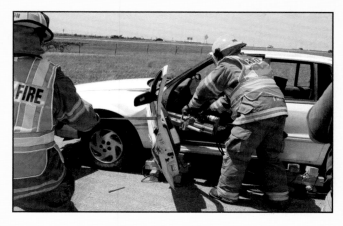

Step 6: Open the spreader until the first hinge fails or can be cut.

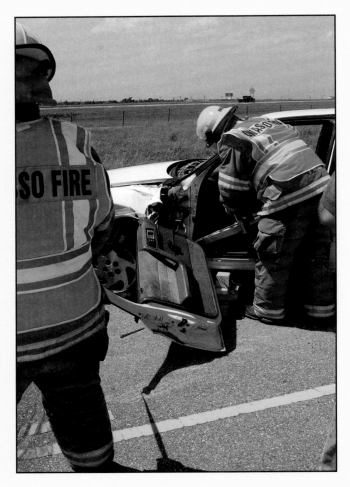

Step 7: If the top hinge was addressed first and the tool has a large enough spreading distance and is properly positioned, it may be possible to continue on and break the second hinge without repositioning. This will depend on the integrity of the doors components. If this is not possible, reposition the tool and repeat the spreading process to break the bottom hinge.

Step 8: If the bottom hinge was addressed first, reposition the spreaders above the top hinge and open the spreaders until the top hinge fails or can be cut. On cars with pressed metal hinges, it may be quicker to cut the hinges. Do not try this on cars with cast metal hinges because it may damage the blades of the hydraulic shears.

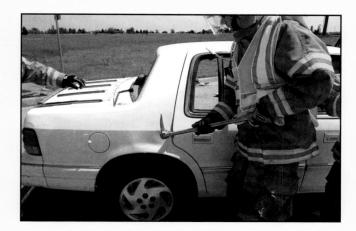

NOTE: Peel interior trim and plastic prior to any spreading or cutting operations. This will allow rescuers to locate any pretensioners, gas cylinders, or other safety devices.

NOTE: One person should maintain control of the side wall using a strap to prevent the door from striking anyone. Never use personnel and the door butt method to maintain control in close proximity when prying the door. A rope, chain, strap, or tubular webbing should be used to tether the door.

Step 1: Create purchase point to access latch on rear door.

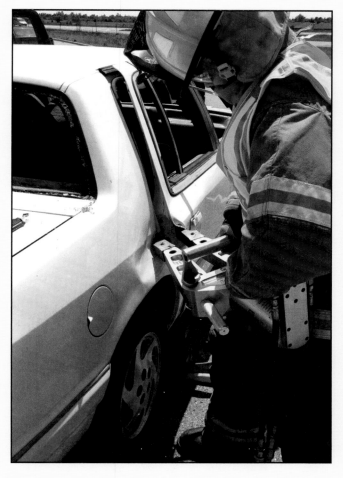

Step 2: Spread or cut the rear door away from the latch.

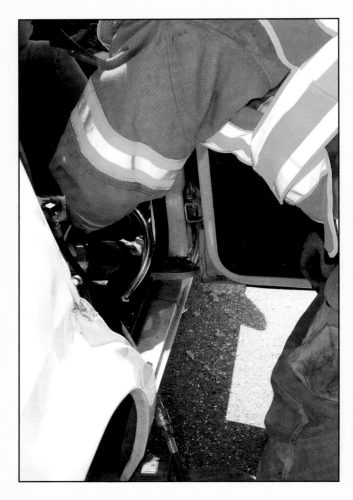

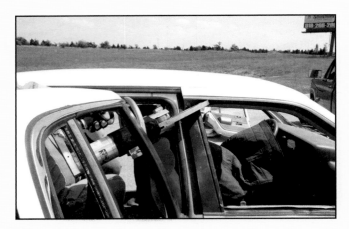

Step 5: Cut the top of the B-post at the roofline.

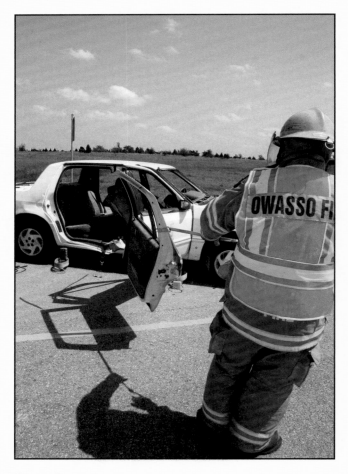

Step 3: After determining the location of the seat belt pretensioner, cut the B-post above or below the pretensioner.

Step 4: Position the tool being used between the rocker panel and the base of the rear door on the hinge side of the door.

Step 6: Operate spreading device until the base of the B-post separates from the rocker panel. The entire side (front door, B-post, and rear door) can now pivot on the front door/A-post hinges.

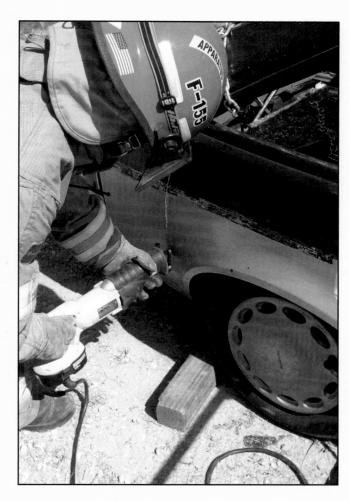

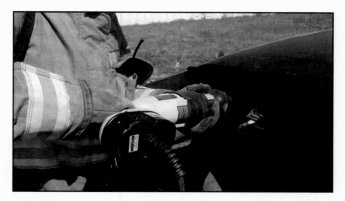

Step 2: Cut the B-post at the roofline.

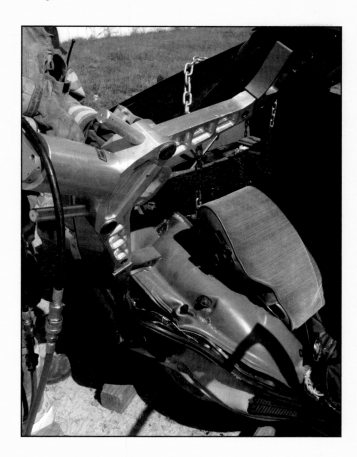

NOTE: Peel interior trim and plastic prior to any spreading or cutting operations. This will allow rescuers to locate any pretensioners, gas cylinders, or other safety devices.

NOTE: This procedure begins the process of creating a "Third Door Conversion" starting from the C-post side.

Step 1: Make a vertical cut from the lower rear corner of the side window down as far as the cutter will go. In the case of a reciprocating saw, the cut may be continued to the rocker panel.

Step 3: The spreading tool can be positioned at either the lower rear corner of the window or between the roof rail and bottom window rail.

Step 4: Operate spreading tool to displace vehicle sidewall down. If the roof is already removed, slowly (without moving the vehicle) pry the section down. As an alternative, cut the entire section out.

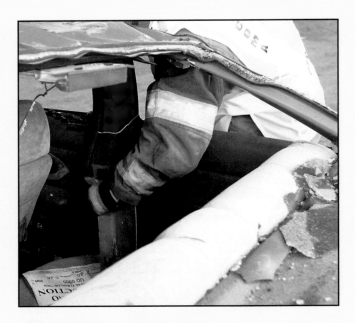

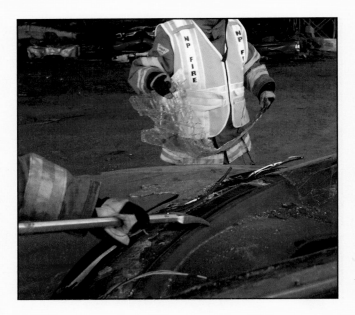

NOTE: Peel interior trim and plastic prior to any spreading or cutting operations. This will allow rescuers to locate any pretensioners, gas cylinders, or other safety devices.

NOTE: There are several different methods to attack a roof: total removal, flapping front to rear, flapping rear to front, or flapping side to side. The method used at an incident will depend on the circumstances found at a particular incident and local procedures and protocols. In some procedures, the windshield may be left in place, scored, or removed as the situation dictates.

METHOD 1 - Total Roof Removal (Removing Glass)

Step 1: Cut the first post at the furthest point from the patient.

Step 2: Remove glass.

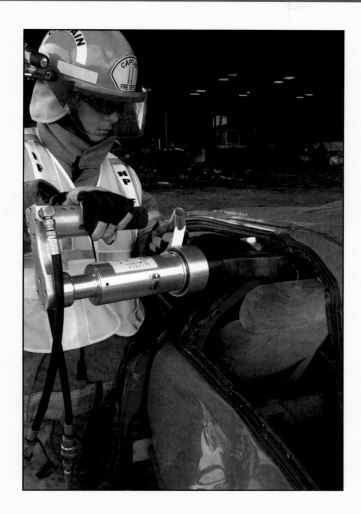

Step 3: Cut the B- and C-posts without cutting into seat belt pretensioners located in the B-posts and any side air bag inflation cylinders that might be located in the C-posts. Assign personnel to support the roof while the posts are being cut so the roof will not fall into the passenger compartment.

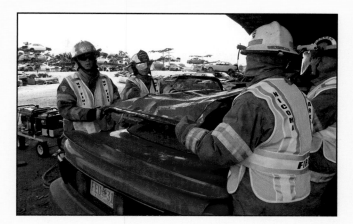

Step 4: Cut post closest to the patient last.

Step 5: Remove the roof.

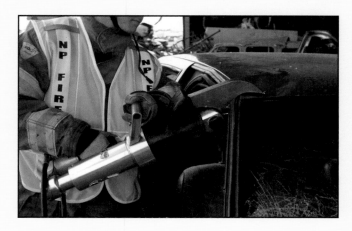

METHOD 2 - Total Roof Removal (Cutting Across Roof)

Step 1: Cut the roof supports/door jams just behind the windshield frame.

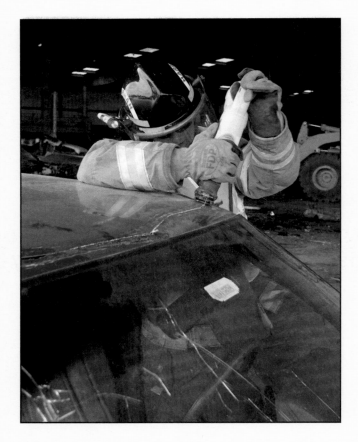

Step 2: Continue the cut across the front of the roof behind the windshield frame.

Step 3: Remove the rear window.

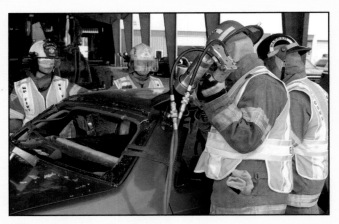

Step 4: Cut the B- and C-posts without cutting into seat belt pretensioners located in the B-posts and any side air bag inflation cylinders that might be located in the C-posts. Assign personnel to support the roof while the posts are being cut so the roof will not fall into the passenger compartment.

NOTE: Cutting through the larger rear posts may be difficult with hydraulic shears. These rear posts may be considerably wider than the opening between the cutting blades of the shears. When this is the case, there are a couple of alternatives that may be used:

Alternative 1: If available, rescuers should use tools that allow continuous cutting (such as reciprocating saws and hacksaws.

Alternative 2: First, cut a triangular section from one side of the post by making two cuts at 45-degree angles. Remove the triangular piece to allow the blades of the shears to be inserted and an additional cut made. Take the shears to the other side of the post and make a cut that will join up with the first cut. Depending on the width of the post, it may or may not be necessary to cut a triangular piece out of the second side.

Alternative 3: Compress the wide post with the hydraulic spreaders. This will compact the metal to such a size that the shears may be able to cut the post in one try.

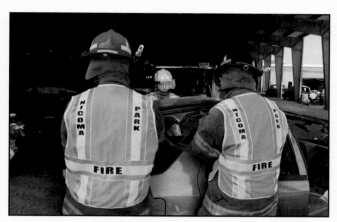

Step 5: Once all the posts have been cut, lift the roof clear and set it aside.

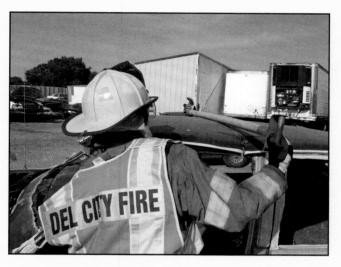

Step 2: Use a pike pole or other long object to push the sheet metal down at the bending point and to push the roof up at the front. Do not use sledgehammers, well-placed boot heels, or other similar devices to strike the roof at the bending point. This creates excess movement to the vehicle and could worsen patient injuries.

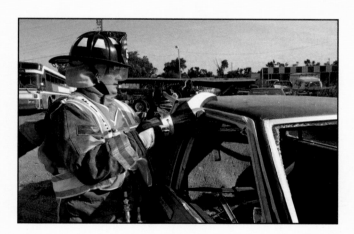

Method 3 - Flapping the Roof

NOTE: If flapping the roof rearward, relief cuts can be made across the roofline in front of the B- or C-posts. If flapping the roof forward, these cuts can be made behind the A-post.

Step 1: Cut seat belts and appropriate posts.

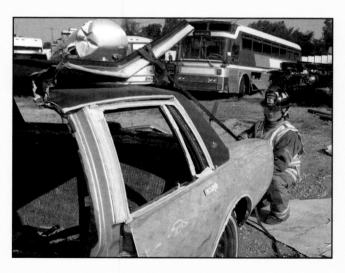

Step 3: Flapped roofs should be secured with ropes, chains, straps, or other appropriate material.

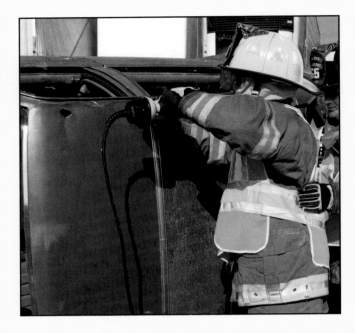

NOTE: Ensure the vehicle has been stabilized prior to beginning this procedure. Cutting posts during this operation can result in instability of the vehicle.

CAUTION: Take care to see that no patients are resting against the portion of the roof being cut. It may be possible to protect against this by placing a backboard or similar object between the roof and the patients.

Method 1

NOTE: This method involves cutting a flap in the sheet metal portion of the roof.

Step 1: Make an entry hole near the top on one side of the vehicle.

Step 2: Insert the cutting tool at this location and drive it horizontally across the top.

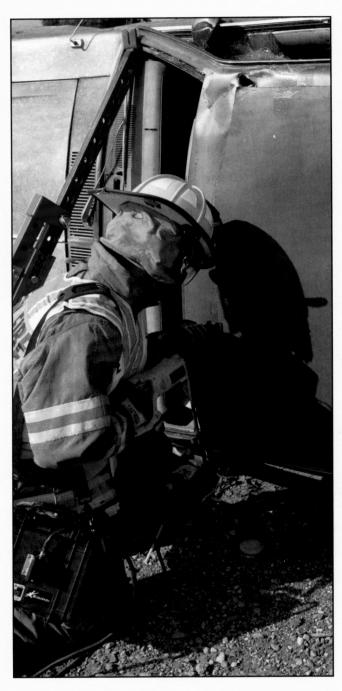

Step 3: Once the horizontal cut is complete, make the first vertical cut toward the ground.

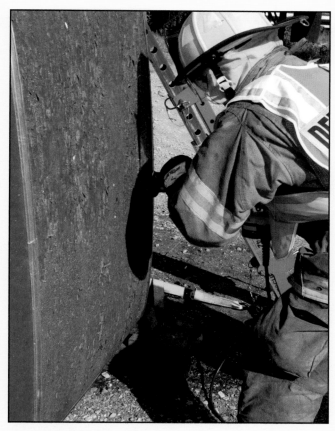

Step 4: Make the second vertical cut from the point of the original entry hole to the bottom of the roof.

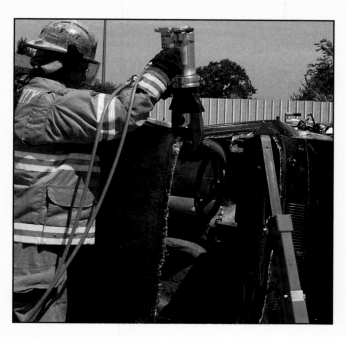

Method 2

Step 1: Cut the roof posts that are easily accessible and lay the roof down in a manner similar to that used on upright vehicles.

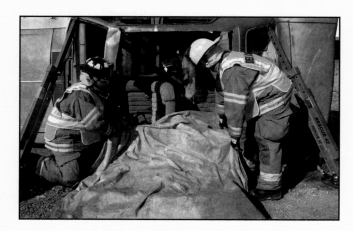

Step 5: Fold the flap down to the ground, remove the head liner and any remaining roof members, and pad the jagged edges. It is always desirable to make the cuts so that the roof folds down to the ground, since this provides a smooth area over which rescue personnel or patients may travel.

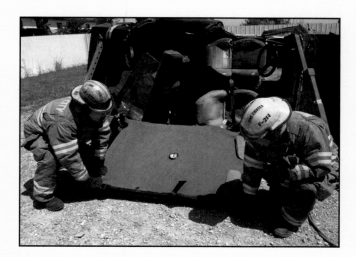

Step 2: Push or pull the roof down to provide access to the passenger compartment. Pad any rough edges.

Step 3: If desired, the roof can be removed entirely by cutting the remaining posts. Again, after the cuts are complete, cover any rough edges.

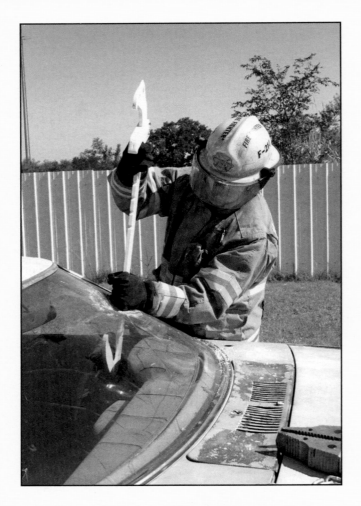

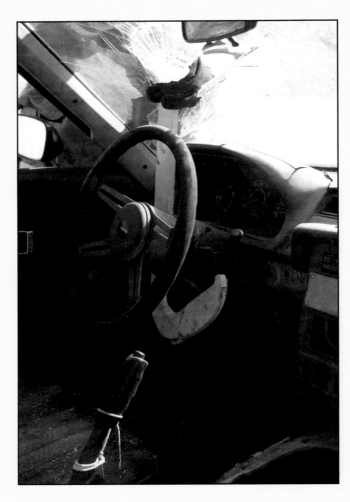

NOTE: This is not to be confused with "Pulling or Rolling a Steering Column and Wheel." Jacking or lifting of a steering column and dashboard is intended to "lift" the steering column and dashboard straight up and off the patient providing the necessary space to relieve respiratory compromise.

WARNING: Steering column should not be severed or jolted due to the potential for air bag deployment.

Step 1: Pierce the windshield above the steering column and wheel with a hook or other tool.

Step 2: Hook a rescue hook or wrap a chain around the steering column (not around or in the steering wheel). Position the hook or wrap the chain under the steering column as close to the dash as possible. This prevents the steering wheel from flying into the patient.

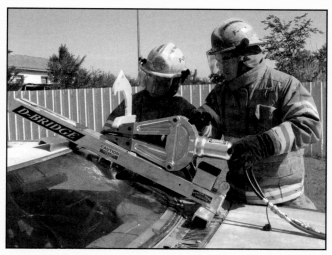

Step 3: Place a bridge device across the windshield, extending from the firewall to the top of the roof.

Step 4: Place the lifting device being used on the bridge in-line with the steering column and dash.

Step 5: Connect the hook or chain to the lifting tool. If a chain is used, the chain's hook should be connected to the chain after it is wrapped around the steering column and over the lifting device that sets on top of the bridge.

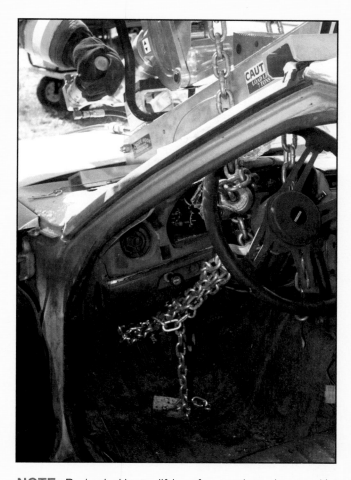

NOTE: During jacking or lifting of a steering column and/or dashboard, if needed, a chain can be wrapped around the pedals to lift them at the same time.

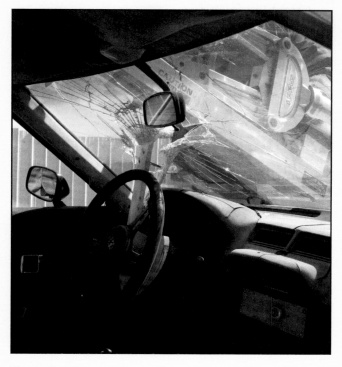

Step 6: Lift the column and wheel to create sufficient space for disentanglement.

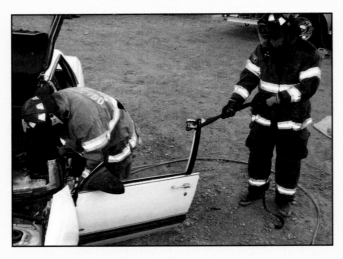

NOTE: Peel interior trim and plastic prior to any spreading or cutting operations. This will allow rescuers to locate any pretensioners, gas cylinders, or other safety devices.

NOTE: Center console connections to dashboards may need to be severed to prevent them from interfering with these operations.

Method 1 – Jacking or Lifting

Step 1: Remove the front door.

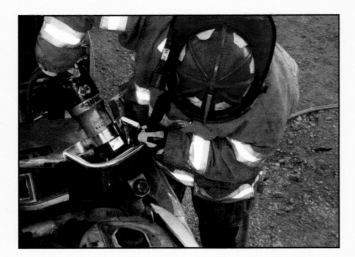

Step 2: Make relief cuts behind the strut mounts to eliminate movement of the front end of the vehicle during this operation and reduce negative energy being transmitted into the passenger compartment. This may include the fender and adjoining gusset supports.

Step 3: Cut the upper portion of the A-post.

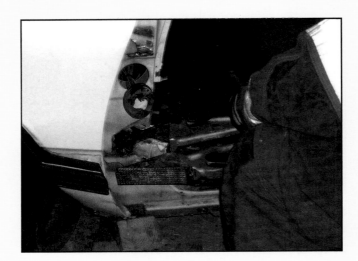

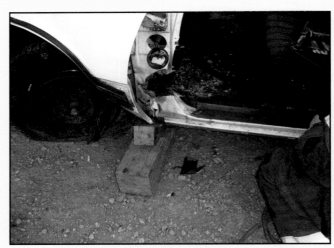

Method 1a - Jacking or Lifting Hydraulically

Step 4: When using a hydraulic tool, make two cuts to the bottom of the A-post. Then use spreaders to pinch the tab between the cuts and fold it towards the front of the vehicle.

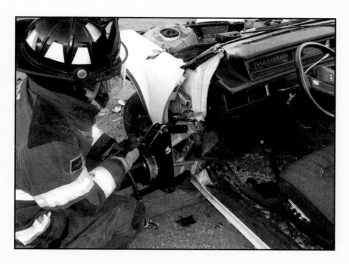

Step 5: Position cribbing under the base of the A-post between the rocker panel and the surface beneath.

Step 6: Insert spreader tips into void made by removing tab.

Step 7: Open spreaders to lift the dash until sufficient clearance is achieved.

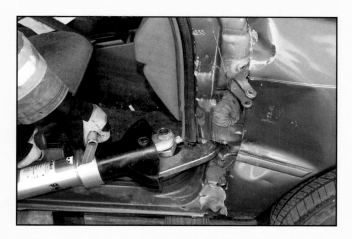

Method 1b - Jacking or Lifting Manually

Step 4: Make one cut to the bottom of the A-post.

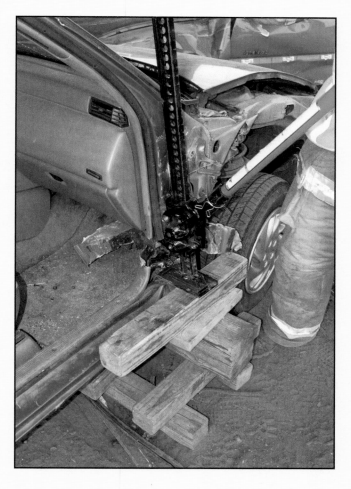

Step 5: Position cribbing under the base of the A-post between the rocker panel and the surface beneath.

Step 6: Position jacking/lifting device base on the rocker panel over cribbing.

Step 7: Place the working end of the jacking/lifting device to the remaining section of the A-post.

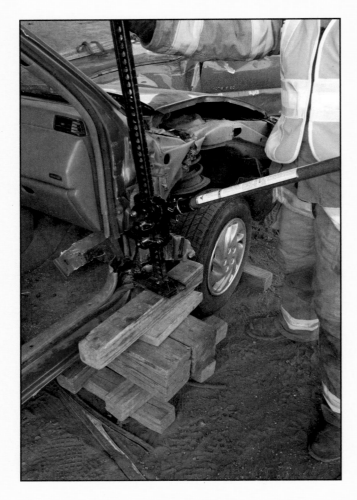

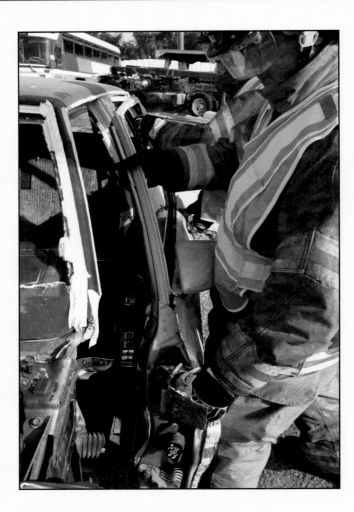

Step 8: Operate the tool until sufficient clearance is achieved.

Step 9: Evaluate and maintain the integrity of the cribbing.

NOTE: Additional relief cuts may be needed during the operation. To remove tools, a wedge can be placed within the void created to prevent the return or lowering of the dashboard.

METHOD 2 - Rolling a Dashboard

Step 1: Remove the front door.

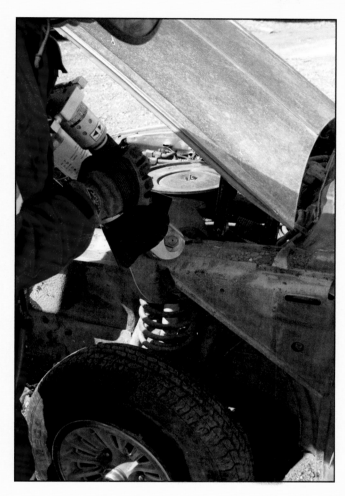

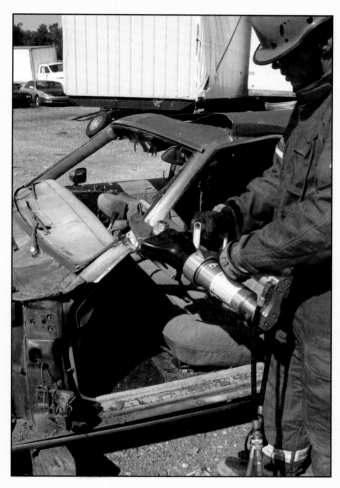

Step 2: Make relief cuts behind the strut mounts to eliminate movement of the front end of the vehicle during this operation and reduce negative energy being transmitted into the passenger compartment. This may include the fender and adjoining gusset supports.

Step 3: Cut the upper portion of the A-post.

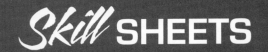
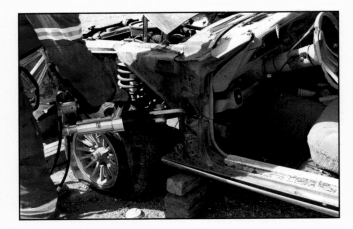

Step 4: Cut the bottom portion of the A-post.

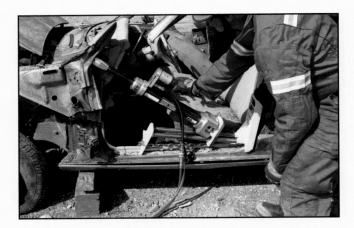

The following steps could be accomplished using a jack or hydraulic ram.

Step 5: Position jacking or ram device between base of the B-post and to an area just above the top hinge on the A-post.

Step 6: Operate the jacking or ram device to move the dashboard.

NOTE: Additional relief cuts may be needed during the operation. To remove tools, a wedge can be placed within the void created to prevent the return or lowering of the dashboard.

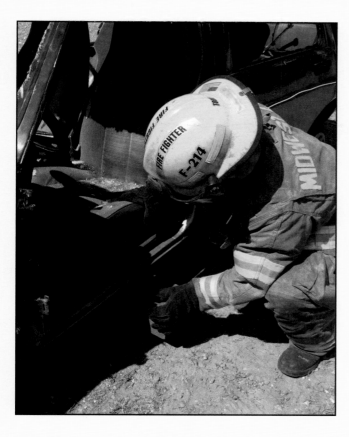

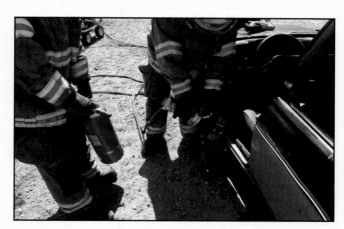

Step 4. Make a cut to the rocker channel parallel to the front of the seat.

Step 1. Remove the door on the side of the vehicle that is to receive the pan drop.

Step 2. Cribbing should be placed in an area that will not restrict the downward travel of the floor pan.

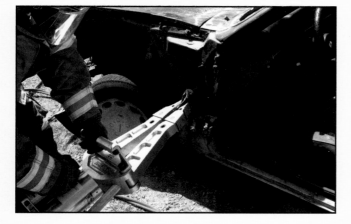

Step 3. Make two parallel cuts to the lower portion of the A-post, approximately one to two inches (25 to 50 mm) apart. Bend or remove the tab created between the two cuts.

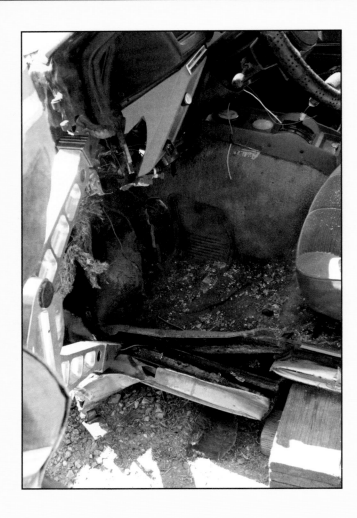

Step 5. Place the end of a spreading device in the opening created by the cuts made in the A-post and push the floor down.

Step 6: Evaluate and maintain the integrity of the cribbing.

NOTE: If using other pushing devices, such as rams or high lift jacks use the upper portion of the A-post or roof rail as the anchor point to push against. This should allow the floor pan to be pushed downward. Additional cutting to the A-post and fire wall area as well as the floor pan itself may be required.

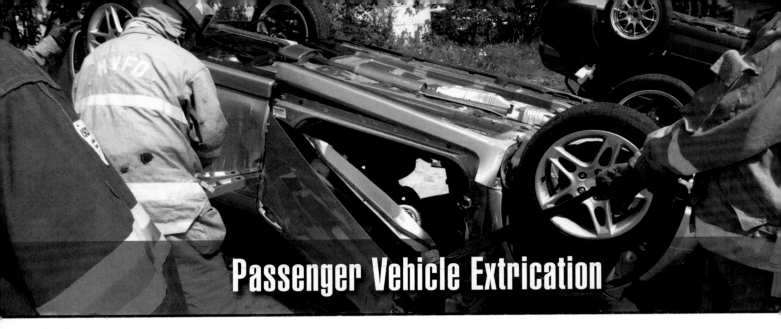

Passenger Vehicle Extrication

Chapter Contents

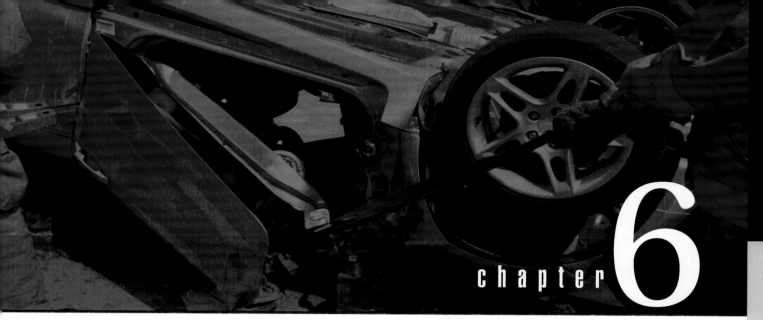

chapter 6

Key Terms

Job Performance Requirements

This chapter provides information that addresses the following job performance requirements (JPRs) of NFPA® 1001, *Standard for Fire Fighter Professional Qualifications* (2008), NFPA® 1006, *Standard for Technical Rescuer Professional Qualifications* (2008), NFPA® 1670, *Standard on Operations and Training for Technical Search and Rescue Incidents* (2009).

NFPA® 1001 JPRs

6.4.1

6.4.2

NFPA® 1006 JPRs

5.2.2	10.1.3	10.1.7
5.2.3	10.1.4	10.1.8
10.1.1	10.1.5	
10.1.2	10.1.6	

NFPA® 1670 JPRs

8.2.3	8.3.4
8.3.3	8.4.2

Passenger Vehicle Extrication

Learning Objectives

1. Describe each class of passenger car and light truck.
2. Identify safety features and concerns relating to passenger vehicles.
3. Explain specific size-up concerns related to passenger vehicle extrication.
4. Describe passenger vehicle stabilization methods.
5. Describe methods for gaining access into passenger vehicles.
6. Identify extrication tactics to be used on passenger vehicles.

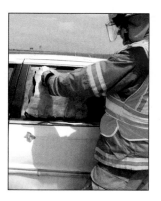

Chapter 6
Passenger Vehicle Extrication

Case History

Rescuers arrived on the scene of a motor vehicle accident involving a mid-size passenger vehicle wrapped around a tree. One patient who was conscious and alert was heavily entrapped within the vehicle. The second patient was partially ejected from the vehicle and was not breathing. Extrication personnel performed a rapid extrication operation and freed the partially ejected patient who was immediately transported to a nearby medical facility. Prompt extrication, transportation, and medical attention saved this patient's life.

It took significantly longer to extricate the more heavily entrapped patient. With the vehicle stabilized, rescuers first removed the roof to allow ALS personnel access to the patient. While one team displaced the driver's seat, the dash board, and the tree away from the patient, a second team removed the vehicle's floor board and the bottom seat cushion. Once freed, stabilized, and packaged, the patient was airlifted to the local trauma center.

The majority of all vehicle extrication incidents involve one or more passenger vehicles. These vehicles may be any of several types — automobiles, station wagons, sport utility vehicles (SUVs), pickup trucks, or minivans. Each vehicle may be occupied by the driver only or by as many as ten or more passengers. To successfully deal with incidents involving passenger vehicles, rescue personnel must know the following information:

- How each type of vehicle differs from other vehicles
- How each behaves in a collision
- How to stabilize the vehicles and the occupants
- How to extricate the occupants quickly and safely

This chapter reviews the various types of passenger vehicles and their anatomy including the following topics:

- Passenger vehicle safety features and concerns
- Mechanisms of injury typical of passenger vehicle collisions
- Operational aspects of passenger vehicle extrication incidents:
- Sizing up these incidents
- Stabilizing the vehicles
- Gaining access to the trapped occupants
- Performing extrication on vehicles that have come to rest in various positions

NOTE: It is the responsibility of individual rescue personnel to make themselves aware of and seek training on a continuing basis in the latest changes in vehicle safety, fuel, drive train, and suspension systems.

Passenger Vehicle Anatomy

Passenger vehicles are all intended for one basic function, to transport people from one place to another in relative comfort and safety. Passengers vehicles each have different designs each of which behaves differently in a collision and presents different challenges for extrication personnel.

NOTE: In the U.S., the National Highway Traffic Safety Administration (NHTSA) classifies passenger vehicles according to wheelbase — the distance between the front and rear axles or vehicle weight. **Table 6.1** describes these vehicle classifications.

Wheelbase — The distance between a vehicle's front and rear axles.

The most common types of small passenger vehicles are as follows:

- Microcars
- Subcompact
- Midsize (Intermediate)
- Full Size
- Station Wagons
- Luxury Cars
- Limousines
- Sports Cars
- Convertibles
- Roadsters
- Kit Cars
- Minivans
- Vans
- Sport Utility Vehicles (SUVs)
- Crossover SUVs (XUVs)
- Utility Vehicles
- Smaller Motor Homes
- Pickup Trucks

NOTE: Medium and heavy trucks, large motor homes, and other recreational vehicles are discussed in other chapters.

Passenger Cars and Station Wagons

Passenger cars and station wagons are available in an incredible variety of sizes, shapes, colors, and capabilities. They range from tiny economy models with few amenities and only those safety features that are required by law, to large luxury models with every amenity imaginable and a host of innovative safety features. It is an ongoing challenge for rescue personnel to stay current on the design and safety features unique to each make and model. The sections that follow provide greater detail on multiple types of passenger vehicles.

Microcars

Microcars (also called station cars) are extremely small vehicles generally less than 10 feet (3 m) in length with interior volumes of less than 85 cubic feet (2.4 cu m). Size restriction limits the vehicles' occupant loads. Some microcars are three-wheel vehicles while others have four. A wide variety of mini-trucks based on microcar designs has also been developed.

Table 6.1
Passenger Vehicle Classification Criteria

Vehicle Type	Size	Criteria
Passenger Cars	Subcompact	Wheelbase: under 100 inches (2 54 0mm)
	Compact	Wheelbase: 100 - 104 inches (2 540 - 2 641 mm)
	Midsize	Wheelbase: 105 - 109 inches (2 667 - 2 768 mm)
	Full-size	Wheelbase: > 109 inches (2 768 mm)
Vans	Minivans	Unibody Vans
	Large Vans[1]	Frame based Vans
SUVs	Midsize	Wheelbase: > 88 inches (2 235 mm) Width: 66 - 75 inches (1 676 - 1 905 mm)
	Full-size	Wheelbase: > 88 inches (2 235 mm) Width: 75+ inches (1 905+ mm)
Pickup Trucks	Compact	Under 4,500 lbs. (2 041 kg)
	Standard	Over 4,500 lbs. (2 041 kg)

[1] Includes vans that are used to transport cargo as well as vans used to transport passengers, i.e., 12/15-Passenger Vans, Conversion Vans, etc.

Adapted from Table 1: Passenger Vehicle Classification Criteria, Traffic Safety Facts Research Note, DOT HS 809 979, January 2006, National Highway Traffic Safety Administration, National Center for Statistics and Analysis.

Subcompact

NHTSA classifies passenger vehicles with a wheelbase of less than 100 inches (234 cm) as subcompact. In general, subcompact cars are primarily economy cars. As such, they are relatively smaller vehicles that typically have unibody construction, they often do not have a trunk, and they may have a third door or a hatchback in the rear. They may only have those safety features required by law.

Compact

Compact cars, according to NHTSA, are those with a wheelbase between 100 and 104 inches (254 cm and 265 cm). They are typically slightly larger versions of those in the subcompact class, with only the required safety features and few amenities. The majority of compact cars also have unibody construction, unlike the subcompacts, some compact cars have four doors, trunks and even station wagon configuration's.

Midsize (Intermediate)

According to NHTSA, midsize or intermediate class vehicles are those with a wheelbase of 105 to 109 inches (265 cm to 278 cm). They are somewhat larger than compacts; many have unibody construction. This size class also includes midsize station wagons, and may have either three or five doors and may or may not have a rigid frame.

Full Size

While still not the largest or heaviest passenger cars and station wagons — full-size passenger vehicles have a wheelbase of 110 to 114 inches (278 cm to 291 cm). This class includes what some call luxury automobiles. Many are built on rigid frames, others have space frame or unibody construction. Their heavy construction can make extrication operations more difficult and time consuming.

Station Wagons

Station wagons are generally modifications of sedan-type automobile bodies designed to carry two to nine passengers. The passenger compartment of a station wagon extends to the vehicle's rear window replacing what would normally be a trunk. The rear space may be used for carrying loads or passengers and may be reached through a hatch, a rear door, or doors. Station wagons are distinguishable from hatchback vehicles, minivans, or SUVs in two ways. First, the height of the passenger compartment remains the same for its entire length. Second, the front body of the vehicle matches other vehicles in the manufacturer's production line.

Limousines

Limousines are some of the largest automobiles and have wheelbases of more than 114 inches (291 cm). The passenger compartment is usually divided between the front and rear seats by a movable glass partition. These vehicles may have extended chassis, multiple doors, and, in some instances, be armored. This category includes those that have been manufactured as or converted into limousines. They are all heavy vehicles built on rigid frames but are still vulnerable in side-impact (T-bone) collisions. Limousine passengers might not wear seat belts, so they can be seriously injured by being thrown about inside the vehicle in the event of a collision.

Side-Impact (T-Bone) Collision — Collision in which one vehicle sustains direct side impact.

Sports Cars/Sports Coupes

This category consists of two-seat roadsters, hatchback models, and muscle cars such as the Chevrolet Corvette and Ford Mustang. Sports cars/coupes can be equipped with various types of rollover protection systems (ROPS). Many of these cars are involved in very high speed collisions, perhaps rolling over numerous times before coming to rest. Manufacturers produce a variety of sports cars based on their various automobile production models.

Muscle Cars — High performance, American cars made from 1964 to 1974 or modeled from cars built during that time; usually 2-door, rear wheel drive, mid-sized vehicles with oversized, V8 engines.

Convertibles

Many manufacturers offer a special variant of their more popular vehicle production lines. These vehicles are called convertibles and have a roof and rear window assembly that is removable or retractable. Many convertibles and sports cars have soft tops and may have ROPS (roll over protection systems) installed in them. Some may be permanently deployed while others may be deployed by crash or roll activated sensors. Unlike roadsters, convertibles are equipped with roll-up side windows.

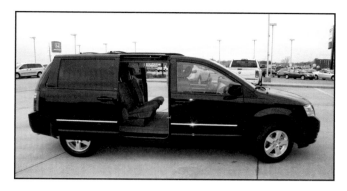

Figure 6.1 A minivan equipped with sliding passenger doors on both sides of the vehicle.

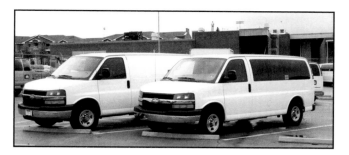

Figure 6.2 Examples of full size cargo and passenger vans.

Roadsters

Roadsters were conversions of popular older vehicles into two-seat open vehicles that offer very limited protection from the weather and collisions because they lacked a roof, rear and side windows, and passenger protection systems. Modern roadsters are two-seat, convertible sports cars.

Kit Cars

Kit cars are automobiles that may be purchased as a kit or set of parts which must then be assembled. Major components such as the transmission and engine are normally taken from other donor vehicles. Kit cars often mirror the appearance of other factory production vehicles. Because these vehicles are often shop built, rescuers need to be aware of the potential presence of additional protection systems or the lack of typical passenger protection systems.

Minivans

Minivans perform the same functions as both station wagons and sport utility vehicles. Their primary function is to transport people; they can often transport an entire family or a children's sports team. While most minivans do not have 4-wheel drive, when the rear seats are removed, they can accommodate cargo that is larger and bulkier than can most other family vehicles. Some minivans have only a driver's door on the left side, and a passenger's door and a conventional or sliding door on the right side. Other minivans are built with a conventional or sliding door on the left side of the vehicle as well **(Figure 6.1)**. They have either a single or double door in the rear of the vehicle. From a safety standpoint, their large profile makes them vulnerable to crosswinds, and their relatively high center of gravity makes them vulnerable to rollovers.

Vans

A van, in North America, is a full frame-based commercial vehicle with an integrated passenger/cargo compartment similar to that of a station wagon. Generally, the passenger version of this type of van has windows along the rear sides of the vehicle while the cargo version (called a panel van) does not **(Figure 6.2)**. In other countries around the world, the word "van" refers to a passenger-based wagon that has no rear side windows. Like minivans, their large profile makes them vulnerable to crosswinds, and their relatively high center of gravity makes them vulnerable to rollovers.

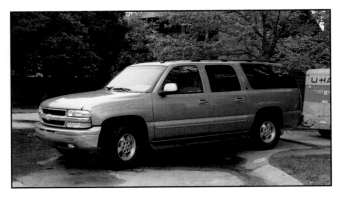

Figure 6.3 Chevrolet Suburbans, once called *truck-based station wagons*, are now considered a type of SUV.

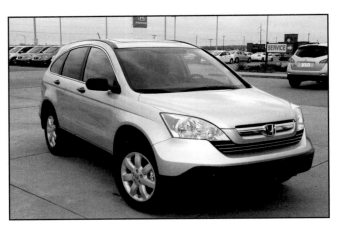

Figure 6.4 The Honda CR-V is an example of a cross-over SUV.

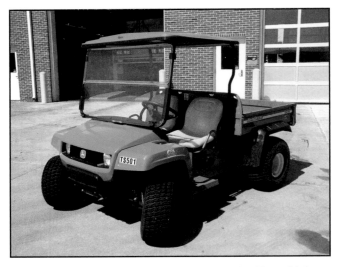

Figure 6.5 A John Deere Gator is a type of utility vehicle.

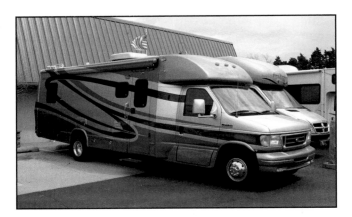

Figure 6.6 An example of a small recreational vehicle (RV).

Sport Utility Vehicles (SUVs)

Sport utility vehicles evolved out of the truck based stations wagons of earlier decades. The older vehicles were basically designed as station wagons but were built on a truck chassis as opposed to a car chassis. The Chevrolet Suburban is an example of a truck-based station wagon that is now considered a SUV **(Figure 6.3)**. Most, but not all, sport utility vehicles have 4-wheel drive capability. Because of their off-road capability, sport utility vehicles may be involved in a greater number of off-highway incidents than any other class of vehicle. The off-road environment can add considerably to the challenges for rescue personnel in these incidents.

Crossover SUVs (XUVs)

A crossover SUV (XUV) is built on car chassis instead of a truck chassis. Crossover SUVs also include those vehicles that combine design elements of SUVs, minivans, and wagons but are not marketed as such **(Figure 6.4)**.

Utility Vehicles

Utility vehicles are designed to carry cargo, passengers, or both. A variety of vehicle beds are available for utility vehicles to include low-walled box, dump beds, or beds with rails **(Figure 6.5)**.

Smaller Motor Homes

Smaller motor homes or recreational vehicles (RVs) are normally on truck or bus chassis. Like their larger counterparts, they are designed to provide self-contained living quarters during recreational travel **(Figure 6.6)**. Their large profile makes them vulnerable to crosswinds, and their relatively high center of gravity makes them vulnerable to rollovers.

These vehicles are often equipped with roof mounted air conditioning units and propane serviced equipment for heating and cooling. If the roof of the vehicle is damaged sufficiently, air conditioning units can fall and strike patients and rescuers. Propane cylinders and lines can create a fire hazard during a vehicle accident.

Pickup Trucks

Pickup trucks are available in a wide range of sizes and styles. Their carrying capacity ranges from ½ to 1 ton, and many have 4-wheel drive capability **(Figure 6.7)**. These vehicles can be equipped with a variety of suspension systems to support the rated carrying capacity. These vehicles are all constructed on full rigid frames.

Safety Features and Concerns

As discussed in Chapter 3, *Vehicle Anatomy and Science*, a variety of safety features and systems have been incorporated into modern passenger vehicles. These include seat belts, seat belt pretensioners, air bags and other restraint

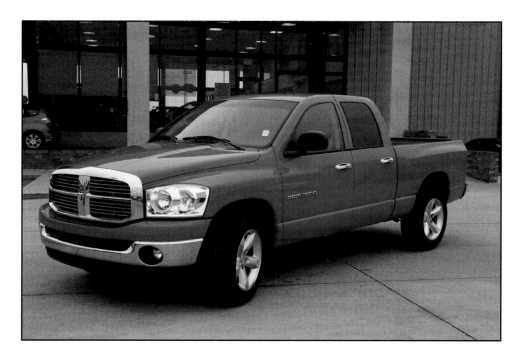

Figure 6.7 A Dodge Ram 1500 pickup.

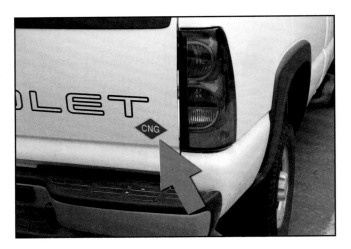

Figure 6.8 Many modern passenger vehicles run on alternative fuels such as compressed natural gas. These vehicles often have decals identifying the alternative fuel system.

systems, roll bars, and energy-absorbing bumpers. The various types of safety features and systems that have been incorporated into modern passenger vehicles include the following:

- Seat Belts and seat belt pretensioners
- Passenger restraint air bags
- Head protection systems (HPS)
- Roll over protection systems (ROPS)

While each of these items is intended to enhance the safety of the vehicle occupants, they can also represent a safety hazard to the occupants and to rescue personnel after a collision.

Other vehicle systems pose a safety concern for rescuers including the following:

- Electrical systems
- Alternative fuel systems (electric, hybrid, LPG, CNG, LNG, hydrogen) **(Figure 6.8)**
- Collision Beams
- Hood and Hatch Pistons/Rods/Struts
- Suspension struts and shock absorbers
- Energy absorbing bumpers

This chapter will address the measures to be taken to protect rescuers from current vehicle systems during extrication operations on passenger vehicles.

NOTE: It is the responsibility of individual rescue personnel to make themselves aware of and seek training on a continuing basis in the latest changes in vehicle safety, fuel, drive train, and suspension systems.

Seat Belts and Seat Belt Pretensioners

Modern seatbelts are designed to include devices called seat belt pretensioners that lock the belt during a crash to prevent further travel of the belt and the person wearing it. Since these seat belt pretenstioners are hidden inside the B-posts or the center console, rescuers cannot easily access them to deactivate them. Rescuers should avoid cutting into these units during extrication operations. Techniques to disable seat belts and seat belt pretensioners include cutting the seat belt webbing, unbuckling, and retracting the seat belts.

Supplemental Passenger Restraint Systems (SPRS)

There are many supplemental passenger restraint systems being installed inside and outside vehicles. There are outside air bag systems, called pedestrian air bags, that are designed to come out of the front bumper and also out of the hood near the firewall. There are also air bags that are under the front driver and passenger seats. There are tubular air bags that extend from the dashboard to the rear of the vehicle on the driver and passengers sides. Another type of air bag is incorporated into the shoulder straps of seat belts for rear seat passengers. There are even motorcycle air bags and an air bag suit designed to be worn by motorcycle riders.

SPRS can prove to be challenging and hazardous to rescuers. Extrication personnel need to understand the hazards relating to these systems and how to overcome them during extrication operations. The safest manner in which to deal with SPRS devices is to give them space! The ABCs of dealing with SPRSs are as follows:

- **A**lways respect the deployment path of any type of air bags, ROPS, or SPRSs.

- **B**e aware that there is no way to make an undeployed air bag, ROPS, or SPRS safe.

- **C**aution must be paramount in cutting or manipulating any vehicle equipped with air bags, ROPS, or SPRSs.

Maintain a safe working distance from all active SPRS devices by using the 5-10-12-18-20 Inch Rule of Thumb. The following are suggested minimum safety zone distances:

- Side Impact Air bags and knee bolsters - 5 inches (127 mm)

- Driver Frontal Air bags - 10 inches (254 mm)

- Impact curtains deploy down from the headliner approximately - 12 - 18 inches (305 - 457 mm)

- Passenger Frontal Air bags - 20 inches (508 mm)

While these distances will not be appropriate for all air bags, it does give the responder a general guideline. Rescuers should also keep in mind the following when mitigating supplemental passenger restraint systems during extrication operations:

- Do not restrain or cut any air bag system

- Do not cut the cushion

- Do not cut inflators

- Pry away trim and interior and look before you cut

- Work with the safety systems not around them

- Do not place body parts through open side windows to access the patient

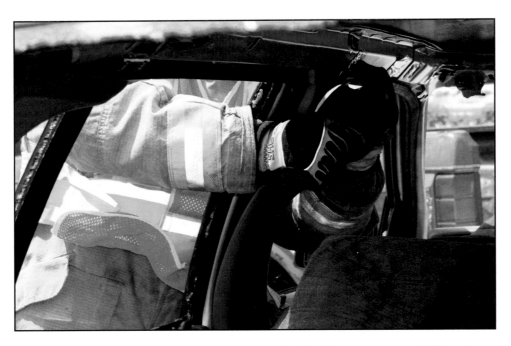

Figure 6.9 Extrication personnel should remove interior trim to expose restraint system components prior to cutting A-, B-, and C-posts.

NOTE: If you strike the air bag it's OK, but if the air bag strikes you it's **BAD!**

Should an accidental deployment occur, having body parts positioned through an open window could result in serious injury. When reaching into the vehicle to remove or turn off the key, rescue members should reach behind the steering hub.

Air bag manufacturers, automobile manufacturers, and the NHTSA do not recommend cutting or restraining any air bag system. If there is an accidental air bag deployment or a failure of a device that a rescuer is using on an air bag system, the rescuer and his or her department will be assumed liable for any injuries that result. Also, the injury from the device may be greater than the injury caused by the air bag its self!

Most air bag systems use hot gases to fill the air bags. Passenger frontal inflators containing sodium azide will reach temperatures in excess of 1,200° F (649 ° C). Cutting the cushion to the air bag system will allow hot gases to be released unrestrained into the ambient atmosphere of the occupant cabin, and could direct them at a responder or patient. Cutting the inflator could result in the two ends becoming projectiles as has been demonstrated in bench tests.

Prying away trim and looking for SPRS devices before cutting will reduce chances of injury by cutting into an inflator pressure chamber **(Figure 6.9)**. Knowing modern vehicle construction and air bag systems and practicing safe distancing should reduce the risk and severity of injury.

SPRS INFLATION MATERIALS

When a vehicle's collision sensor signals a SPRS to inflate, an igniter starts a rapid chemical reaction that generates gas to fill and deploy the air bag. Some systems employ gases such as nitrogen or argon gas while others may use a variety of energetic propellants. Early inflators used sodium azide but many of these were phased out during the 1990s.

When a SPRS deploys, the interior of the vehicle and all those inside may be covered with a dusting of fine white powder. This powder contains sodium azide residue and the talcum powder or cornstarch that was used to lubricate the bag during deployment. In the chemical reaction that deploys an air bag, the sodium azide converts to sodium hydroxide, a highly alkaline powder that becomes ordinary lye when wet. The eyes and any open wounds should be protected from contamination by this residue or any other foreign material. This powder may cause some minor irritation of the throat and eyes in most people. Minor irritation may occur if vehicle occupants remain in the vehicle for several minutes. The powder may cause asthma attacks in people who have asthma.

NOTE: Rescuers should exercise caution if the sodium azide canister has been opened without the air bag deploying. Sodium azide that has not been converted to sodium hydroxide is extremely toxic. Refer to the latest edition of the Emergency Response Guidebook for information on handling sodium azide.

A partial list of supplemental passenger restraint and roll over protection systems and components can be found in **Table 6.2, p. 280**. The sections that follow focus on the most common SPRS that rescuers will encounter.

Passenger Restraint Air Bags

Since their inception, many falsehoods, myths, and half-truths have developed about passenger restraint air bags. Understandably, these systems have been the source of endless discussions among rescue personnel. Based on test data from controlled crashes, and the investigative results from actual collisions, the information in the following sections is the most reliable available regarding air bags.

Driver and front passenger air bags can be single- or dual-stage systems. Single stage air bags can deploy only once. Dual-stage air bags are equipped with two inflator devices for one air bag that can be deployed twice. Rescuers should always use caution when working around these air bags. Rescuers won't be able to differentiate between single or dual stage air bags just by looking at them therefore they should all be treated as if they could deploy.

Undeployed air bags are a serious potential safety threat. Front-impact air bags deploy deploy in 0.05 seconds at speeds in excess of 200 mph (322 km/h) with an inflating force of over 3000 psi (20 684 kPa). Side-impact air bags deploy at even higher rates. The reason that side-impact air bags are designed to deploy faster than front-impact bags relates to the differences in the volume of structural material between the passenger compartment and the exterior of the vehicle. The rate at which front-impact air bags deploy takes into account that there is considerable mass — the engine, radiator, front fenders, and front bumper — between the front, exterior of the vehicle and the passenger compartment. However, the mass between the passenger compartment and

Table 6.2
Examples of Supplemental Passenger Restraint Systems, Roll Over Protection Systems, and Components
(as of date of publication)

AIR BAGS
Driver's single and dual stage (frontal)
Passenger single and dual stage (pyrotechnic inflated)
Passenger single and dual stage (compressed gas inflated)
Front side impact in the door (torso style)
Front side impact in seat (head and torso types)
Front side impact in seat (torso type)
Front side impact (extending up from door)
Rear side impact in the door
Rear side impact in the seat (torso type)
Rear side impact in seat (head and torso types)
Rear occupant frontal in back of front seat
Side curtain (front windows)
Side curtain (full length)
Head protection tube type
Third row side curtain (Chevy Suburban)
Driver's knee (bolster)
Passenger knee (bolster)
Carpet
Seat belt
Seat position
Front bumper (experimental)
External windshield (experimental)
Motorcycle (Honda Goldwing)

ROLL OVER PROTECTION
Full bar
Dual bar

PRE-TENSIONERS
Pyrotechnic seat belt (spool and buckle types)
Pyrotechnic seat belt (buckle type)
Dual pyrotechnic seat belt

OCCUPANT POSITION SENSORS
Strain gage
Sonogram (Jaguar)
Wireless antenna (Honda)

SEAT POSITION SENSORS (OCCUPANT WEIGHT SENSORS)
Blatted
Matt
I-bolt strain gage

OTHER
Back lash protection headrests
Seat belt tension sensors
Air bag cut-off switches
Pre-accident sensing systems
Post-accident reporting systems
Multiple batteries
Multiple battery locations
Windows and door locks operated by air bag module

the side exterior of the door is minimal; therefore, the amount of time needed for the energy of a side-impact collision to be transmitted through the door is measurably less than for the energy of a front-impact collision to reach the passenger compartment. Consequently, side-impact air bags must deploy in a much shorter amount of time than front-impact bags if they are to be effective in protecting the occupants. The sound of air bag deployment is very loud, in the range of 165 to 175 decibels for 0.1 second. Hearing damage can result in some cases.

Electrically activated air bags continue to be armed as long as the vehicle's battery is connected — and even after it has been disconnected until the reserve power has drained. The amount of time needed for the reserve power to drain varies from 1 second to 30 minutes depending upon the make and model of vehicle involved. The current average time is 5 minutes. All rescue vehicles should carry a chart listing the latest information from vehicle manufacturers regarding air bag deactivation times for various vehicles. Many vehicles have after-market energy capacitors or amps installed for other electronic devices; such as entertainment systems, computers, and video games. These may take longer to drain. Some of these devices may discharge or "backfeed" electricity through the vehicle's electrical system.

If air bags or other supplemental restraint systems did not deploy during a collision, the occupants and rescue personnel must respect those systems and give them space. Attempting to shield the occupants with hard protection or by wrapping the air bag housing with duct tape or air bag safety covers, will have little likelihood of success and can be extremely dangerous. Air bag manufacturers, automobile manufacturers, and NHTSA do not recommend cutting or restraining any air bag system.

Mechanically activated air bags and supplemental restraint systems respond to shock or pressure. If rescue personnel strike the sensor unit or put too much pressure on it during extrication operations, the bag can suddenly and unexpectedly deploy. Some air bags are mechanically activated. Side impact bags that are mechanically activated can have the sensor units located in various

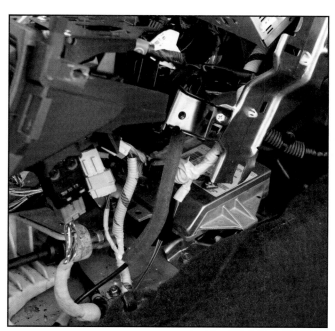

Figure 6.10 Electrical wiring for air bag systems is usually identified by yellow tape, insulation, or tags.

WARNING!
Do not cut yellow colored or yellow-tagged cables in an air-bag system. Doing so may deploy armed air bags (Figure 6.10).

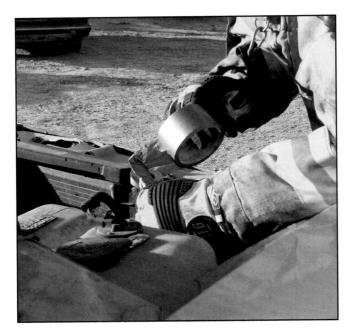

Figure 6.11 When isolating a vehicle's battery, rescuers should tape the ends of the battery cables once they have been disconnected. *Courtesy of Alan Braun, University of Missouri Fire and Rescue Training Institute.*

locations throughout the vehicle. Enough pressure to activate the air bag can be produced if some object is between the sensor unit and the inside of the door as the door is closed. Each air bag operates independently, so accidentally activating one of them does not activate both. The same precautions must be used with knee bolsters as with other front-impact air bags.

Both fire suppression and extrication activities are capable of accidentally activating either electrical or mechanical restraint systems. In electrically operated systems, an electrical impulse as small as .5 volts (such as a static discharge from an extrication tool) during the extrication process may cause the air bag to deploy. In mechanically operated systems, a sharp blow to the sensor or excessive pressure on the inside surface of the vehicle door can accidentally activate them. Also, water intrusion into the SRS electrical components can cause activation. NHTSA reports that static electricity generated at an extrication operation can possibly deploy a vehicle's air bags even if the vehicle's battery is disconnected. Also, mechanically-operated side air bags can be deployed accidentally by the use of rams or prying open parts of a vehicle's body. Therefore, it is recommended that all air bag systems be treated as if they are live!

On many vehicles, the only way to isolate electrically operated air bags is to turn the ignition switch to the "off" position, disconnect both battery cables (negative cable first), and wait for the reserve power supply to drain. In addition, it is good practice to tape the ends of the battery cables after they have been disconnected from the battery **(Figure 6.11)**. Some agencies also advocate grounding the vehicle to prevent static buildup and discharge. Some vehicles are equipped with a key-operated switch that disables and drains the reserve power from the passenger-side air bag.

NOTE: Before isolating a vehicle's battery, it may be desirable to use its power to operate adjustable seats, electric door locks, electric windows in the vehicle, adjustable pedals, and open the trunk.

Head Protection Systems (HPS)

One danger with both types of HPS is that if a rescuer is working through the window opening, the rescuer is in the deployment path of the air bag. This danger can be mitigated by a complete roof removal. However, when cutting the posts for roof removal, rescuers must be careful not to cut into high-pressure cylinders and other devices used to support supplemental passenger restraint systems.

Extendable Roll Over Protection Systems (ROPS)

An effort must be made by the rescue team to discover the presence of extendable ROPS and the potential for their deployment if not already deployed. Some will be behind the front seats of the smaller sports cars and some will be found in the rear window deck. Responders must be aware of the need to be in a safe position within a vehicle equipped with an active ROPS when stabilizing a patient's cervical spine.

Extendable ROPS can be deployed rapidly when the vehicle exceeds 23 degrees from the horizontal, a lateral angle limit of 62 degrees, or a longitudinal angle of 72 degrees. Additionally, these systems can deploy if the vehicle experiences a 3G acceleration force, or becomes weightless for at least 80 milliseconds (such as during a collision or lifting operations). To safety these devices, it is recommended that the rescuers power down the vehicle as soon as possible. Under some circumstances, it may be necessary to deploy these ROPS to prevent them from being a hazard to rescuers.

NOTE: Some vehicles are equipped with a ROPS shut off system that may be equipped with a dedicated power source.

Collision Beams, Hood and Hatch Pistons/Rods/Struts, and Suspension Struts and Shock Absorbers

Other vehicle components that can prove difficult or hazardous during a vehicle accident and/or fire include collision beams, hood and hatch pistons/rods/struts, and suspension struts and shock absorbers **(Figure 6.12, p. 284)**. Descriptions of these vehicle members are as follows:

- **Collision Beams** — heavy-gauge steel members (reinforced panels, pipes, or I-beams) that are strategically located inside vehicle doors to limit penetration of an object into the passenger compartment. Because of their structural strength, these beams can add to the difficulty of breaching vehicle doors during extrication operations.

- **Hood and Hatch Pistons/Rods/Struts** —commonly found under hoods and in hatchbacks; however, they can be found in other locations of some vehicles. They are two piece tubular devices that contain fluid or gas and are pressurized. Others are spring operated. The rods are attached to the pistons, and they move in and out under pressure as a hood or hatchback is opened or closed. Because they are under pressure, these devices can pose serious hazards following an accident of if the vehicle is involved in fire.

- **Suspension Struts and Shock Absorbers** —components of a vehicle's suspension system. They are designed to operate in a similar manner to the hood and hatch struts and thus present similar hazards.

> **CAUTION**
> Under adverse conditions, all of the previously mentioned devices may fail and rods can be explosively ejected becoming dangerous projectiles. It is recommended that rescue personnel avoid cutting struts.

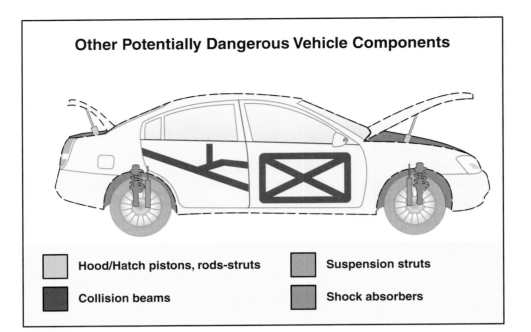

Figure 6.12 Locations of various dangerous vehicle components in passenger vehicles.

Energy Absorbing Bumpers

As discussed in Chapter 3, *Vehicle Anatomy and Science*, all vehicles manufactured in North America since 1974 are equipped with some form of energy absorbing bumper system **(Figure 6.13)**. Therefore, if an automobile or other small passenger vehicle is involved in fire, rescue personnel should avoid the area directly in front of or behind the vehicle, and a distance from the vehicle's front or rear corners equal to the length of the bumper. Also, if the vehicle is equipped with a crushable bumper system, the involved bumper should be flushed with large quantities of water after the fire is out, and personnel should avoid skin contact with any clear liquid that may form on the surface of the bumper as it cools. These bumper struts can jettison up to 300 feet (91

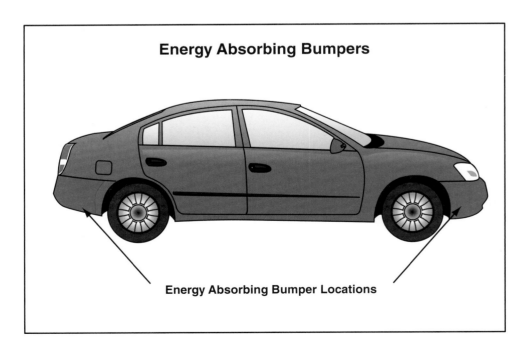

Figure 6.13 Locations of energy absorbing bumpers on passenger vehicles.

m). They can go through the lights and through the newer plastic or fiberglass bumpers that are on the market today. It is also recommended to approach vehicles at a 45° angle if fire is involved.

Specific Size-Up Concerns for Passenger Vehicle Extrication

In addition to the size-up objectives covered in Chapter 2, *Extrication Incident Management*, there are size-up concerns unique to passenger vehicles. The sections that follow cover size-up of electrical systems and alternative fuels systems found in passenger vehicles.

Electrical Systems

Electrical systems can range from 6 volts to 42 volt systems in more modern vehicles. Modern passenger vehicles may also have onboard power inverters that provide electricity to remote power outlet (RPO) sites. These allow the use of AC power for the operation of electrically powered equipment such as drills, saws or other devices at various locations on or in the vehicle. Vehicles on the road today may be equipped with more than one battery. These vehicles use one battery for only part of the vehicle's electrical needs and another for the rest of the vehicle's electrical needs.

It is important that passenger vehicle electrical systems be isolated as soon as possible. When disconnecting batteries, the negative terminal should be disconnected first. Some agencies advocate taping the terminals to further isolate them.

Remote Power Outlet (RPO) — An AC power receptacle mounted on or in a vehicle and powered by an inverter from the vehicle's DC electrical system.

Alternative Fuel Systems

Because the propane or other liquefied petroleum gas (LPG) fuel cylinder is most likely to be installed in the trunk of an automobile or the bed of a pickup truck, checking these areas should always be part of the vehicle size-up process **(Figure 6.14)**. Obviously, adding highly flammable gaseous products to a vehicle crash increases the potential danger for everyone involved.

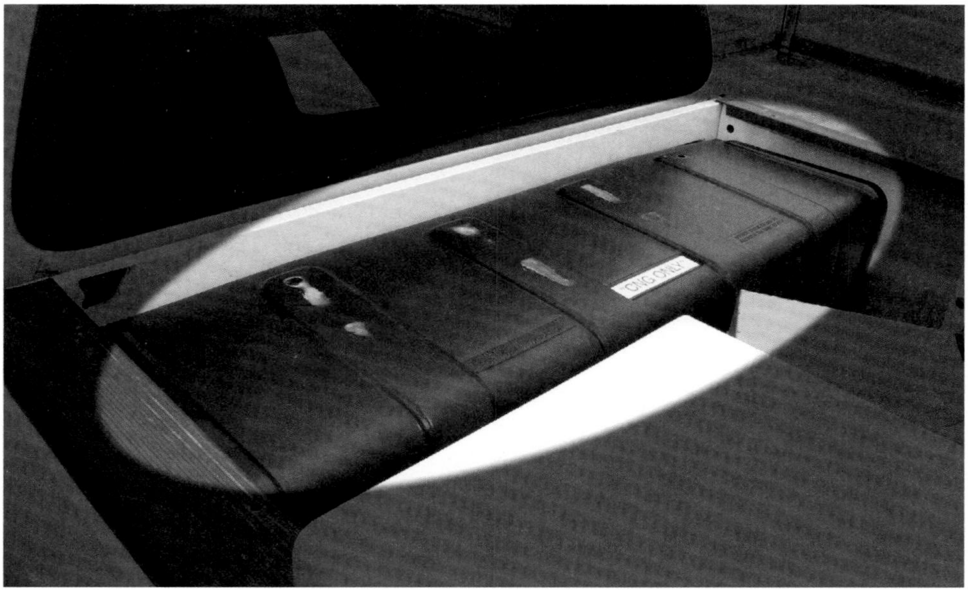

Figure 6.14 Cylinders for LPG and CNG may be enclosed in plastic containers in the bed of alternative fuel pickups.

Passenger Vehicle Stabilization

Before rescue personnel can enter a crashed vehicle to conduct a more thorough assessment of the victims inside and properly package them for extrication, it is imperative that the vehicle be stabilized first. The essence of vehicle stabilization is to prevent sudden and unexpected movement of the vehicle by creating a sufficient number of points of contact between the vehicle and a stable surface — the ground or the pavement — that prevent it from moving in any direction. While the equipment used remains the same, the techniques employed to stabilize a passenger vehicle will vary depending upon the position in which the vehicle is found. The sections that follow discuss the stabilization techniques used for a passenger vehicle that is upright, on its side, on its roof, and in other positions. Possible patient access areas should be left open when stabilizing vehicles.

NOTE: The stabilization instructions described in this section can best be accomplished using the tools and techniques described in Chapter 4, *Extrication Equipment*, and Chapter 5, *Extrication Techniques*.

Upright/On Wheels: Stabilization

The majority of vehicles involved in collisions will be found upright. However, just because a vehicle is resting on its wheels does not mean that it is stable. The inflated tires allow a certain amount of movement, especially laterally. Also, the vehicle's suspension system is designed to allow the vehicle's chassis to move in various directions. Even these small amounts of bounce and sway are enough to aggravate a trapped patient's injuries. Therefore, the vehicle must be stabilized as quickly as reasonably possible.

In many cases, chocking the wheels and doing a four-point crib by installing one step chock aft of the front wheel well (forward of the door) and one forward of the rear wheel well on both sides of the vehicle will suffice. Once the chocks are shimmed into a tight fit, the vehicle should be stable enough to start the next phase of the operation **(Figure 6.15)**.

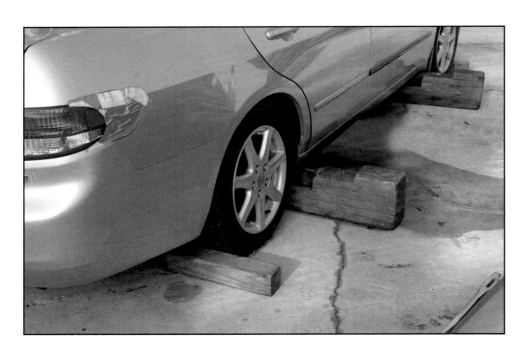

Figure 6.15 This vehicle has been chocked to prevent horizontal movement and step chocked to prevent vertical movement.

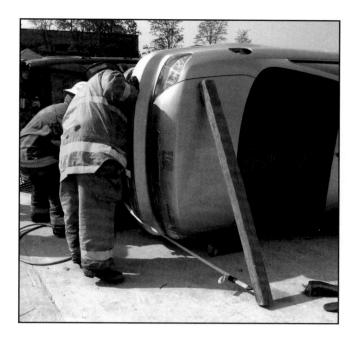

Figure 6.16 Extrication personnel often used a combination of cribbing, shoring, and struts to stabilize passenger vehicles resting on their sides.

On Side: Stabilization

A passenger vehicle on its side can sometimes be a challenge to stabilize. This is because the contours of the side of the vehicle are usually more rounded and offer fewer positive purchase points than a vehicle that is upright. The sheet metal or plastic fenders and side panels are not as strong as other structural members, and they tend to simply bend when supports are wedged under them. As a precaution, chocks or other supports should be installed at the door posts. Depending upon how stable the vehicle is after cribbing is installed as just described, it may be advisable to shore the floor pan of the vehicle to prevent any possibility of the vehicle rolling back onto its wheels. This shoring can be accomplished using Hi-Lift® jacks, manufactured metal shores, or pieces of 4-x 4-inch (100 mm x 100 mm) shoring secured with webbing **(Figure 6.16)**. Securing the vehicle with rope, chain, or webbing in addition to the shoring is also recommended.

On Roof: Stabilization

A passenger vehicle on its roof can be even more of a challenge to stabilize than one on its side. The roofs of most passenger vehicles are rounded and offer few if any positive purchase points. Initially, a four- or six-point crib with step chocks installed at the door/roof posts will prevent most movement. To prevent the vehicle from rocking fore and aft, and to prevent further roof collapse, the front and rear of the vehicle should be supported with cribbing, stabilization struts, struts and chain cradles, or Hi-Lift® jacks **(Figure 6.17, p. 288)**.

Other Positions: Stabilization

Stabilizing vehicles found in positions other than those already described will test the ingenuity of rescue personnel assigned to perform this task. Regardless of what technique is used to stabilize a vehicle, the emphasis must be on safety. While speed and efficiency are highly desirable, the security and effectiveness of the stabilization measures are far more important. A rapidly installed crib that fails is far worse than one that takes longer to install but does the job.

/////////

CAUTION

Loaded bumpers could be activated if they have been damaged or if fire is involved.

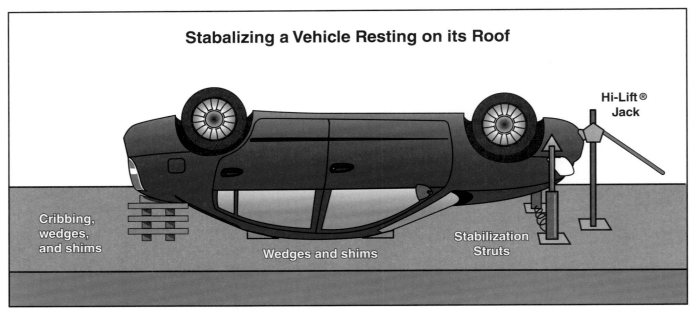

Stabalizing a Vehicle Resting on its Roof

Hi-Lift® Jack

Cribbing, wedges, and shims

Wedges and shims

Stabilization Struts

Figure 6.17 The rounded shape of a vehicle's hood, roof, and trunk can present a challenge in stabilizing an upside down vehicle.

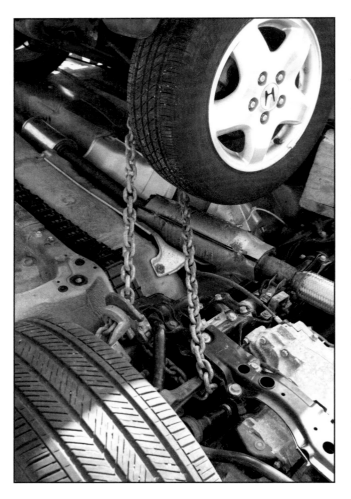

Figure 6.18 Chains, straps, and rope can be used to "marry" two vehicles together and prevent movement.

When deciding how to stabilize a vehicle that has come to rest in an unusual position, rescue personnel should remember the discussions in Chapter 3, *Vehicle Anatomy and Science*, regarding center of gravity, mass, and vehicle integrity. These basic, physical principles will dictate how a vehicle is likely to move when its components are manipulated or removed during extrication operations. If a vehicle is on a steep slope or hanging over the edge of a bridge or cliff, shoring and/or rigging can be used to offset the forces of gravity and secure the vehicle in place. If the vehicle is wedged under another vehicle or other object, the goal is to limit if not eliminate the vehicle's reaction when the overlying object is removed. Exactly how this is done will be dictated by the specific situation. In many cases, it is best to attach (or "marry") the two vehicles together as well as using standard stabilization techniques to prevent them from moving **(Figure 6.18)**. This attachment should be done prior to performing any rescue operations.

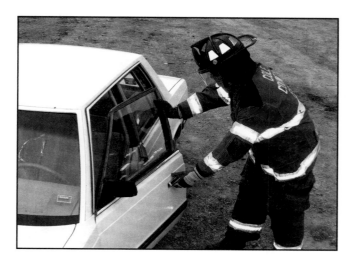

Figure 6.19 Just as in structural entry situations, rescuers should try to open doors normally before resorting to prying them open.

Gaining Access Into Passenger Vehicles

Once a crashed passenger vehicle has been stabilized, the next step is to gain access to the interior of the vehicle. As mentioned earlier, entry may be as simple as opening the doors in the normal way — as in all forcible entry, try before you pry **(Figure 6.19)**. However, in many cases, the doors are either locked or jammed, or both.

NOTE: The instructions for gaining access to the interior of passenger vehicles described in this section can best be accomplished using the tools and techniques described in Chapter 4, *Extrication Equipment*, and Chapter 5, *Extrication Techniques*.

Windows

If the doors are either locked or jammed, removing the side windows to allow access to the door locks/handles is often necessary. Once the windows have been removed, the door lock/handle can be reached through the window opening. Depending upon the specific situation, it may or may not be necessary to remove the vehicle's windshield.

Doors

When the door has been unlocked, the door handle should be tried. If that allows the door to be opened, the door handle can be held in the open position by inserting a short piece of angle-iron — cut specifically for this purpose — between the handle and the door handle recess **(Figure 6.20, p.290)**. Holding the door handle in the open position prevents the door from latching again if it closes when released.

If the doors are jammed, they must be forced open. Whether the doors need to be removed or merely opened will be dictated by the specific situation. In two-door passenger vehicles, even opening or removing the doors may still not provide sufficient working room for safe and efficient extrication operations. In these cases, a third-door conversion may be needed.

Third-door conversions involve cutting and spreading tools to flap back the side panel between the B-post and the rear fender well **(Figure 6.21, p. 290)**. This creates an unobstructed opening from the A-post back to the rear fender well.

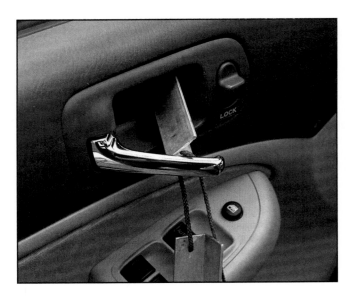

Figure 6.20 Angled metal wedges can be inserted into door handles to prevent doors from latching closed.

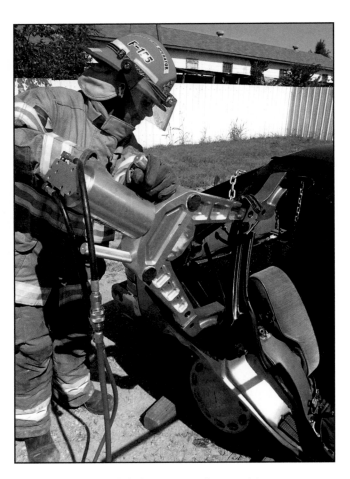

Figure 6.21 The third-door conversion provides rescuers with greater access to patients in the back seat of a vehicle.

Roofs

When victims are trapped inside a vehicle that has come to rest on its side, one of the fastest and most efficient ways of gaining access to them is by opening the doors that are on the top side of the vehicle. However, this is usually not the best route to use for extricating the patients. Removing all or part of the vehicle's roof is generally more effective **(Figure 6.22)**.

Shears or other suitable cutters can be used to cut through the door/roof posts that are accessible, depending upon how the vehicle is lying. If the vehicle is lying on its side doors, but the door/roof posts are accessible, all the posts can be cut and the entire roof removed. If the vehicle is lying on the door/roof posts on one side of the vehicle, the other posts can be cut and the roof flapped down to the ground. A cut around the edge of the roof and removing of the sheet metal and any cross members will create a relatively large opening through which patients can be extricated. However, compared to roof removal, cutting through the roof will probably take longer.

Floor Panels

Some vehicles use the floor panels and the undercarriage as structural elements and thus do not require a full chassis to provide body support. Because of their strength and configuration, these floor panels may be more difficult to penetrate and remove in order to gain access to the interior of the vehicle.

> **⚠ CAUTION**
>
> Flapping or removing the roof of a passenger vehicle on its side may compromise the vehicle's stability.

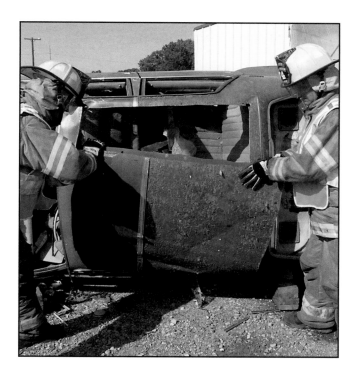

Figure 6.22 Extrication personnel can flap down the roof of a vehicle on its side in order to gain access to patients inside the vehicle.

Passenger Vehicle Extrication Tactics

Once the vehicle has been stabilized and access to its interior has been gained, all that remains of the extrication phase of the operation is the sometimes challenging process of disentangling the trapped patients and removing them from the vehicle. As mentioned earlier, the techniques and procedures involved in medically stabilizing and properly packaging an injured patient for extrication are beyond the scope of this manual. Therefore, in the extrication techniques that follow, it is assumed that medical stabilization and packaging have been or are being done. As with the other phases of the process, the extrication techniques used will vary depending upon the position of the vehicle — upright, on its side, on its roof, or in other positions.

NOTE: The passenger extrication tactics described in this section can best be accomplished using the tools and techniques described in Chapter 4, *Extrication Equipment*, and Chapter 5, *Extrication Techniques*.

Vehicle Extrication Progression

The following is a progression that works well for the average passenger vehicle extrication and may need to be modified due to the specific situation encountered.

A- Assess the scene (starts at dispatch, inner and outer evaluation, etc.)

Access patients verbally (Do not enter the vehicle until stabilized! Gain EMS info)

Account for all patients (ejections, patient count and EMS priority)

Advance a hoseline

Abate hazards (bystanders, fuel leak, etc.)

Vehicle Extrication Progression (continued)

B- Balance (stabilize) the vehicle

Break (control) the glass

Back out any intrusion

C- Cut or remove the roof, if required (lowers patient anxiety, gives more room to work)

D- Displace or remove the doors, if necessary

E- Enlarge openings (third door, dash displacement, pedals, etc.)

Extricate patient

F- Finish (prepare tools for the next call, critique/after action review, assist other agencies as appropriate)

Upright/On Wheels: Extrication

Regardless of where the trapped victims are located within the vehicle, rescuers must focus their efforts on disentangling the patients — that is, removing the vehicle from the patients. And, they must do so in a way that will not aggravate the patients' injuries. The extrication team must closely coordinate their efforts with those who are stabilizing and packaging the patients.

Disentanglement may involve cutting the brake and/or clutch pedals or bending them out of the way to free the driver's feet. It may involve removing the front seat backs or the entire seats. Or, it may involve removing or flapping the roof or doing a third-door conversion and/or a dashboard roll-up. Caution must be used when cutting brake and/or clutch pedals, these are made of metals that often break and shatter instead of cutting; thus, propelling them in an unknown direction.

Once the vehicle has been removed from the patients, and they have been properly packaged, the extrication team should work with the medical team to secure each patient to the appropriate size backboard. Then, working together, the team members carefully lift each patient and remove them from the wreckage. Once clear of the wreckage, the patient can be transferred to those responsible for transporting them to a medical facility.

On Side: Extrication

Disentangling and extricating patients from a vehicle on its side can sometimes be very challenging. However, because the patients may still be belted into their seats or piled on top of each other at the bottom of the wreckage, the greatest challenge may be for the medical team responsible for stabilizing and packaging the trapped patients. As described in the preceding section on gaining access, roof removal is probably the best option for creating a clear opening through which the patients can be extricated — provided that it can be done without compromising the vehicle's stability. Given a well-trained and equipped extrication team, the roof of a passenger vehicle can be flapped down or removed in less than a minute.

On Roof: Extrication

When a vehicle has come to rest on its roof, the occupants may be in dire need of extrication — and as quickly as safely possible. Unconscious patients hanging upside down from their seat belts will not survive very long, even if their injuries are not otherwise life-threatening. In addition, the possibility of the vehicle catching fire is greater than when in other positions because of the fuel and other hazardous fluids that are almost surely to be leaking from the vehicle. Therefore, time is of the essence. However, the safety of rescue personnel and patients should not be compromised to expedite the extrication.

Depending upon the structural condition of the vehicle, members of the extrication team may be available to assist the medical team in freeing patients hanging from their seat belts and with packaging them for extrication. As in all extrication operations, all rescue personnel must work together cooperatively for the good of those in need of their help.

Disentanglement and extrication from a vehicle on its roof may be complicated by the fact that removing door posts or other components may weaken the vehicle's structural integrity. This removal could cause the vehicle to suddenly and unexpectedly move in some way, perhaps aggravating the patient's injuries. Therefore, rescue personnel must anticipate the consequences of each of their actions before it is taken. If removing a structural component will weaken or destabilize the vehicle, steps must be taken to counteract those effects or another option must be considered. Otherwise, disentangling and extricating patients from a vehicle on its roof are no different than from vehicles in the other positions already discussed.

In those cases where the roof posts have collapsed to form what is known as a pancake roof collapse, one proven method of gaining access through the door opening is as follows:

Step 1: Create a purchase point between the rocker panel and the bottom of the door midway between the A- and B-post.

Step 2: Insert the spreading device into the access opening and slowly spread the center of the door outward.

NOTE: If it becomes necessary to reposition the spreading device during this operation, insert cribbing into the opening before removing the spreading tool to prevent the opening from closing or the metal from recoiling and possibly striking a patient.

Step 3: When the upper edge of the door has been pulled away from the chassis, use the opening thus created to look inside the vehicle to determine the patients' locations and assess their conditions. As the vehicle's interior will be quite dark, use a flashlight to illuminate the interior. If available, a search camera can be used.

Other Positions: Extrication

When a vehicle has come to rest in a position other than those already discussed, rescue personnel may have to use all of their ingenuity and skill to safely and efficiently disentangle and extricate the patients trapped inside. For example, if the patients are trapped inside a vehicle that is wedged under a collapsed bridge or other structure, the working room inside the vehicle may be extremely limited. The space limitation may render the most reliable extrication techniques impractical, if not impossible, to perform. Members of the medical and extrication teams may have to work in either the prone or supine position inside of the vehicle. They may also have to take turns working inside the vehicle. Regardless of how innovative the situation forces rescuers to be, they must never forget that the techniques employed must be safe for them to apply and as safe as possible for the patients. While the goal of extricating all patients without doing further injury still applies, these unusual situations may not allow that to happen. In some extremely rare instances, it may be medically necessary to sacrifice a limb to save a life. Such a decision must be made according to local protocols and through consultation between the incident commander (IC) and a physician at the scene.

Secondary Vehicles

Secondary vehicles are those that collide with vehicles that were already involved in the accident or with a vehicle that was not initially involved in the accident. The final resting position of these vehicles will depend upon their speed and angle that they strike the other vehicle.

Overrides and Underrides

The vehicle in motion (the striking vehicle) not the vehicle being struck will determine the underride/override condition. In cases of override or underride, one vehicle ends up under the other. Should the striking vehicle end up over the other, then the crash is considered an override. If the striking vehicle ends up under the other, then the crash is considered an underride.

Tunneling Through a Trunk

If a vehicle's roof has been crushed but the trunk lid is accessible, rescuers may be able to tunnel into the passenger compartment through the vehicle's trunk. This would require opening the trunk lid and removing the contents of the trunk. Any structural supports located between the front of the trunk and the back of the rear-most seat(s) of the vehicle would need to be removed carefully. Then the back of the rear-most seat(s) can be removed or pushed into the passenger compartment. **Skill Sheet 6-1** describes the procedures for tunneling through a trunk.

Summary

Rescue personnel should be well trained and adequately equipped to safely and efficiently handle extrication incidents involving passenger vehicles of all types. Rescue personnel must be familiar with the types of passenger vehicles, their anatomy, and their individual safety features and concerns. They must also be familiar with how and why vehicle occupants are injured in collisions. When sizing up a passenger vehicle incident, the IC must assign a priority to each vehicle involved in the collision based on the potential for saving lives. In general, this potential relates to the condition of the trapped patients and the time that will be required to extricate them. Rescue personnel must then be capable of stabilizing the involved vehicles, gaining access to the trapped patients, and extricating them as quickly as possible. Finally, an orderly process for terminating these incidents must be used.

Review Questions

1. What is used by the NHTSA to classify passenger vehicles?

2. What distinguishes station wagons from hatchbacks, minivans, and SUVs?

3. What steps should rescuers take in mitigating supplemental passenger restraint systems?

4. What can cause an active ROPS to extend?

5. What hazards or difficulties can be caused by collision beams, hood and hatch pistons/rod/struts, suspension struts, and shock absorbers during a vehicle incident?

6. What hazards are created by vehicle electrical and alternative fuel systems during passenger vehicle extrication operations?

7. What stabilization methods should be used during passenger vehicle extrication operations ?

REMINDER: Not all agencies advocate the following procedures and practices. The following skill sheets present a snapshot of various procedures utilized during extrication operations. As always, local agency procedures and protocols must be followed.

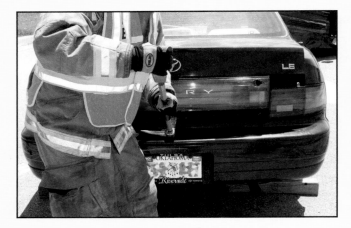

Step 1: Select the tools to be used to open the trunk lid.

Step 2: Open the trunk lid. If the vehicle is not in its normal orientation, use caution when opening the trunk as objects may fall out and injure rescuers.

Step 3: Remove the contents of the trunk.

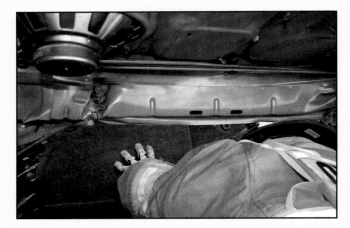

Step 5: Carefully remove the seat back by pushing it into the passenger compartment or pulling it out through the trunk opening, if possible.

CAUTION: It may be difficult to move the back seat due to the presence of structural components within the trunk and patients in the rear seat area.

Step 6: Make entry into the passenger compartment by crawling through the opening. Remove any objects that may interfere with patient care and removal.

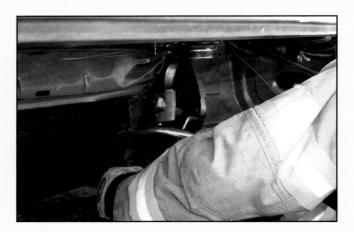

Step 4: Cut and remove any seat back support structures to allow a greater opening.

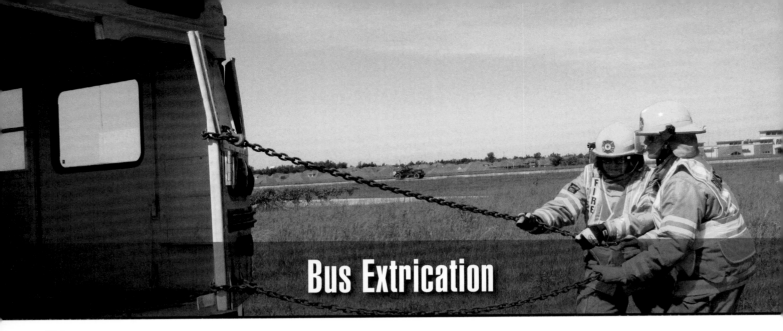

Bus Extrication

Chapter Contents

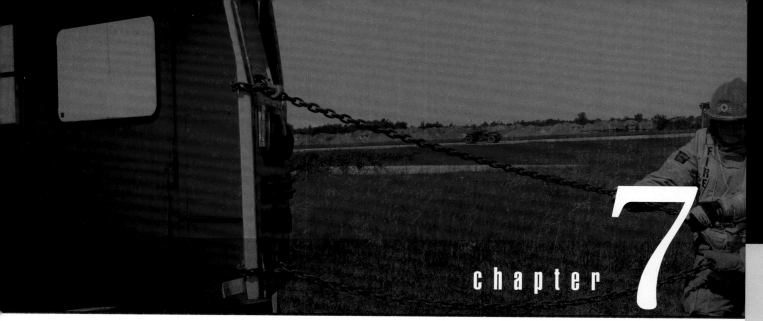

Key Terms

Job Performance Requirements

This chapter provides information that addresses the following job performance requirements (JPRs) of NFPA® 1001, *Standard for Fire Fighter Professional Qualifications* (2008), NFPA® 1006, *Standard for Technical Rescuer Professional Qualifications* (2008), and NFPA® 1670, *Standard on Operations and Training for Technical Search and Rescue Incidents* (2009).

NFPA® 1001 JPRs
6.4.1

6.4.2

NFPA® 1006 JPRs

5.2.2	10.1	10.1.5	10.2	10.2.4
5.2.3	10.1.1	10.1.6	10.2.1	10.2.5
5.3.1	10.1.3	10.1.7	10.2.2	
5.3.2	10.1.4	10.1.8	10.2.3	

NFPA® 1670 JPRs

8.2.3	8.3.4
8.3.3	8.4.2

Bus Extrication

1. Describe anatomical features of each type of bus.

2. Identify bus fuels and their related hazards.

3. Explain specific size-up concerns related to bus extrication.

4. Describe bus stabilization methods.

5. Describe common hazard control procedures related to bus extrication.

6. Describe methods for gaining access into buses.

7. Identify extrication tactics to be used on buses.

Chapter 7
Bus
Extrication

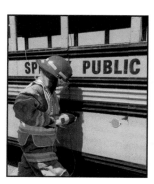

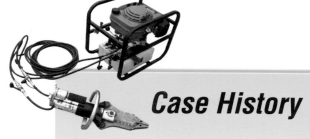

Case History

A county emergency dispatch center received a call of a motor vehicle accident involving a school bus. The fire department initially dispatched an engine and a medic unit. Upon arrival at the scene, the captain of the engine company discovered the bus lying on its driver side in a creek about one foot deep. The bus had fallen from a bridge 49 feet above. Aboard the bus were 27 high school students and 4 adults (including the driver). The captain requested an additional response of three engine companies, an aerial unit, a medic unit, and a battalion chief.

Upon arrival, the battalion chief assumed command of the incident, declared it to be a mass casualty incident, and requested an additional five medic units and a medical helicopter. The majority of the students were found within the bus with numerous patients pinned by their arms and legs between the bus seats and bus interior wall. One female student had been ejected and was pinned between the bus and the bank of the creek. One male student was pinned face down within the bus and drowned.

The responders at the scene had limited knowledge of bus construction and extrication techniques which hampered extrication efforts. Attempts to create purchase points in the bus roof for extrication tool insertion proved ineffective due to the roof's construction. The hydraulic spreaders carried by the department were too large to fit between the seats in the bus, so rescuers had to use hack saws to cut through the bus seat legs and free the patients. The patients were moved to a park where they were triaged and received emergency medical treatment prior to being transported to local hospitals by ambulances. Six of the student patients were airlifted to an area trauma center for more critical care.

With the exception of railroad passenger cars, buses are the largest passenger vehicles with which rescue personnel may have to contend. Like other passenger vehicles, buses are manufactured in a variety of shapes and sizes. They range from 10-passenger commuter vans, to transit and commercial buses capable of carrying more than 40 passengers, to school buses capable of carrying in excess of 90 passengers, to a variety of specialty buses. No matter what the size, buses are all designed for the same purpose — to convey a relatively large number of passengers from one point to another in relative safety and comfort. The fact that a large number of vehicle occupants may be trapped in a bus collision sets this type of extrication problem apart from those involving automobiles and trucks. If emergency response organizations are to function safely and effectively during bus extrication incidents, pre-incident planning and realistic training exercises involving mass casualty scenarios are imperative.

This chapter reviews the following aspects of bus extrication:

- Bus anatomy
- Bus Fuels
- Size-up concerns at bus incidents
- Bus stabilization
- Hazard Control
- Access to bus interior
- Extrication tactics involving buses

Bus Anatomy

There are four main classifications of buses are as follows:

- School buses
- Transit buses
- Commercial buses
- Specialty buses

Even though all buses are intended for the same purpose — transporting a relatively large number of passengers from one point to another safely — there are significant differences in how the various types of buses are constructed. The level of familiarity that rescue personnel have with the anatomy of any particular type of bus will dictate how effectively they can handle extrication problems in that type of vehicle. Therefore, it is important that rescue personnel learn as much as possible about the common and unique features of each type of bus as discussed in the following sections.

School Buses

Federal Motor Vehicle Safety Standards define a school bus as "a passenger motor vehicle designed to carry more than 10 passengers in addition to the driver, and which the Secretary of Transportation determines is to be used to transport preschool, primary, and secondary school students to or from such schools or school-related events." While this definition limits this type of vehicle to school functions, the rescue procedures for these vehicles are the same regardless of who is using the vehicle.

School buses have the following characteristics:

- Variety of sizes and configurations
- At least one entry/exit door
- At least one additional emergency exit, usually at the rear of the vehicle, that may or may not be an exit door.

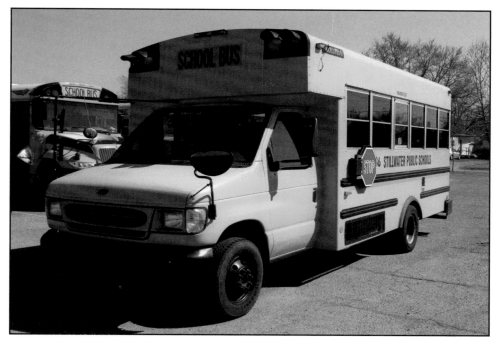

Figure 7.1 An example of a Type A-2 school bus.

According to the National Standards for School Buses and School Bus Operations, school buses are divided into four types: A, B, C, and D. In the United States, approximately 85 to 90% of all buses on the road are either Type C or D. The types are further described as follows:

- Type A — smallest type of bus; Suburban-type or van conversion built on a heavy duty, van-type front section chassis; carries 10 to 20 passengers; entry/exit door aft of the front wheels; has driver-side door; engine is under windshield or between front seats; 2 varieties:

    1. A-1 — gross vehicle weight rating (GVWR) of more than 10,000 lbs. (4 450 kg)

    2. A-2 — GVWR of less than 10,000 lbs. (4 450 kg) **(Figure 7.1)**

- Type B — conversion or body constructed on a front-section vehicle chassis; GVWR of more than 10,001 lbs. (4 450 kg); passenger capacity 16-24; engine beneath the windshield and/or beside the driver's seat; entry/exit door aft of front wheel **(Figure 7.2, p. 304)**

NOTE: The Thomas built Vista model has a capacity of 33-78 passengers, yet is still considered a Class B bus.

- Type C — the model Americans usually think of when they think of a school bus; passenger body installed on a flat-back cowl chassis; GVWR of more than 10,000 lbs. (4 450 kg); engine compartment protrudes from the front of the vehicle; no driver-side door; entry/exit door aft of front fender; carries 30 to 78 passengers; average weight of 20,000 to 30,000 lbs. (8 900 to 13 350 kg) **(Figure 7.3, p. 304)**

- Type D — full-size vehicle with a "boxy" appearance; no driver-side door; entry/exit door forward of front wheels; engine locations front, midship, or rear; authorized carrying capacity of 66 passengers **(Figure 7.4, p. 304)**

Gross Vehicle Weight Rating (GVWR) — The maximum allowable total weight of a road vehicle or trailer when loaded to include the weight of the vehicle itself plus fuel, passengers, cargo, and trailer tongue weight.

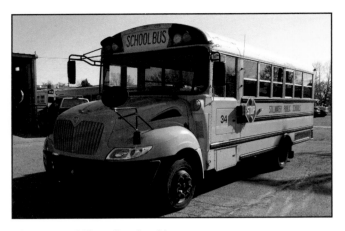

Figure 7.2 A Type B school bus.

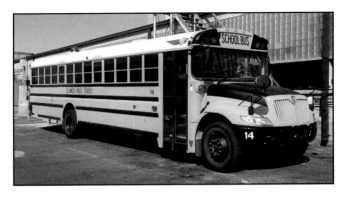

Figure 7.3 This bus is an example of a Type C school bus.

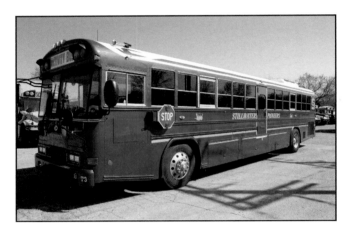

Figure 7.4 An example of a Type D school bus.

"Super" School Bus

Although most of the full-size school buses have an authorized carrying capacity of up to 66 passengers, changes in the technology of school bus construction have resulted in school buses with larger carrying capacities. All U.S. school bus manufacturers now offer a "super" school bus, 8 x 40 feet long (2.4 m x 12.2 m). The engine in a super bus is located inside, at the front or rear of the bus. The front engine position is similar to the engine location in a typical van-type vehicle.

In the typical super bus, the interior of the bus has been extended forward to the front bumper. By lengthening the body of the vehicle, the flat-nosed bus now has a legal seating capacity of 90 passengers plus the bus driver. A legally permissible overflow of standees equal to 20 percent of the seating capacity is also permitted in some states. In addition to the usual door exits, roof hatches may also be provided, one toward the front of the bus and a second toward the rear.

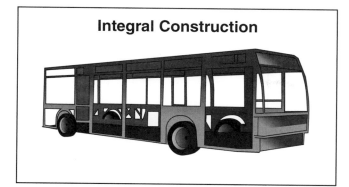

Integral Construction

Figure 7.5a In integral construction, the body and chassis are built as one unit.

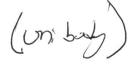
(uni body)

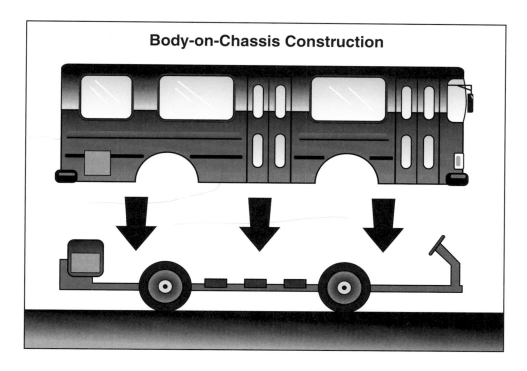

Body-on-Chassis Construction

Figure 7.5b In body-on-chassis construction, the body and chassis are built separately and then connected together.

There are two basic construction methods used by major school bus manufacturers:

1. **Integral Construction.** The body and chassis are formed as a unit. The manufacturer assembles the vehicle starting with the frame and chassis assembly and proceeds item by item to the finished vehicle (**Figure 7.5a**).

2. **Body-on-Chassis.** The body and chassis are manufactured as separate units and joined by the bus manufacturer. (**Figure 7.5b**).

The sections that follow highlight some of the common elements found on most school buses manufactured in North America.

School Bus Skeletal System

All school bus body units are comprised of a roof, a floor, two sidewalls, and front and rear assemblies (**Figure 7.6, p. 306**). The finish and trim components of each area of the body are supported by a skeletal system beneath. This skeletal system forms the basic structure of the entire bus. It dictates how the vehicle will respond during a collision and forms the basis of the protective envelope designed to provide occupant safety and survival.

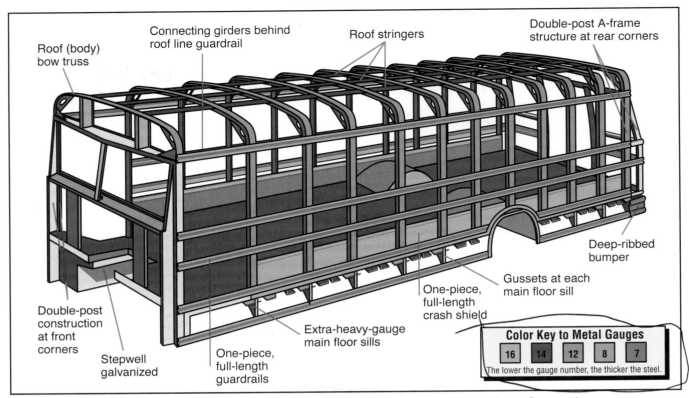

Figure 7.6 An in-depth look at the skeletal system of a school bus body. *Courtesy of the Wayne Corporation.*

Sidewalls are comprised of vertical load-bearing frame members and in some models, the roof bows extend down to form the support members. These vertical members serve as partitions between window openings. Running horizontally along the base of each sidewall is a framing element referred to as a collision beam. This heavy-gauge steel member is strategically located to limit penetration of an object into the passenger compartment.

Finish panels of 20-gauge steel are typically mounted on the exterior and 22-gauge on the interior of the sidewall frame members. To meet requirements for interior noise attenuation and temperature control, insulation materials may be sandwiched between the interior and exterior panels.

Additional impact resistance is added to the exterior sidewall. Formed rub rails (4 3/4-inch [120 mm] wide) of 16-gauge steel run the full length of the sidewalls. They are intended to minimize penetration during collision and can also be used for identifying occupant location from the exterior. One rub rail will indicate the seat cushion level; if a second rail is present, it will identify the floor level **(Figure 7.7)**. Some school buses have as many as four rub rails from the bottom of the windows down to the bottom of the skirts.

The rear skeletal system is similar to the sidewall, with additional reinforcement installed to provide protection from rear-end collisions. The additional reinforcement may be a double-post A-frame structural member built into the rear corners of the bus.

The skeletal framework of the school bus roof commonly consists of 11- to 14-gauge steel frame members called roof bows. These members span the roof structure from side to side. Within this frame are 14- to 16-gauge girders

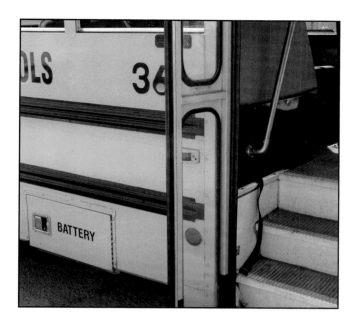

Figure 7.7 The bottom rub rail indicates the level of the floor while the upper rub rail indicates the level of the seat cushions inside the school bus.

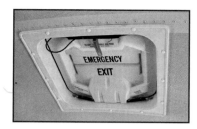

Figure 7.8a An emergency escape hatch in the roof of a school bus as seen from the interior.

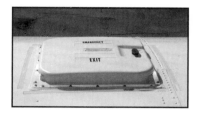

Figure 7.8b An exterior view of a roof mounted emergency escape hatch on a school bus.

(known as stringers) running from front to rear, strengthening and spacing the bows. There may be as many as three of these longitudinal members in the roof skeleton.

Insulation material and electrical wiring are located within the framework of the roof. The outside and inside of the framing members are generally covered with sheet metal panels. If breaching the roof structure becomes necessary, the location of the roof bows and stringers can be determined by the rows of rivets used to secure the roof panels.

Emergency escape hatches may also be located in the roof structure. These hatches are made of fiberglass or other lightweight materials, and they open by the activation of a release mechanism from inside or outside **(Figure 7.8a and b)**. If necessary, they may be forced open using conventional prying techniques. These hatches open fully to provide a clear opening of at least 11 x 14 inches (275 mm by 350 mm). Some buses may have larger hatches, especially if they are used to transport physically disabled passengers.

School Bus Floor and Undercarriage

The floor of a school bus consists of several components. In most of the full-size buses, a heavy-duty vinyl or rubber floor covering is typically applied over plywood decking and 14-gauge metal flooring panels. The smaller conversion-type vehicles may have 1/2- or 5/8-inch (13 mm or 16 mm) plywood sheets placed on top of the existing vehicle floor. Structural members, acting as floor joists, are spaced as close as every 9 inches (225 mm) along the underside of the floor.

NOTE: Because of the amount of time needed to breach a floor, floors SHOULD NOT be considered as a primary entry point.

The undercarriage of a typical school bus is substantially reinforced with 8-gauge angle bar, 12-gauge channel stock, and 14-gauge sheet metal. There are guard loops around the entire length of the driveshaft to prevent the driveshaft from falling to the ground if it breaks or becomes disconnected. As mentioned earlier, forcible entry through the floor is difficult and time consuming — any other available entry route should be used.

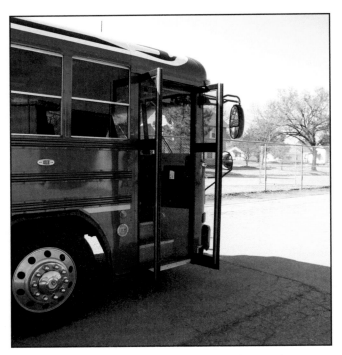

Figure 7.9 Outward opening, two-part, split-type doors on a Type D school bus.

School Bus Front Doors

There are various types of entry doors on school buses, each serving a specific function. The doors are strategically located to maximize exit paths during an emergency.

Entry doors on some Type A and Type B buses are stock versions provided by the original manufacturer. The latch and lock mechanism is the Nader safety lock found on most motor vehicles since 1973.

The passenger side front door may be drastically altered to suit the needs of the school bus owner/operator. The passenger door may have the same general design as a standard passenger vehicle door, but the window glass is typically permanently fixed in a closed position. The door handles, armrests, and window cranks may be removed.

The passenger side front doors on the full-size Type C and D school buses open in a variety of ways. Some are two-part, split-type doors that open inwardly or outwardly, with outward being most common. When operated, these doors split in the middle, with each half of the door swinging to its respective side **(Figure 7.9)**.

Another common type of door is a center-hinged type door that opens by folding forward or rearward **(Figure 7.10)**. Regardless of the type of door, the most common way to open it or secure it in the closed position is with the manual control arm mechanism. When open, school bus front doors typically have a horizontal opening of between 22 and 24 inches (550 mm and 600 mm) and a minimum vertical opening of approximately 68 to 72 inches (1 700 mm to 1 800 mm).

On older buses, the only means of opening or closing the front passenger exit door is a manual control arm operated by the driver. Newer buses have a powered door opening mechanism operated by the driver and an emergency release handle mounted on the inside of the door. Some of these buses may also be equipped with the same type of split, folding doors that are typically found on larger buses. School buses of all types used to transport handicapped passengers may be equipped with electric lifts at the side doors.

Some school buses use air-operated mechanisms to control the front door. The main switch is usually located to the left of the driver on the instrument console. There will also be a backup emergency release mechanism in the exit stairwell inside the vehicle. The readily identifiable release button or switch causes the air lock device to release the door. Rescue personnel can then manually move the door through its normal path of travel. There may not be an air override release mechanism if there are two similar doors located along the same side of the bus.

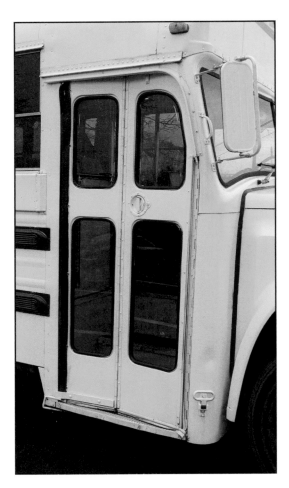

Figure 7.10 A center hinged, forward folding door.

School Bus Rear Doors

The rear exit door is designed to give occupants inside the vehicle a way to exit if the front door does not function or is blocked. On Type A school buses, there may be either one or two rear exit doors. On Type B and C, and some D school buses, there is usually one large rear exit door **(Figure 7.11)**. There is no locking device on these rear doors, and they open outwardly by manipulation of a lever to release a latch mechanism. These doors may be opened from the exterior as well as from the interior.

The rear exit door is secured by a one-point or three-point latch system. The main latch is at the edge of the door near the control handle and the other two latches, if present, are found at the top and bottom of the door, engaging the bus body and the floor assembly.

NOTE: Rear-engine Type D buses do not have a rear exit door but are required by U.S. Motor Vehicle Safety Standards to have a rear emergency window exit.

In some states, buses with larger capacities are required to have an additional exit door along the driver's side of the vehicle. This door, known as the "third door" or the "left-hand door," provides an opening of 24 x 48 inches (600 mm by 1 200 mm) and is secured with the same one- or three-point latch mechanism as the rear door. Access is easier from the exterior, since the interior access to the latch mechanism may be obstructed by the passenger seats.

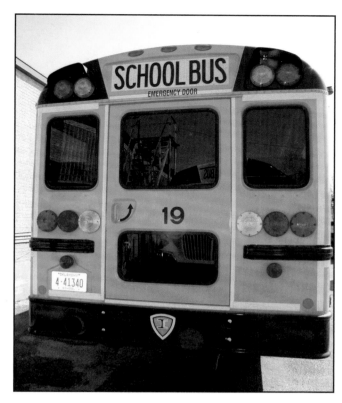

Figure 7.11 A rear exit door on a Type C school bus.

School Bus Windows

The openings for the side and rear windows are defined by the vertical frame members, the roof edge, and the top of the sidewall. The vertical posts between the windows are either extensions of the roof bows or are hollow tubular structures consisting of several layers of sheet metal. These posts can be removed with power shears or reciprocating saws.

The windows may be laminated or tempered safety glass framed in extruded aluminum. The windows are of the split-sash design and are affixed to the rough openings with screws, rivets, or similar fasteners. Typical school bus windows open from the top down, providing an opening of approximately 9 x 22 inches (225 mm by 550 mm), or one-half the total size of the window area **(Figure 7.12, p. 310)**.

To provide a larger opening, some states have regulations requiring that certain side windows be designed as emergency exits and labeled as such inside the vehicle. From the exterior, rescuers can identify these exits by the hinges located along the top side of the window frames. Once opened, these windows provide a larger opening through the side of the vehicle than do standard windows.

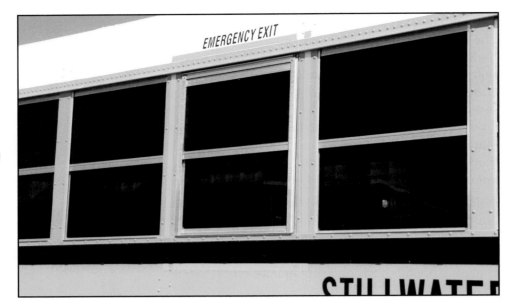

Figure 7.12 Examples of school bus windows. The center window with the silver colored frame can be removed and the opening used as an emergency exit.

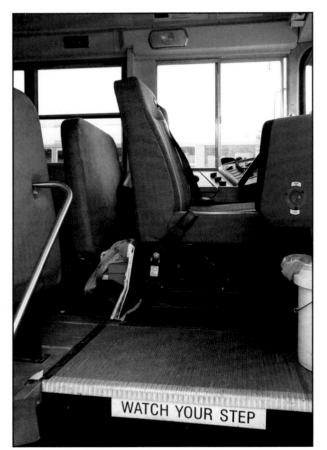

Figure 7.13 The driver's seat of a standard school bus.

On the smaller conversion-type school buses, the stock one-piece laminated safety glass windshields are set into the vehicle body with a multipiece rubber mounting gasket. Windshields on full-size buses consist of two or more sheets of laminated safety glass. These sheets are also secured into the vehicle body with a multipiece rubber mounting gasket.

Rear windows are flat sheets of laminated safety glass and are also mounted with removable rubber gaskets. The mounting components for both the windshield and the rear windows are similar to those described in the preceding chapter on passenger vehicle extrication. Types C and D may also be equipped with fixed windows and air conditioning systems.

School Bus Seats

The two types of seats found in school buses are driver's seats and passenger seats **(Figure 7.13)**. The driver's seat is an adjustable bucket-type seat with a floor-mounted seat belt and/or shoulder harness assembly. Passenger seats are framed with 1-inch (25 mm) tubular steel. The seats are bolted into the bus floor and into the sidewall area. Detachable foam rubber seat cushions and seat backs are covered with a vinyl upholstery material. Since 1977, school bus seat backs have been required to be of the high-back style, 24 inches (600 mm) high.

School bus passenger seats may be equipped with lap-style seat belts if mandated by local ordinance or state law, but all Type A buses under 10,000 pounds (4 450 kg) GVWR must have lap belts. In buses used to transport physically or mentally handicapped persons, positive body restraint harnesses may be found in specially designated seats.

School Bus Aisles

The position of the seats inside the school bus dictates the width of the vehicle's center aisle **(Figure 7.14)**. The aisle of Suburban-type buses can be as narrow as 10 inches (250 mm). Aisle space in van-conversion buses increases to approximately 12 inches (300 mm). Full-size school buses may have aisle widths between 12 and 15 inches (300 mm and 375 mm). Since the width of a typical backboard is 18 inches (450 mm), a narrow center aisle can make the process of removing patients more difficult. Wheelchair-equipped vehicles generally have a 30-inch (750 mm) wide aisle in the area where the chair will be maneuvered; however, the aisle may not be that wide throughout the entire vehicle.

School Bus Batteries

On Type A and some Type B buses, the batteries are usually located in the engine compartment. On most Type B, C, and D buses, the batteries are typically located in a separate compartment on the driver's side of the vehicle **(Figure 7.15)**. If the bus is equipped as a handicapped transport with an electric lift, a separate battery may be provided for the lift. This battery is usually located in a separate compartment on the driver's side of the vehicle. Disconnecting this battery will not interrupt power to the engine.

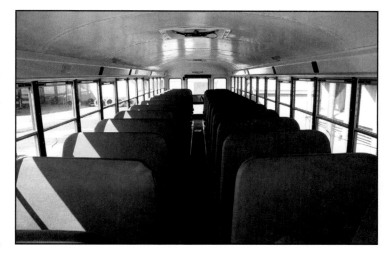

Figure 7.14 An example of the aisle space provided between passenger seats on either side of a school bus.

Transit Buses

Transit buses are designed to move a large number of people over relatively short distances. They are most commonly found in urban or metropolitan areas that operate mass transit systems **(Figure 7.16, p. 312)**. In some cases, these systems may have bus routes that extend far into the suburbs that surround the core coverage area. Transit buses have capacities for more than 60 seated passengers — plus a number of standees. Similar types of buses are often used as parking shuttles at airports, large amusement or entertainment facilities, or as employee shuttles within large business or industrial complexes. Because transit buses generally operate in heavy traffic, the potential for involvement in accidents is very high. The potential for a large number of casualties is also present because of the high passenger load and the fact that people may be sitting in an irregular and unrestrained manner or may even be standing.

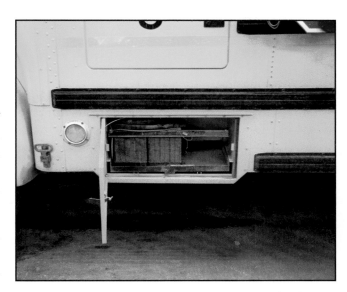

Figure 7.15 The battery compartment on a Type C school bus.

Also included in this classification are articulated transit buses. In some areas, budget limitations have forced transit systems to reduce the frequency of bus service. To offset this reduction, some now use larger buses that can transport more passengers per trip. Because it is impractical to design a single

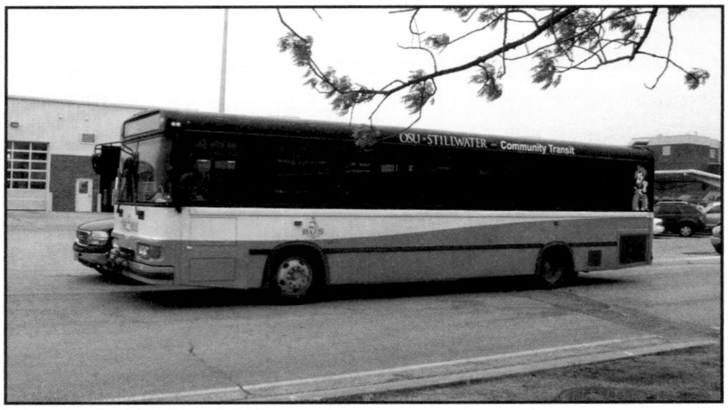

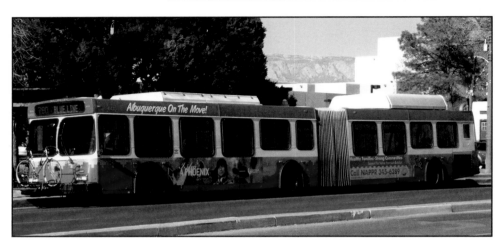

Figure 7.16 An example of a transit bus.

Figure 7.17 An example of an articulated transit bus. *Courtesy of John Perry, Albuquerque, N.M.*

Articulated Transit Bus —
A passenger carrying bus constructed with two sections (a tractor and a trailer) which are connected by a pivoting joint.

chassis vehicle longer than about 40 feet (12 m), some transit authorities have switched to articulated buses **(Figure 7.17)**. The advantages in maneuverability offered by these buses are similar to those that the tractor-tiller aerial apparatus offers to the fire service. The vehicle's ability to flex in the middle makes it able to maneuver extremely well in areas that single-chassis vehicles of comparable size could not.

The articulated transit bus consists of a tractor section and a trailer section. The two are connected by a pivoting joint that is enclosed by a large, bellows-like seal. The tractor section is nearly the size of a standard transit bus. The trailer section is considerably shorter. Older articulated buses had two separate engines, one located in the middle of the tractor section and the other engine located in the rear of the trailer section. This is known as the puller configuration. Newer models have a single engine located at the rear of the trailer section. The longitudinal stability of the vehicle is controlled by hydraulic cylinders mounted near the joint. This configuration is called a pusher. **(Figure 7.18)**. This rear engine will also power the air-conditioning system. Aside from these specifically mentioned features, articulated buses are constructed in the same manner as conventional transit buses.

In general, transit buses are of integral body construction. This construction combines the chassis framing and the body understructure into one integral module. The main undercarriage structure consists of longitudinal beams that support horizontal and vertical beams made of carbon steel, mild steel, and other materials. All other structural components are made of either galvanized or stainless steel or aluminum. These include tubular support members, cross bracing, inner or outer panels, plates, and any other formed members.

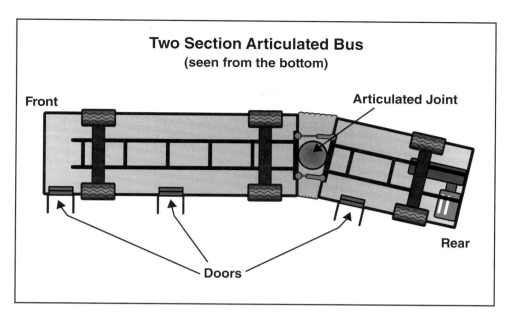

Figure 7.18 An illustration showing how the longitudinal stability of an articulated transit bus is controlled.

Formed tubular members are used to support the upper body portion of the bus. This upper body structure is welded to the vertical carline supports located near the floor of the bus. Carline supports are gussets that strengthen the side wall of a bus at the level most likely to be struck by a car. The roof is constructed of inner and outer panels that sandwich insulation and electrical wiring and fixtures between them. The most common material used for transit bus floor decking is 3/4-inch (19 mm) plywood. The decking may be covered with any of a variety of floor coverings, most of them rubber or linoleum type **(Figure 7.19)**. The sections that follow offer details about specific portions of transit buses.

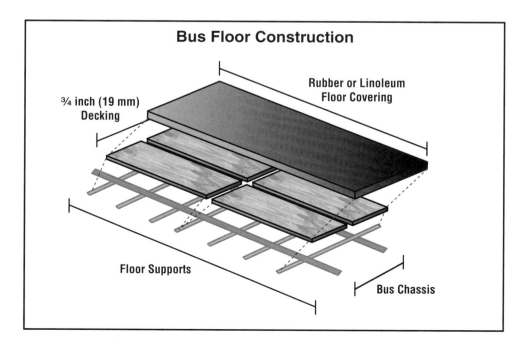

Figure 7.19 An exploded view showing how bus floors are constructed.

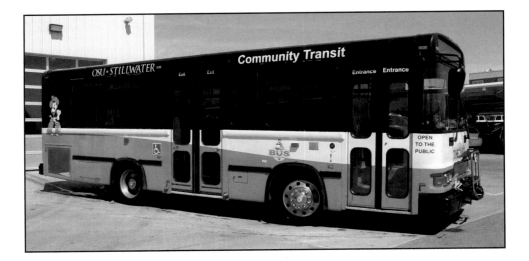

Figure 7.20 Midship and front doors on a transit bus.

Transit Bus Doors

Nearly all transit bus doors are of the two-piece, center-opening type. While most swing toward the outside, some slide laterally. The opening mechanism may be pneumatic, hydraulic, or electric, depending upon the manufacturer. The operating control is usually located at the driver's left side. Most transit buses are constructed with two passenger side doors. One is at the very front of the vehicle, directly opposite the driver; the other midship, or slightly aft of midship **(Figure 7.20)**. Both doors are intended for normal entry and exit by passengers. Normally, these doors will open and close simultaneously. Unlike school buses, transit buses generally do not have a specific emergency exit door. The two standard doors are considered to be sufficient for most emergencies. All buses are equipped with window exits in addition to the regular exits.

Some transit buses are designed to accommodate disabled passengers. These buses may be equipped with one or a combination of features that allow easier access for passengers with limited mobility or those confined to wheelchairs. One such feature is a hydraulic lift designed to raise passengers in wheelchairs from curb height to assist them onto the bus and to lower them back to curb height when they wish to exit. The lift may be located at the front, middle, or rear of the vehicle, however, the lift may have its own access point **(Figure 7.21)**. By operating a control next to the door, the bus driver is able to convert the stairway into a lift. When the control is operated, the stairs fold out into a lift platform. From that position, the platform may be lowered or raised.

Another feature allows the front end of the bus to be lowered to curb level, often referred to as "kneeling," so that a passenger is not required to step up to get into the bus. By controlling the air in the suspension system bellows, the driver can lower the level of the step from its normal height of about 12 inches (300 mm) down to about 6 inches (150 mm) **(Figure 7.22)**. This feature demonstrates how important it is that rescuers stay clear of an unsupported bus with an air suspension system. If the air suspension system fails, anyone underneath would be crushed.

Transit Bus Windows

Laminated safety glass is the most common type of glass used in transit bus windows, but some transit buses have side windows of tempered glass, Plexiglas®, or other synthetic material. Transit bus windshields and rear windows are

Kneeling — The ability of some buses to lower the front end of the bus to curb level for ease of passenger boarding.

WARNING!
Never put any part of your body beneath an unsupported bus with an air suspension system.

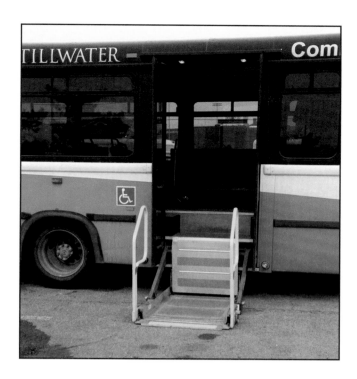

Figure 7.21 A hydraulic lift system on a transit bus.

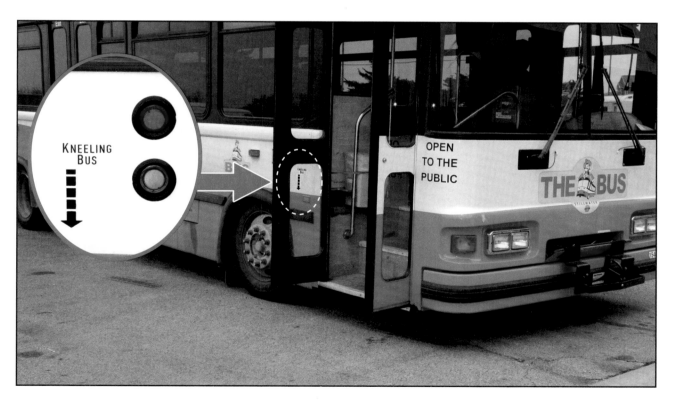

Figure 7.22 A transit bus in the "kneeling" position.

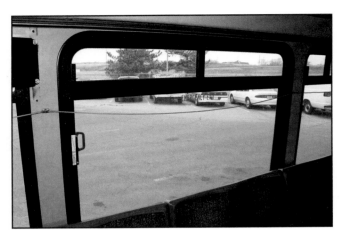

Figure 7.23 An example of a transit bus window as seen from the interior.

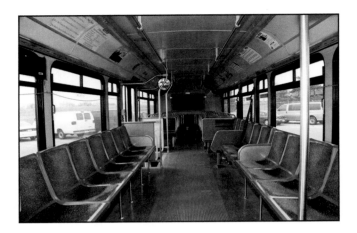

Figure 7.24 The front seats in this transit bus face the center while those in the back of the bus face forward.

similar to those in school buses or other large vehicles. The large windshields are typically of two-piece design. Transit bus windshields are held in place by a simple locking rubber filler strip.

The type of transit bus side windows varies greatly, depending on the age of the bus and the manufacturer. Older buses — those without air conditioning — may have windows that can only be opened by sliding the window to one side or the other. The glass is set into an aluminum or other lightweight metal frame designed to slide open a distance equal to one-half the width of the entire window unit. Transit buses are now commonly equipped with windows that are hinged at the top and are designed to tilt out when the latch on the lower side is released **(Figures 7.23)**. Some transit buses have windows that are designed to slide open during normal operation; however, they still tilt out to provide an emergency exit. These windows will not stay open by themselves and have to be propped open.

Transit Bus Seats

Nearly all passenger seats found on transit buses are molded from some type of plastic. They may be further covered by a vinyl or plastic covering or cushions. The seats are supported by a metal framework that is bolted to the floor and the sides of the bus. In some cases, the supporting framework of the seats is combined with handrail systems that are also bolted to the ceiling of the bus.

A major difference between transit bus seating and that in other types of buses is the layout of the seats. Most transit buses do not have the standard, uniform front-facing seat arrangement. The seats in a transit bus may be arranged facing forward, towards the center aisle, or towards the rear of the bus **(Figures 7.24)**. The layouts will vary depending on the owner/operator's specifications. They may even vary within the same transit fleet, depending on the age of individual buses and prevailing trends at the time the vehicles were purchased. The driver's seat in a transit bus is similar to those described in the school bus section of this chapter.

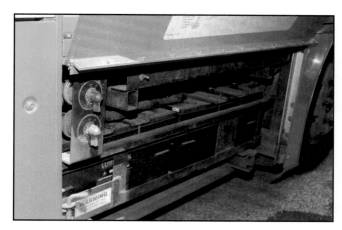

Figure 7.25a The battery compartment on a transit bus.

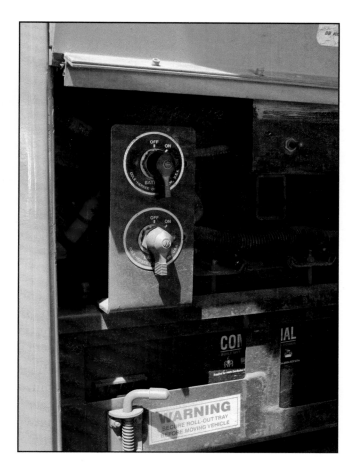

Figure 7.25b The battery shut off switch located in the upper left corner of the front of the battery compartment.

Transit Bus Aisles

In most transit buses, the width of the center aisle is considerably wider than those in typical school buses. This is because transit buses are designed for adults who may be carrying packages, briefcases, etc. The wider aisle also results from different seating arrangements. Depending on seat layout, transit bus aisles vary in width from about 20 inches (500 mm) to about 5 feet (1.5 m). This makes transit buses somewhat easier than school buses for rescue and EMS personnel to work and maneuver in.

Transit Bus Batteries

The battery banks on nearly all transit buses are located on the driver's side of the vehicle, just forward of the rear wheels. For ease of access, the batteries are grouped together on a tray that can be pulled out when the compartment door is open. However, sliding out the tray is usually unnecessary because most transit buses are equipped with a battery shutoff switch located in the battery compartment. Power from the batteries can be interrupted by simply moving this switch to the "off" position **(Figures 7.25a and b)**.

Commercial Buses

Commercial buses (also called "motor coaches," "charter buses," and "touring buses") are primarily designed to transport large numbers of people over relatively long distances. These buses may travel regularly scheduled routes or may be chartered by groups to travel to a specific location **(Figure 7.26, p. 318)**. Because charter buses travel through almost every region and area, every organization responsible for extrication must be prepared to deal with this type of vehicle. Typically, these buses carry up to about 50 passengers. Some buses may have bathrooms, kitchen, and sleeping areas. The kitchens may have propane fueled equipment.

Most manufacturers of commercial buses construct the entire frame of the vehicle as one integral unit. This method of construction is sometimes referred to as "bird cage" construction, since the assembled frame resembles a

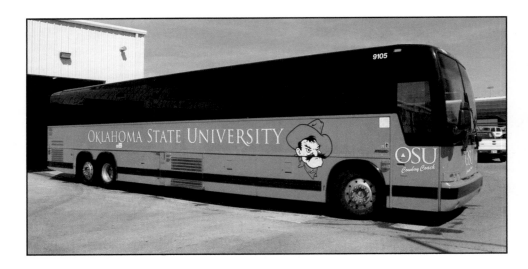

Figure 7.26 An example of a commercial bus, also called a motor coach, charter bus, or touring bus.

large bird cage. The majority of the frame is constructed of low carbon, square steel tubing 1 to 2 inches (40 mm to 50 mm) in diameter. The frame is covered with either aluminum or stainless steel sheeting. On some buses, the panels covering the front and rear modules are made of fiberglass.

Framing members that support the roof are generally separated by about 24 to 26 inches (600 mm to 650 mm) on center. Wiring and insulation are sandwiched between the outer (roof) and inner (ceiling) panels. A major difference in roof construction between commercial buses and other types of buses is that the panels in a commercial bus may not be riveted to every structural member. Some manufacturers rivet the panels to every other roof rafter; therefore, there is a structural member about halfway between each row of rivets. If the rows of rivets are more than about 2 feet (0.7 m) apart, a rafter is likely to be located between the two riveted members.

Commercial bus floors are constructed in a manner similar to those on transit buses. Most are ½- or ¾-inch (13 mm or 19 mm) plywood covered with a composite rubber or other synthetic covering.

Commercial Bus Doors

All commercial buses have a single door at the front, opposite the driver's position. This door is usually a one-piece, single-hinged door with hinges located on the forward edge of the door. A few models have a two-piece center-opening door, similar to those on a transit bus, or a folding door. The folding door is not a center opening door like those found on school or transit buses; rather, it has a hinge along one edge and in the center allowing it to fold to one side. The door folds toward the front of the bus instead of swinging open like a one-piece door.

Many commercial bus manufacturers use air-operated opening mechanisms on their doors. When the driver operates a dash-mounted control device, compressed air pressure opens the door. In the event of air compressor failure, or any other emergency, the driver can open these doors by operating an emergency release that dumps the air pressure from the system and allows the door to be manually operated. Emergency releases are located inside the bus near the top of the door. Exterior releases are usually located either in the right front wheel well, under or to the left of the door itself on the outside of the

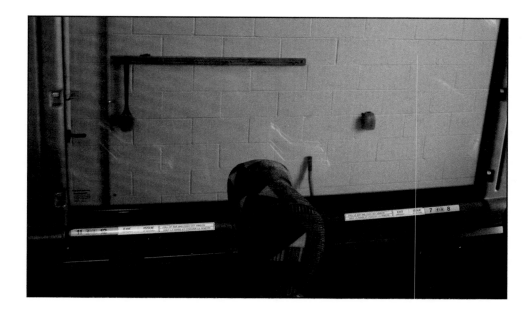

Figure 7.27 A commercial bus window as seen from the interior. The red and white decals at the base of the window explain how to open it in an emergency.

vehicle, or directly below the center of the windshield. Some motor coaches have mechanical pivot arm openers similar to those used on school buses. The emergency release for doors with a mechanical arm is a knob or latch located directly under the center of the windshield on the front of the bus.

Most commercial buses do not have emergency exit doors, although a few import models do. Most rely on window exits for emergencies. Window exits are covered in more detail in the next section.

Commercial Bus Windows

Because most commercial buses are air-conditioned, there is little or no need for windows that open. Because of this, all modern motor coaches are designed with single-piece side windows, some of which can be opened in emergencies. These exit windows are set in metal frames that are hinged at the top. Typically, these windows are opened by lifting a horizontal bar located across the bottom of the window frame. When the mechanism is released, the bottom of the window can be pushed out to provide an exit path. These emergency exit window openings are at least 20 x 48 inches (500 mm by 1 200 mm), with many being considerably larger **(Figure 7.27)**. These window exits will not stay open by themselves, so if it is necessary to keep them open, they will have to be propped. Pike poles are well suited for this purpose.

Commercial bus windshields and rear windows are set in a rubber molding. Windshields and rear windows are usually constructed of laminated automotive safety glass. Side windows may be laminated glass, tempered safety glass, Lexan®, or other synthetic material.

Commercial Bus Seats

Commercial buses are generally equipped with individual bucket-type seats for each occupant, similar to those on commercial airliners. These seats have high backs, can be inclined, and may or may not have armrests between the seats. They are usually mounted four to a row, two on each side of the center aisle **(Figure 7.28, p. 320)**. How the seats are mounted varies from manufacturer to manufacturer. Some seats are connected and mounted like the bench

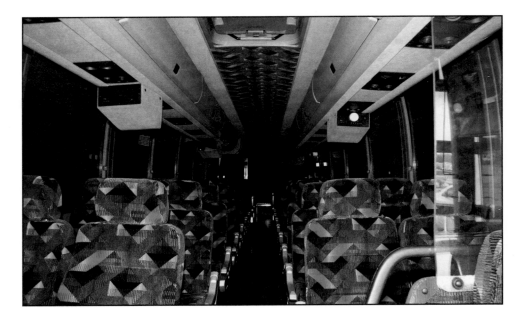

Figure 7.28 Commercial bus seats are designed for passenger comfort.

seats in a school bus. The legs on the aisle side are bolted to the floor, and the window side of the seat is bolted to the floor and/or the sidewall. Other seats may be mounted on an individual pedestal that is bolted to the floor. Most drivers' seats are pedestal mounted. Some motor coaches have a bench at the rear of the bus; this bench is usually molded into the rear frame design and removing anything other than the cushions is extremely difficult.

Commercial Bus Aisles

Most commercial buses have a uniform aisle width for most of the length of the seating area; however, there may be some variation in aisle width toward the rear of the bus near the restroom. The center aisle is usually between 13 and 18 inches (325 mm and 450 mm) wide. This narrow width creates problems for rescuers trying to remove patients on backboards, scoop stretchers, or other litters. The ceiling height in most motor coach aisles is generally 75 to 78 inches (1 875 mm to 1 950 mm). Because of the high seat backs and low overhead luggage racks, it may be difficult to carry the litters over the seat tops. In some cases, seats may have to be removed to make passage possible.

Commercial Bus Luggage Compartments

Most commercial buses are equipped with overhead storage compartments located directly above the seats. These compartments are designed for passengers to stow small articles of carry-on luggage. The compartments may be either open shelves or enclosed cabinets similar to those on commercial airliners. These storage areas reduce the ceiling height directly above the seats and may present some working space difficulties for rescuers.

Commercial buses also have large luggage compartments located below the seating area of the bus that open from the outside. While these compartments are primarily designed to carry large pieces of luggage, in many cases motor coaches also haul common freight. No matter what is hauled, there is a heavy fuel loading near these storage compartments and any ignition in this area could result in a serious fire. Because these lower compartments

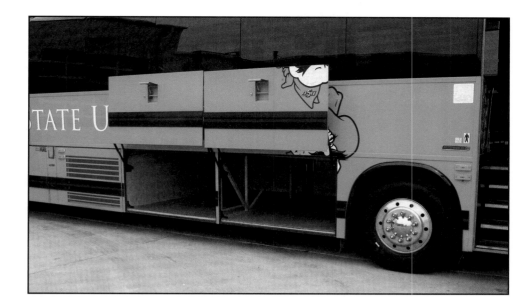

Figure 7.29 The luggage and cargo compartments along one side of a commercial bus.

extend completely through to the other side of the bus, firefighters may be need to open the doors on both sides of the bus when attacking a fire in this area **(Figure 7.29)**.

Once the fire has been knocked down, pike poles can be used to either pull or push the cargo out of the storage area and onto the ground. Emptying the cargo compartment will lessen the overall damage to the bus and make extinguishment and overhaul much quicker and easier. As with any other vehicle fire, firefighters should wear self-contained breathing apparatus.

Commercial Bus Batteries

The location of the batteries on commercial motor coaches varies depending on the manufacturer of the bus. Many are found just aft of the front wheel on the passenger side of the bus.

Regardless of the location of the batteries, all manufacturers place an electrical disconnect switch in the battery compartment. This switch will either be directly above or below the batteries. Electrical service to the bus's 24-volt systems (power plant, air-conditioning systems, etc.) can be interrupted by operating this switch **(Figure 7.30, p. 322)**. In some cases, interior emergency lights will still have power even though the battery switch is off. To de-energize these systems, it will be necessary to disconnect or cut the battery cables. When isolating the battery the negative terminal should be disconnected first.

Specialty Buses

Some specialty buses are similar to Type A and B school buses but have been converted into vehicles for transporting those with disabilities. Others are commercial buses that have been converted into mobile living quarters, offices, and recreational vehicles.

Transporters of those with disabilities may have fewer passengers than school buses of the same size but the occupants may be less able to help themselves in an emergency. Commercial bus conversions present the same extrication problems and challenges as any other commercial bus, but usually with fewer passengers.

CAUTION
While buses should not be used to transport hazardous materials, the operator does not check the contents of passengers' bags.

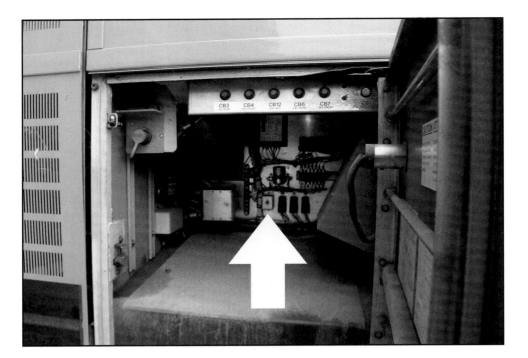

Figure 7.30 The disconnect switch for a commercial bus' electrical system.

Converted buses have the same general construction features as the conventional vehicles from which the conversions were made — with a few exceptions. The following sections discuss some of the exceptional features of bus conversions.

Type A/B School Bus Conversions

Many Type A/B school buses have been converted into transports for those with disabilities. These conversions are different from the conventional Type A/B units in several ways. First, they are usually designed to carry fewer total passengers because of the space requirements for wheelchairs and other devices. Secondly, the center aisles in these buses are significantly wider than those in conventional buses so there is more room for EMS personnel to maneuver inside the vehicle **(Figure 7.31)**. Finally, many of these units are equipped with double entry/exit doors located midship on the passenger side. The entry/exit stairs also convert to an electrically operated wheelchair lift. When equipped with a wheelchair lift, a separate battery box for supplying power to the lift is usually located on the driver's side of the vehicle. Disconnecting this battery will not interrupt power to the engine.

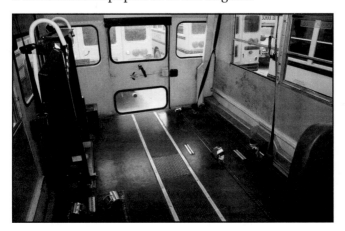

Figure 7.31 This section of a Type B school bus was converted to provide space for passengers in wheelchairs. A hydraulic lift can be seen folded into the travel position on the left side of the picture.

Commercial Bus Conversions

Commercial buses have been converted for a variety of purposes. Some have been converted into transports for prisoners. Others have been converted into large mobile field hospitals and ambulances. Some have been converted into mobile command posts and communications vehicles by fire departments and other public safety agencies **(Figure 7.32)**. Others have been converted into mobile living quarters for entertainers and offices for others whose jobs require them to relocate with relative frequency.

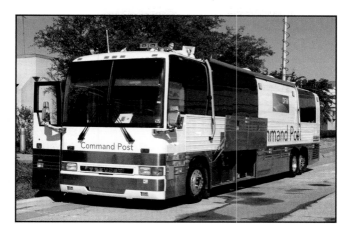

Figure 7.32 An example of a commercial bus converted into a department of public safety mobile command post.

In most cases, since these are conversions of conventional buses, the basic construction will remain the same as other conventional buses of that type. The major differences will be in how the interiors of the converted buses are configured. Those converted as prisoner transports may have more-or-less conventional seating but the windows may be covered with bars, heavy gauge wire screens, or even metal plates with louvers to allow for air circulation. Those converted for use as mobile offices may have most of the original seating removed and typical office furniture in its place. There may or may not be separate sleeping quarters. Those that have been converted into mobile living quarters may be more like motor homes than buses, but their basic structure is still that of a commercial bus, and rescue personnel should follow the protocols and procedures recommended for that type of bus. These conversions can often be identified by their blacked-out windows and the sometimes garish cosmetics on the vehicle's exterior.

Bus Fuels

Modern buses run on a variety of fuels. Many use common fuels such as gasoline or diesel while others use alternative fuels such as compressed natural gas (CNG) or liquefied petroleum gas (LPG). Hybrid systems are also becoming more popular on buses.

Gasoline and Diesel

Most school bus fuel systems use either gasoline or diesel fuel. Nearly all transit and commercial buses are powered by diesel fuel, although some are powered by a mixture of diesel fuel and kerosene. Depending upon their size and weight, motor homes may use any of these fuels. Fuel tanks on Type A and B buses are commonly in the rear of the vehicle. The fuel tank(s) on school buses, transit buses, and commercial buses may be as large as 180 gallons (720 L). In Type C and D school buses, as well as most transit and commercial buses, the fuel tank is located in the midship portion of the bus or slightly ahead of midship, just behind the front wheels. The fuel filler is usually located on the passenger side, just behind the front wheels, although some commercial buses may be equipped with fillers on both sides of the vehicle.

Alternative Bus Fuels

Many transit buses and motor homes are powered by engines using alternative fuels — those other than gasoline or diesel. Some are powered by CNG and others LPG. The presence of an alternative fuel system may be evident because of decals or other signs on the exterior of the vehicle indicating the type of fuel in use. Otherwise, the presence of a fuel filler and main supply valve at some point on the lower half of the vehicle body may be the only indication. In any case, the fuel filler and main supply valve will be located at the same point, and this point should be relatively easy to access because it is where the filler hose connects.

Alternative fuels behave differently when released into the atmosphere because of their differing vapor densities. At this point, it is sufficient to remember that CNG is lighter than air, so it will rise when released, perhaps filling the passenger compartment. LPG is heavier than air, so it will fall when released and will collect in depressions and other low areas. In both cases, at the point of optimum fuel/air mixture, these are both highly flammable gases and represent significant safety hazards.

Other buses are powered by alternative fuels such as hydrogen. These fuels and fuel systems are considered experimental, and their use is still limited to a very small number of vehicles. When buses using these or any other alternative fuels are introduced into an area, the rescue personnel in that jurisdiction should familiarize themselves with the fuels and their characteristics.

Hybrid Buses

Numerous cities in the United States and around the world have begun using hybrid propulsion systems for transit buses. Yosemite National Park has begun using hybrid buses as part of their shuttle service. These buses are designed to reduce hydrocarbon fuel consumption and improve air quality in these locations.

These systems contain a vehicle propulsion system (a diesel or gasoline powered internal combustion engine), a battery system to store electricity, and an electric motor. The electrical motor is frequently used to run the bus on level terrain or in tunnels while the internal combustion engine is used to provide power while on surface streets and when climbing grades.

There are two primary hybrid propulsion system configurations: series and parallel. In the series configuration, the internal combustion engine runs a generator that provides power for the battery or electric motor. In the parallel configuration, the electric motor and the internal combustion engine are both connected to the vehicles transmission to individually or simultaneously provide power to move the vehicle. Some hybrid buses are equipped with a larger, secondary battery storage system that can be recharged at night from the local electrical grid.

Hybrid buses physically resemble conventional buses and most construction features are similar. The major difference is that hybrid buses are constructed to include the battery storage system, electrical motor, and the wiring to connect them together. Extrication personnel must be cautious while isolating the power supplies on these vehicles because of the high voltage carried in these systems.

Electricity

Some local transit buses do not have liquid or gaseous fuel because they are powered by electricity supplied from overhead wires through a rooftop apparatus called a pantograph **(Figure 7.33)**. As discussed in greater detail in Chapter 9, *Rail Car Extrication*, rescue personnel should avoid working on the roof of any vehicle powered in this way — even if the pantograph is disconnected from the overhead wires.

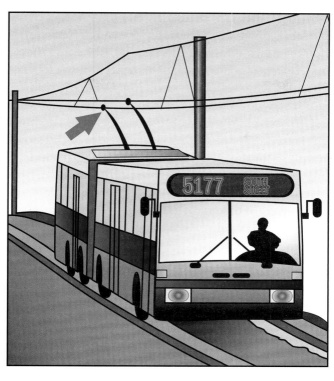

Figure 7.33 Some buses are powered by electricity that is supplied from overhead wires through a pantograph.

Specific Size-Up Concerns for Bus Extrication

Given the possible number of trapped patients and the potential for loss of life in a serious collision involving a fully loaded bus, the importance of performing a rapid but thorough size-up cannot be overstated. There may well be dozens of patients trapped inside, outside, or under a crashed bus — many of them needing immediate medical intervention to save their lives — so the first-arriving resources at this type of incident can easily be overwhelmed. Therefore, it is critical that the Incident Commander (IC) develop an incident action plan (IAP) and order any other needed resources as soon as possible. Additional cribbing, airbags, and other lifting equipment might be needed to safely and efficiently stabilize or lift the vehicle.

Because buses are large and designed to carry a large number of passengers, an accident involving a bus may result in a large number of injured personnel. More ambulances and EMS personnel may be required to provide first aid and life support to those injured during a bus incident than at a car accident. Multiple patients aboard a bus can also create a patient removal problem. It may be necessary to clear less injured patients out of access ways first, prior to moving other, possibly more seriously injured patients.

Bus Stabilization

In every vehicle extrication incident, one of the first tasks is to stabilize the vehicle. Stabilization must precede gaining entry to evaluate or extricate patients trapped inside the vehicle. Stabilizing buses upright and in various other positions is discussed in the sections that follow.

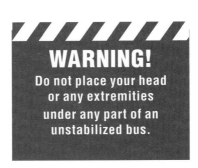

WARNING!
Do not place your head or any extremities under any part of an unstabilized bus.

Bus Upright/On Wheels: Stabilization

If a bus is upright, the task is to prevent it from moving in the most likely directions — horizontally and vertically. Chocking the wheels usually prevents any bus, regardless of type or size, from moving forward or backward. Whenever possible, wheel chocks — and not pieces of cribbing — should be used. Manufactured wheel chocks are usually more effective, and it saves the cribbing for use in stabilizing the vehicle. However, if the bus is on a slope — especially if it is in danger of rolling sideways down the slope — it may be necessary to supplement the wheel chocks with a chain, cable, or webbing attached to the bus and a "bombproof" anchor point. The term bombproof is taken from rope rescue and it means any object that absolutely, positively cannot be moved by the weight of whatever is attached to it. Stabilizing a bus horizontally may require a heavy-duty tow truck, a huge boulder, or a large, fully mature tree as an anchor point.

In general, vertically stabilizing a school bus is no different from vertically stabilizing any other bus. Most school buses built by either integral construction or the body-on-chassis method all have conventional heavy-duty suspension — that is, leaf and/or coil springs. Most transit, commercial, and some newer school buses are equipped with air suspension systems. In these systems, the conventional metal springs are replaced with compact rubber air bags that are similar to a bellows. At each wheel, there are two air suspension bags — one on each side of the axle. An on-board compressor maintains the air pressure within the bags as high as 120 psi (840 kPa). Depending upon the load of the vehicle and the condition of the road, the pressure within each bag is automatically increased or decreased to maintain the bus in a level state. If the pressure in an air suspension bag is lost because of damage to the bag or its associated piping, the chassis of the bus can suddenly drop without warning to within 3 to 3½ inches (76 mm to 89 mm) of the roadway surface.

Some transit and commercial buses are equipped with an air inlet valve on the front end. This valve allows the bus to be hooked to an air compressor or cascade system to reinflate a collapsed suspension system in a controlled environment by trained vehicle service technicians. Reinflation of the suspension system by emergency response personnel should not be considered due to the potential for catastrophic failure of the system that could cause further injuries to patients and rescuers.

Even though a small percentage of transit and commercial buses are equipped with a standard mechanical suspension system (similar to that of a school bus), unless rescuers are positive that the bus being worked on has a mechanical suspension system, the bus should be treated as one that has an air suspension system.

Because most transit and commercial buses do not have a rigid frame, they are equipped with specially designed jack plates for use as contact points for cribbing or jacks. On transit buses, these plates are located slightly behind each axle, near each wheel. On commercial buses, the jack plates are located under the body between the two rear axles and in back of the front axle. Again, cribbing may be used on these points, although they are designed more for use with hydraulic jacks. All four jack plates should be supported to completely stabilize the vehicle. If rescuers are unsure of the location of jack plates on a particular bus, cribbing the body at any solid frame member can stabilize the vehicle. If possible, the middle axle (also known as the "bogie" or "tag" axle) should also be cribbed.

When cribbing is used to stabilize a bus, the cribbing must be large enough to hold the weight of the bus. Generally, 6- x 6-inch (150 mm by 150 mm) wooden cribbing is the minimum size that should be used. If hydraulic jacks are used to stabilize or lift the bus, they should be of at least 8-ton (7 250 kg) capacity. On many buses, each axle is equipped with a piece of tubing welded on the axle near each wheel. This tubing is designed to accept the shaft of a jack to prevent the jack from slipping.

In some cases, the engine supports can be used as jack points. However, this should be done only if there is no other alternative and if it is possible for rescuers to access these supports without having to place themselves beneath the unsupported bus. Because of their location beneath the bus, using these engine supports as jack points can be dangerous.

As mentioned earlier, rescuers should never place any part of themselves under any portion of an unsupported vehicle. Cribbing or jacks should be pushed into position using another piece of cribbing, a pike pole, or some similar device. Jacks should be equipped with handles that allow them to be operated from outside the perimeter of the vehicle.

To stabilize a bus, cribbing and wedges or shims should be installed at a sufficient number of points to prevent the bus from settling any further. If jacks are used, they should be extended only to the point where they would begin to lift the bus. If the objective is to lift the bus, the jacks should be extended slowly and evenly. As the bus is raised, cribbing should be added to minimize the distance the bus will fall should the jack(s) fail. The bus should be raised only as much as necessary to stabilize it — and no more.

NOTE: Always follow this standard rule when lifting: Lift an inch, crib an inch.

Bus on Side: Stabilization

Stabilizing any bus that has come to rest on its side is virtually the same regardless of whether it is a school bus, transit bus, or commercial bus. Because the sides of most buses are large flat surfaces, buses in this position tend to be relatively stable. However, if the crash that caused it to roll has drastically altered its original shape, or if it came to rest on an uneven surface, a bus on its side may be anything but stable. Just as in any other vehicle extrication incident, the goal is to create as many points of contact between the bus and the surface on which it rests as are necessary to prevent sudden and unexpected movement of the bus in any direction. This stability is usually achieved through the use of cribbing, step chocks, shoring, jacks, or a combination of these. These devices should be installed as described in earlier chapters. The bus may also need to be secured to a solid object with chains, cables, or webbing.

Depending upon the dynamics of the crash and other variables in the situation, a bus on its side may leak fuel and other flammable fluids — and access to the means of controlling these and other hazards may be difficult if not impossible. The battery compartment may be on the underside of the

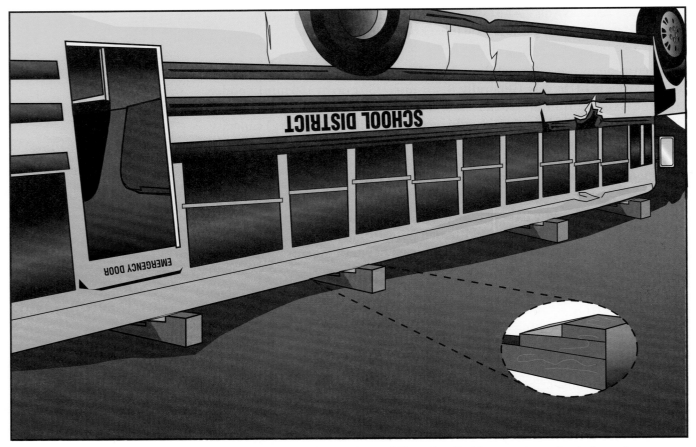

Figure 7.34 This illustration shows how step chocks can be used to stabilize a bus that has overturned onto its roof.

vehicle. The fuel supply valve on an LPG- or LNG-fueled vehicle may likewise be inaccessible. These situations make the need for fire protection a very high priority. When fire protection is indicated, it should be provided with no less than two 1½-inch (38 mm) hoselines with foam capability.

Bus on Roof: Stabilization

Just as with automobiles, most buses have rounded contours along the junction between their roof and sides. In addition, the roof itself is usually rounded to a greater or lesser extent. Unless its roof was significantly flattened during the crash, a bus that has come to rest upside down on a flat surface may be very unstable and will require the installation of multiple step chocks or other similar devices along both sides of the bus, and perhaps both ends **(Figure 7.34)**.

The amount of fuel and other fluids leaking from a bus that is on its roof may be even greater than that from a bus on its side. Liquid fuels will almost certainly leak from the fuel filler. Engine oil will drain from the crankcase, and battery acid may drain from the batteries. This combination of uncontrolled fluids can drain into electrical components causing short circuits and increasing the danger of fire ignition. Therefore, fire protection is a very high priority.

Buses in Other Positions: Stabilization

Just as with automobiles, buses can come to rest in any of a variety of positions other than those already described. A bus may be still on its wheels but on such an angle that it is in danger of falling onto its side — or even worse — rolling over and over down a steep hillside. The lives of those trapped inside the bus may depend upon fast and efficient work by the first rescuers on scene to stabilize the vehicle. Buses in these unusual situations can tax the ingenuity and resourcefulness of these rescuers. The situation will dictate the means by which rescuers can stabilize the bus. Therefore, rescuers must be thoroughly trained in the use — and adaptation — of all available tools and equipment, both from within the agency and from outside sources.

When a bus loaded with passengers has come to rest in an unusual position, rescuers may have to use a combination of cribbing, jacks, shoring, and other devices. They may have to secure the vehicle with chains, cables, or webbing attached to a secure anchor point. Or, they may have to employ tow trucks or cranes to stabilize the vehicle.

Secondary Vehicles, Overrides and Underrides

Other, smaller vehicles are often involved in accidents with buses. The amount of damage incurred by these vehicles will depend upon size of the smaller vehicle or vehicles and the type of impact made with the bus. As in other motor vehicle accidents, rescuers must search each vehicle involved in the accident as well as the area surrounding the accident scene to locate any potential patients.

Accidents involving buses can and do include override and underride situations. Bus over rides tend to result in extreme damage and injury to other, smaller vehicles and their passengers. Often, it is extremely difficult to gain access to the patients in the smaller vehicle because of the size and weight of the bus. Underride situations, while rare, can cause severe damage and injury to the bus and its passengers.

Hazard Control

Another very important part of incidents involving buses is controlling and mitigating the other hazards that may be present. Among these other hazards are the vehicle's engine, its electrical power supply, leaking fuel or other hazardous substances, and downed power lines.

Power Shutoffs

As in the crash of any type of motor vehicle, one of the most important functions rescuers must perform as part of stabilizing a bus is to disconnect the vehicle's batteries. This eliminates a possible ignition source for flammable vapors and also de-energizes any power equipment that may still be functioning. Operating the battery shutoff switch located in the battery compartment, disconnecting the battery cables, or cutting the cables are all methods for interrupting the electrical power supply.

Before switching off or disconnecting the batteries, rescuers should first shut off the engine, if it is still running. A running engine causes vibration that may further injure patients, may add noise that can upset patients and hinder communications and could cause the bus to move. Rescuers should first attempt to turn the ignition key or push the ignition system switch to the "off"

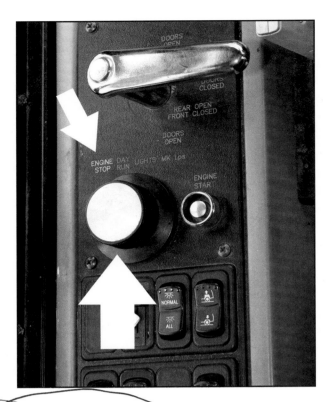

Figure 7.35a A driver's engine stop switch located on a panel to the driver's left.

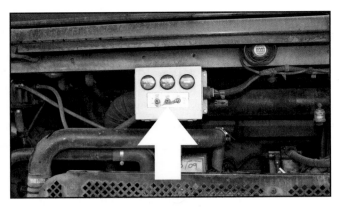

Figure 7.35b An engine stop switch mounted in a bus' engine compartment.

position. This will minimize the chance of an electrical system malfunction and will shut off the vehicle's engine. On buses equipped with an alternate fuel system, such as LPG or propane, shutting off the fuel system main supply valve will also stop the engine.

Transit and commercial buses have engine stop switches located on the driver's console, usually to the left of the driver's seat. In addition, a stop switch is located in the rear engine compartment. It should be clearly marked and is usually found in the top left or right corner of the compartment. The stop button may have either an on/off position or it may be a push button that has to be held in until the engine comes to a complete stop **(Figures 7.35a and b)**.

NOTE: Use extreme care when opening the engine compartment door(s). There are no safety guards around the fans and their speed of rotation makes them difficult to see. Contact with a moving fan may result in serious injury.

If these methods do not stop a running engine, CO_2, Halons, or halon replacement agents can be discharged into the air intake located at the rear corner of the vehicle. Air intakes may be located on either or both sides of the vehicle. Rescuers should discharge the extinguishing agent into the air intake screen area, aiming the main stream of it inward and toward the front of the vehicle. Because this method is dangerous, it is to be used ONLY if all other attempts to stop the engine have failed.

Batteries on Type A and B school buses are usually located in the engine compartment. If the bus is equipped as a handicapped transport with an electric lift, a separate battery may be provided for the lift. This battery is usually located in a separate compartment on the driver's side of the vehicle. However, disconnecting this battery will not interrupt power to the engine.

On Type C and D school buses, the batteries will be located either under the hood or in a separate compartment on the driver's side of the bus. In some buses, a hex key or Allen wrench must be used to unlatch the compartment door. The required key is usually located inside the school bus near the driver's area. In the absence of a key device, battery compartment doors may have to be forced open. Just as with school buses, the batteries of transit buses and commercial buses should be disconnected to interrupt the flow of electrical power to the rest of the bus.

Fuel Leaks

Many Type A, B, and C school buses, and other buses of similar size, have gasoline-powered engines. Other buses of all sizes operate on alternative fuels such as LPG or LNG. Because of the volatility and flammability of these fuels, it is critically important that any leaks be controlled and any spilled fuel be covered with Class B foam. As mentioned earlier, shutting off the main fuel supply valve on those buses operating on alternative fuels will interrupt the flow of fuel. Because of the possibility of LPG or LNG becoming trapped in and around a crashed bus, it may be necessary to ventilate the area using intrinsically safe fans.

Downed Power Lines

A relatively small percentage of bus crashes involve downed power lines. However, if they are involved, they add another potentially life-threatening dimension to the incident. One of the most frustrating and most dangerous vehicle extrication scenarios is that in which an injured vehicle occupant can be seen through the vehicle's windows but rescuers cannot touch the vehicle because it is in contact with a downed power line. Because rescue personnel are trained to help those in need, the temptation to assume that the power line is no longer energized — or to attempt to move the power line off the vehicle — becomes almost overwhelming. But it must be resisted! Until power has been shut off by utility service personnel, rescuers must assume that all power lines are energized.

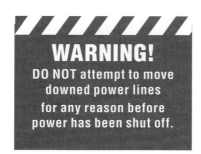

WARNING!
DO NOT attempt to move downed power lines for any reason before power has been shut off.

While waiting for utility service personnel to arrive at the scene, rescuers should cordon off the area of the downed power line to protect themselves and others at the scene. The presence of a downed power line should be announced over the radio to alert all emergency personnel and over public address systems or bull horns to alert others.

Bus Interior Access

Once a crashed bus has been stabilized, rescuers can begin the task of gaining access into the interior of the vehicle. Access is necessary before rescue personnel can perform the remaining functions: patient triage and initial treatment, disentanglement, and extrication. In any extrication incident involving a bus, there are three primary access routes: doors, windows, and other openings.

Doors

Assuming that the bus has come to rest in a position that allows access to the front service door, this is the preferred starting point. Rescuers should always first attempt to open doors in the normal, operating manual. Most front doors

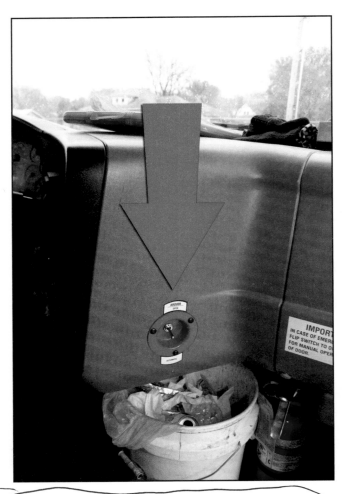

Figure 7.36 An emergency door opening button located on the bottom edge of the driver's console in the center of a school bus dashboard.

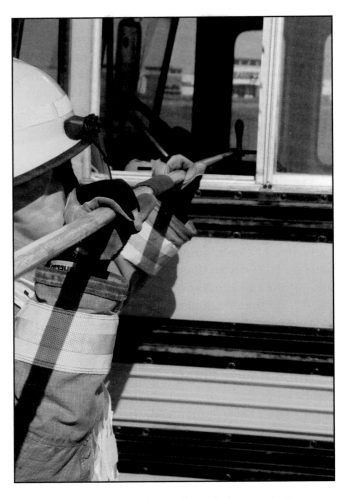

Figure 7.37 A rescuer using a pike pole to operate the manual door opening pivot arm control.

on buses are designed to operate only from the inside, while rear emergency doors are operable from both the inside and outside. Rarely are all doors inoperable following a collision.

Operable Front Doors

Entry may be somewhat difficult if the front door is the "operable door" but is in the closed position. However, the door will often be open because passengers will have escaped through it, leaving it open.

On buses so equipped, the quickest way to open front doors is to use the emergency opening button located below the center of the windshield **(Figure 7.36)**. Some newer buses have this button located on the exterior of the A-post in front of the door. On other buses, the fastest way is to create an avenue of access to the center pivot arm control and operate the door in the normal manner in one of the following two ways:

Remove the windshield so that a rescuer can reach through the opening and manually operate the control.

Reach in through the driver's side window with a pike pole to operate the control **(Figure 7.37)**.

If the door is operated by an alternate method, such as an air-actuated control mechanism, it can be opened by reaching in through the driver's side window and operating the main switch. This switch is usually located to the left of the driver's instrument console. There will also be a backup emergency release mechanism in the stairwell just inside the door. The readily identifiable release button or switch permits the air lock device to release the door. Then, rescue personnel can manually move the door through its normal path of travel. The air override release mechanism may not be required if there are two operable doors located along the same side of the bus.

Stair Removal

Removing the entrance steps from a bus may be performed by utilizing hydraulic cutters in combination with reciprocating saws or pneumatic tools to cut the material away from the bus. This can be a lengthy process because of the materials involved in the construction of the steps.

Inoperable Front Doors

If it is necessary to force the doors, any type of power spreading tool may be used. First, rescuers should identify the type of door by locating the hinges. If there are hinges on either side of the door and an overlapping rubber seal in the middle, it is a center opening door. This type of door can be pried open by inserting a power spreader between the two overlapping seals about half way up the door and forcing each half to its respective side. It may be necessary to repeat this procedure at the top and bottom of the door to maximize the size of the opening.

A jammed center opening door can also be cut apart, disconnected, or disassembled. It is often possible to remove the door by breaking the hinges (usually piano hinges) that connect it to the bus. Breaking the hinges can usually be done by driving the wedge end of a Halligan into the hinge area with a sledgehammer. This will usually fracture the hinge, enabling rescuers to remove the door. The pivot control arm will also have to be cut or detached to completely remove the door.

If the door has hinges in the middle and on one side, during normal operation it will open toward the side with the hinges. When using spreaders on this type of door, they should be inserted between the nonhinged side and the frame. The entire door can then be forced toward the hinged side. Depending on the circumstances, it may also be necessary to completely remove the door.

Because of the narrowness of the front door area on some older buses, it may be difficult to maneuver litters and/or immobilized patients through that area. To create a wider space near the front door, rescuers should perform the following procedures:

1. Cut through the A-post at the top of the windshield opening.

2. Make a relief cut in the bottom of the A-post at floor level.

3. Insert an extension ram between the A- and B-posts parallel to the ground at the top of the dashboard level.

4. Extend the ram to push the front wall forward.

Rear Doors

If it is necessary to use the rear emergency exit door for access following a rear-end collision, it may be necessary to force this door open. The rear exit door is held secure by one or three latch points. The main latch is at the edge of the door near the control handle. The other two latches, if present, are found at the top and bottom of the door, locking into the bus body and the floor assembly. This door may be forced open by inserting a prying or spreading tool between the door and the frame and separating the two.

Inserting a spreading tool on the hinged side of the door and operating it to rip the hinges off the frame will remove the door. If a spreading tool is not available, the rear door can also be disassembled, disconnected, or cut apart with a variety of other rescue tools. **Skill Sheet 7-1** describes the procedures for forcing the rear door.

One reason that removing a rear door is slightly more difficult than removing other doors is that the rear door is normally higher above the roadway surface. Rescuers will have to stand on something to effectively operate the rescue tool. Any object that provides solid footing will suffice.

Sometimes opening or removing the rear door still does not provide a large enough opening to remove immobilized patients. In these cases, it may also be necessary to remove part of the rear wall of the bus.

If the bus comes to rest on its side with the hinge side up, it may be difficult for small children to push the rear door open because of its weight. Rescuers should first try to open the door using the handle. Once the door is open, it must be propped open with a pike pole or similar tool. If time permits, remove the door. Removal of the rear wall is a good idea when a bus comes to rest on its side **(Figures 7.38a, b, and c)**. Rear wall removal eliminates the need to step over the wall every time someone goes through the exit. The procedure for removing the rear wall is the same as that described for upright buses.

Windows

The windshield and side and rear windows can be used as access points for gaining entry into a bus. Each provides different advantages and disadvantages for the rescuers.

Windshield Access

Entry through the windshield can be advantageous when the front exit is unusable or the bus has come to rest on its side. Removing the windshield will give rescuers quick access to the interior of the bus and will also provide a route for removing patients.

Unlike automobile windshields, bus windshields are often divided into two or more parts, which may be separated by posts. Bus windshields are mounted with gaskets that are somewhat different than those used for automobile windshields, although removal methods are basically the same. To remove a bus windshield, rubber mounting gasket should be cut with a knife, baling hook, or other similar tool.

Once the gasket is removed, a rescuer should next remove each piece of the windshield. If no rescuer is inside the bus yet, rescuers can sometimes reach through the gasket gap with the end of a baling hook and gently pull the glass

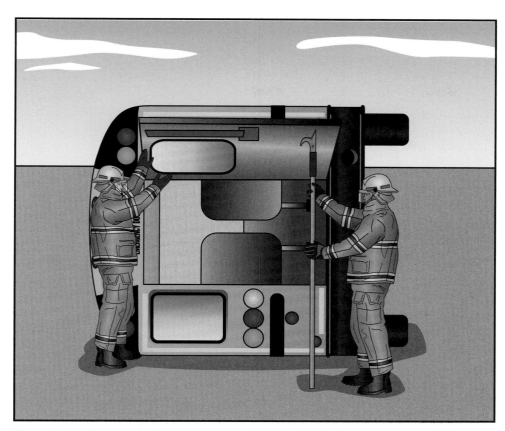

Figure 7.38a Rescuers using a pike pole to hold a rear exit door open.

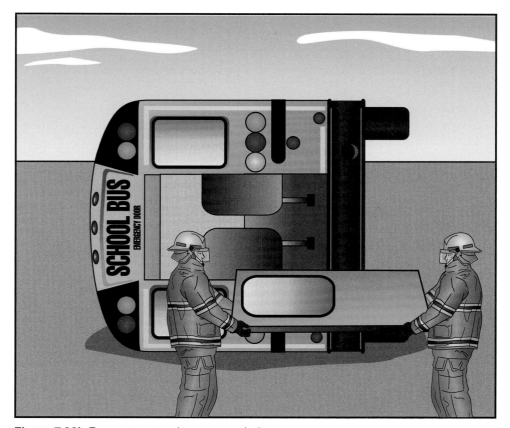

Figure 7.38b Rescuers removing a rear exit door.

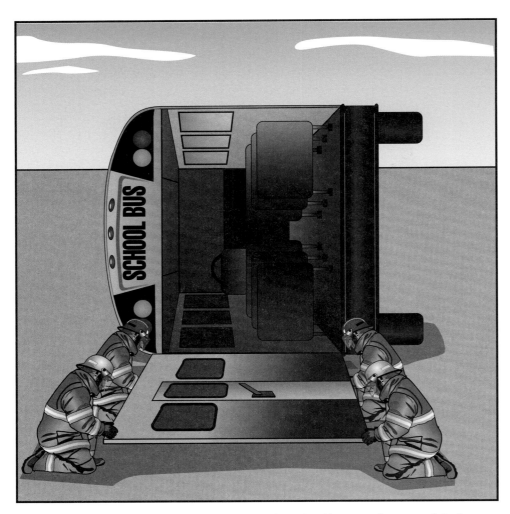

Figure 7.38c Rescuers removing the rear wall of a school bus to gain access into the vehicle.

toward them. If a rescuer is already inside the bus, a gentle push on the glass should loosen it enough that the rescuers on the outside can remove it. After the glass has been removed, removing the center windshield post will provide rescuers with a full width opening through which they can work.

NOTE: Rear windows can be removed in a similar manner; however, it is preferable to use the rear exit door or completely cut away the rear walls whenever possible.

Side Window Access

Gaining access through the side windows may be difficult for two reasons: (1) they are small, and (2) they may be 6 to 8 feet (2 m to 2.5 m) above ground level. Rescuers must work from ladders or platforms which makes it more difficult to handle tools and patients.

Even with the positive latching systems found on many transit and commercial buses, the side windows can be pried open from the outside with a screwdriver or other rescue tool. Many buses have a small access hatch that rescuers can reach through to open a window from the inside. This hatch is usually level with the bottom of the last window on the passenger side of the bus. On commercial buses, it is located directly outside the restroom. It will be necessary for the rescuer to stand on a ladder or other object to reach this hatch. Once the hatch is opened, the rescuer can reach in and operate the window latch to open the window. Then, rescuers can enter and open more windows as necessary.

Most school buses have side windows that only slide down part way. They provide an opening of about 9 x 22 inches (225 mm by 550 mm), which is too small to be useful. Therefore, it will be necessary to enlarge the window opening. To double the size of the window opening, rescuers should break the glass and remove the aluminum frame from the opening. Almost any cutting tool can be used to cut away the soft aluminum window frame.

NOTE: Remove the glass using standard techniques described in Chapter 5, *Extrication Techniques*.

Removing two adjacent windows and the post between them followed by removing the same section of sidewall can enlarge the opening of a window that is too small for extrication purposes. If necessary, more windows can be removed and the posts cut. However, removing too many posts may compromise the structural integrity of the bus.

Side Wall Access

Even though forcing entry through the sides of a bus can be time consuming because of the extensive amount of skeletal structure and the obstructions posed by the seats, it may sometimes be necessary. It becomes necessary when the bus has remained upright but the front and rear exits are unusable. If the proper equipment is available, a large hole can be cut that will provide maximum access to the passenger area.

Forcible entry through the side of a bus will require considerable work to cut a usable opening. The heaviest beams in bus construction are located on the floor, where the seats bolt to the wall, and above and below the windows. The seats should be removed before opening a side wall.

If time allows, the seats can be unbolted from the floor. If not, the steel tube seat frame can be cut with any number of cutting tools. Cutting the legs or supports may leave sharp stubs, and they should be covered with duct tape to prevent additional injuries.

Once the seats have been cleared away and the windows and posts removed, cutting on the side wall may begin. The best tool for this operation is the reciprocating saw with a 6-inch (150 mm) metal cutting blade. This combination will cut through any of the structural components found in the side wall of the bus. See **Skill Sheet 7-2** for the steps in cutting through the side wall of a bus.

Another way to remove a portion of the side wall is to remove entire sheets of metal by using an air chisel to pop the rivets or welds that hold the sheets. Once the sheets are removed, the individual beams in the side of the bus can be cut. However, this method is considerably slower and noisier than using a reciprocating saw and should only be used as a last resort.

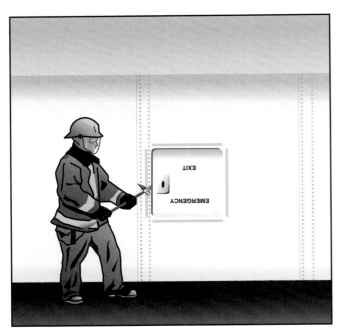

Figure 7.39 A rescuer using a halligan bar to pry open a roof emergency hatch on an overturned bus.

Roof Access

In some cases, it may be necessary to gain access through the roof of a bus. A roof opening may be needed when a bus has come to rest on its side, and occasionally on an upright bus. When a bus lands on its side, the front door may be virtually useless. It will either be under the bus, making it inaccessible, or it will be on top, making it difficult to use for evacuation purposes. Access may still be possible through the rear emergency door or windshield; however, these openings may not be sufficient or may themselves be blocked. Any of these situations may require rescuers to make entry through the roof.

The first choice for removing patients through the roof should be to use any roof escape hatches with which the bus may be equipped. These hatches are easy to force from the outside. Most can be pried off with any standard prying tool or power spreading tool **(Figure 7.39)**. However, these hatches only provide a clear opening of up to about 2 feet (0.6 m) square. They may be too small to allow the removal of immobilized patients requiring rescuers to enlarge the opening.

Before beginning to cut, rescuers must determine the best location for the roof opening. The location of the patients inside the bus, the position of the bus, and the type and amount of damage to the bus all combined determine the best location for a roof opening. If there are patients located throughout the entire length of the bus, the opening should be cut where it will be most effective. Each situation will dictate where the best location is.

Cutting an opening in the roof of the bus can sometimes be difficult and time consuming. However, the overall benefits can easily justify the time involved. Cutting an opening in the roof can provide rescuers with more or less complete access to the interior of the bus. However, cutting an opening in a bus roof can be time consuming because of the multiple layers of materials that are used in the roof's construction. The roof is comprised of two layers of sheet metal with supports, insulation, and wiring sandwiched between them.

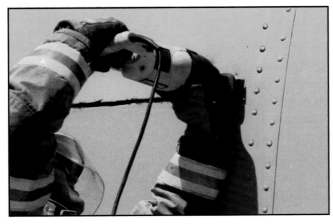

Figure 7.40 Rescuers can use a reciprocating saw to cut through a bus roof.

While an air chisel can be used if that is all that is available, it is not ideal. Because an air chisel can only cut one layer of metal at a time, the layers have to be cut one at a time. This virtually doubles the amount of time needed to cut the opening.

The most effective tool for cutting roof panels is a reciprocating saw with at least a 6-inch (150 mm) blade. The reciprocating saw will produce a smooth cut through all layers of material at one time, and with little chance of igniting any flammable vapors in the area **(Figure 7.40)**. The procedures for cutting an access hole in a bus roof are listed in **Skill Sheet 7-3**.

Sometimes access through the front of the bus is needed. In these cases, it may be useful to flap a portion of the roof backward. While this procedure is possible with the proper equipment, it will be difficult. **Skill Sheet 7-4** covers the steps for "flapping" a bus roof.

Floor Access

Gaining access through the floor of a bus should only be considered as a last resort. Fortunately, this will rarely be necessary. Any attempt to breach this area will require a considerable amount of time because of the many layers of materials that are combined to construct the floor. Bus floors consist of a heavy frame to support the entire bus, plus sheet metal, plywood, and a vinyl or rubber floor covering. The beams and other framework are often placed as close as 9 inches (225 mm) apart. One factor helping rescuers is the fact that, depending on the manufacturer of the bus, only every third or fourth beam is a solid, supporting member. The beams in between are only welded to the underside of the floor and provide little support or hindrance to rescue operations. Because through-the-floor access is likely to be attempted only when the bus is on its side or roof, the fuel tank, which is mounted under the vehicle, will be inverted and probably leaking fuel near the cutting area. This makes the risk of a flash fire very high.

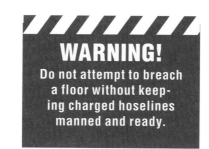

WARNING!
Do not attempt to breach a floor without keeping charged hoselines manned and ready.

Regardless of the type of bus, the steps involved in cutting an access opening are virtually the same. **Skill Sheet 7-5** lists the steps for cutting an access hole in a bus floor.

Because of the massive understructure associated with transit buses and commercial buses, access through the undercarriage and floor is a difficult and tedious job. When a storage area is located between the bottom of the bus and the actual underside of the floor, an access opening must first be cut through the storage area floor and then through the main floor of the bus. The other methods of gaining access previously described in this section should be used as alternatives to access through the floor of a bus.

Rear Wall Access

Sometimes opening or removing the rear door still does not provide a large enough opening to remove immobilized patients. In these cases, it may also be necessary to remove part of the rear wall of the bus. The rear glass should be removed and center two pillars cut high. A rescuer can then use a suitable tool to cut along the bottom edge of both side panels of the rear of the bus. Next a rescuers should cut the outer two pillars on the outside edge from the window edge allowing the door and both rear sides of the bus to open up for a full rear access or egress point. Removal of one or two rows of the rear seats will allow greater access to the interior of the bus. The procedures for removing the rear wall were described in **Skill Sheet 7-6**.

If the bus comes to rest on its side with the hinge side up, it may be difficult for small children to push the rear door open because of its weight. Rescuers should first try to open the door using the handle. Once the door is open, it must be secured in the open position. If time permits, remove the door. Removal of the rear wall is a good idea when a bus comes to rest on its side. This eliminates the need to step over the wall every time someone goes through the exit. The procedure for removing the rear wall is the same as that described for upright buses.

Bus Extrication Tactics

Once a crashed bus has been stabilized and access has been gained, rescuers can enter the bus for triage, disentanglement, and extrication of the patients trapped inside. While many of the required tools and techniques are the same regardless of the position of the bus, the extrication process is discussed with the bus upright, on its side, on its roof, and in other positions.

Bus Upright/On Wheels: Extrication

When a bus has been involved in a front-end or rear-end collision, the bus often remains in an upright position. In front-end collisions, the driver is sometimes trapped by the steering wheel. Bus drivers often must tilt the steering wheel down into their laps when they take the driver's seat. In the event of a collision, the wheel in this lowered position virtually traps the driver even before any impact. After impact, the driver usually cannot move the steering wheel into its original position and, therefore, cannot get out of the driver's seat even if he or she is able. A first instinct of rescuers might be to pull the steering column and steering wheel up and away from the driver as might be performed in a vehicle extrication. This technique is not recommended, however. Just as in an automobile, tilting the steering wheel or cutting the steering wheel ring puts the driver at less risk of being injured by the end of the steering column pivoting into his or her torso. In many cases, it is possible to free the driver by simply tilting the steering wheel toward the windshield. In some older buses, cutting the brace between the steering column and the front wall of the bus may be necessary. Otherwise, cutting the steering wheel ring may be the next best option.

The steering wheel on a bus is constructed in a manner similar to that of an automobile. A hardened steel ring is molded inside a covering of rubber or plastic. The quickest method of freeing the patient is to cut away the bottom half of the steering ring. While a hacksaw or reciprocating saw can be used to cut the ring, a power shear is the tool of choice. Often, this alone will free the driver, thus eliminating the need for further action. A bridge system can be set up in front of the dash, and a hook or chain assembly used to lift the steering column up and off of the driver.

However, if cutting the steering wheel ring is not possible, or if cutting it does not free the driver, it may be because the driver's seat is pneumatically controlled. These seats automatically adjust to changes in weight or pressure on them. The seat's automatic adjustment can hold the driver against the steering wheel and make him or her appear to be trapped. Operating the seat adjustment control may release enough air to lower the seat and free the driver. If this does not free the driver, the seat may have to be unbolted from the floor and moved rearward. It may also be necessary to remove the partition behind the driver's seat to create enough room to lay the driver's seat back.

Similarly to freeing a bus driver, it may be necessary to move or remove interior features of the bus to facilitate removal of patients. The narrow aisles in buses create a limited working space. Most litters and backboards are too wide to fit in the aisle and have to be placed on the top of the seat cushions or across the tops of the seat backs. Seat frames are easily bent during a collision and can entrap a patient.

Deciding whether to simply move a seat or to remove it will depend on the position of the patient and the rescuers' need for operating space. In many cases, it is advantageous to remove the seat and get it out of the way. There are several effective ways to do this. The seats may be pulled from their moorings by using a winch, come-along, or power spreader. A seat should not be removed if any patients are still trapped close to the seat being pulled because the seat may suddenly dislodge and aggravate their injuries.

There are several good methods for removing seats. One method is to use a power spreader to dislodge the legs connected to the floor and then break the seat-to-wall connection. Another method is to cut the legs of the seats. The legs are made of tubular steel and can be cut with power shears. The legs should be cut as close to the floor as possible and the sharp stubs taped or covered with duct tape. If patients are in close proximity, rescuers may have to use hand tools to remove seat mounting hardware.

Many school buses also have partitions in front of the first row of seats, on either side of the aisle. These dividers are usually made only of thin sheet metal attached to a tubular steel frame. The whole unit is connected to the bus in a manner similar to the seats. These partitions can be removed in the same manner as a seat.

Likewise, most of the objects inside transit or commercial buses are either seats or partitions. Both of these assemblies are bolted to the floor. Partitions may also be connected to the ceiling. If it becomes necessary to remove either of these objects, it is best to unbolt them and remove them from the bus. If time does not permit them to be unbolted, most can easily be cut with any number of cutting tools. The legs or supports are generally constructed of tubular steel that can easily be cut. Cutting these legs or supports will result in sharp stubs being left behind and, if possible, rescuers should cover them as described earlier.

Commercial buses also have overhead storage bins. If it is necessary to remove them to facilitate extricating immobilized patients, rescuers may need to cut or chop them out. Any type of saw or air chisel will work. If a saw is not available, a crash axe or standard fire axe may be used. Rescuers should be cautious when chopping inside of a bus as the space will be very confined and the potential for striking oneself or another person is high. They should use short, controlled strokes. To reduce the slip and fall hazard for those working inside of the bus, debris should be removed as soon as it is cut or chopped away.

Motor Coaches

As mentioned earlier in this chapter, some motor coaches are not designed to transport large groups of people. Rather, they have been converted into mobile living quarters and/or offices. They are used as campers or mobile living quarters by entertainers on tour and others whose jobs require them to relocate frequently. It is usually easy to distinguish these vehicles from commercial buses by their blacked-out windows and sometimes ornate cosmetics on the vehicle's exterior. The interior layout of some of these vehicles will vary considerably from that of standard motor coaches. Some of these vehicles may have fully equipped galleys for meal preparation and may carry one or more LPG tanks for cooking and for heating water. All of these alterations can complicate the disentanglement and extrication processes.

CAUTION

Use of power tools in close proximity to patients increases the chances that extrication operations will result in further patient injuries.

Bus on Side: Extrication

When an occupied bus has come to rest on its side, the occupants will be concentrated on the bottom side. Their general condition will depend upon the event that caused the bus to roll over and whether it slowly rolled onto its side or if it rolled over several times and came to rest on its side. In either case, access from either end of the bus will be extremely difficult because the center aisle is now horizontal and movement within the bus will involve climbing over each row of seats. Therefore, it may be more efficient to cut a large opening in the roof of the bus near its middle. Such an opening reduces the distance that occupants need to travel in order to escape and that rescuers need to travel to reach trapped patients.

The cost/benefit of removing seats and other interior obstructions will be affected by the number of trapped patients, their locations within the bus, and their conditions. If it is determined that the benefit of removing these objects outweighs the time and resources needed to do so, the techniques described in the previous section can be used.

Even though most bus passengers do not wear seat belts, the likelihood of them being ejected in a rollover is relatively low. However, bus rollovers may still result in passengers being trapped beneath the vehicle when it comes to rest. There are two primary methods for removing a person trapped beneath a bus. First, if the bus is resting on soft ground, it may be possible to dig the patient out. The second and most common method of removing a patient from beneath a bus is to lift the bus off the patient. Any one of a number of lifting tools can be used to perform the actual lifting. Regardless of the tool used, the method for performing the rescue will be essentially the same.

The rescue device best suited to perform this operation is the pneumatic lifting bag. The flatness of the uninflated bag allows it to be inserted beneath the bus in a position to achieve the maximum lift possible **(Figure 7.41)**. The procedures for using high-pressure pneumatic lifting bags to free a patient trapped beneath a bus are described in **Skill Sheet 7-7**.

If low-pressure bags are used, they should be placed in the same locations as high-pressure bags would be. However, when using low-pressure bags, it is not necessary to stack the bags.

As mentioned earlier, other tools may be used to do the lifting if pneumatic lifting bags are not available. Power spreaders or hydraulic jacks can be used to lift a bus. When lifting on soft ground, it will be necessary to place a board beneath the bottom tip of the spreader or the base of the jack. Because of the overall height of most jacks, it may be necessary to dig a hole beneath the intended lifting area in order to place the jack. Once a jack is in position, one rescuer can operate it while the other rescuers concentrate on building the box crib or adjusting the chocks.

Another option would be to use a Class C wrecker. These wreckers have long booms and the necessary straps to lift a bus or large vehicle quickly and safely. Personnel using a wrecker must be well trained with the equipment before allowing them to participate in a life safety situation. A rescuer should be assigned to the wrecker operator to ensure proper communications during the extrication.

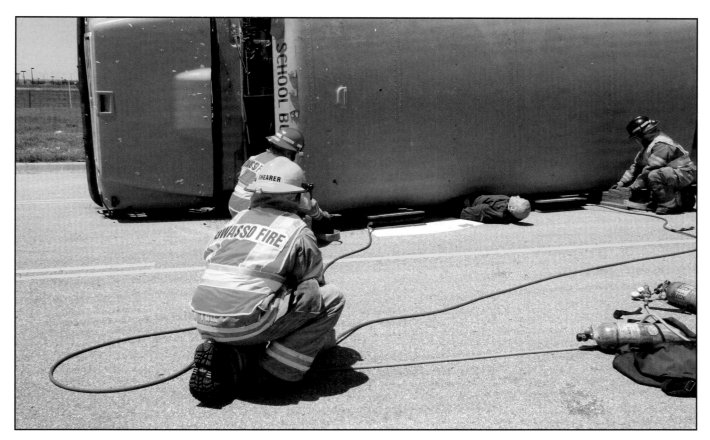

Figure 7.41 Pneumatic lifting bags can be used to lift a bus off of a patient pinned beneath the vehicle.

Bus on Roof: Extrication

When an occupied bus has come to rest on its roof, the occupants will be concentrated on the ceiling because that is now the lowest point. Just as in the preceding discussion, how the bus came to be in that position will largely dictate the condition of the occupants. If the bus rolled over several times, there can be significant distortion of the seats, partitions, and other interior features. The dynamics creating this distortion can result in many occupant injuries and entrapments.

Unlike a bus on its side, one on its roof can allow easier movement within the bus — provided that the roof did not collapse in the rollover. If the roof is still more or less intact, removing the windshield and the rear and side windows will allow uninjured passengers to crawl out and rescuers to crawl in. Ultimately, it may be advisable or necessary to remove portions of a side wall and to remove seats and other features to facilitate movement inside the bus. Removing too much of the side wall may weaken the side of the bus and allow the bus to collapse. If a large area of the wall must be removed, additional stabilization may be required.

Buses in Other Positions: Extrication

In every vehicle extrication operation involving a vehicle in a position other than those already discussed, the ingenuity and resourcefulness of the on-scene rescue personnel can be severely tested. However, regardless of whether the bus was teetering on the edge of a precipice, dangling from a bridge or overpass, or partially submerged in a body of water, the work of stabilizing the vehicle and gaining access to its interior has already been done. What remains are the critical tasks involved in triaging and treating the trapped patients, disentangling them, and extricating them from the wreckage. Therefore, the tools, equipment, and techniques described in the preceding sections apply equally to buses in any position, however unusual.

Summary

There are a number of different types and sizes of buses traveling the streets and highways of the world. They range from school buses to local transit buses to commercial buses that travel great distances. These vehicles all share certain characteristics, but each type is also unique in some way. Conducting safe and efficient extrication operations at bus collisions depends largely upon the extent to which rescue personnel know these vehicles and what to expect when they are faced with a collision involving one.

Collisions involving an occupied bus can present rescue personnel with the same physical and psychological challenges associated with any other vehicle extrication incident — compounded by the possibility of a massive number of patients. However, if rescuers remain calm, view the situation objectively, and apply their training and experience to the situation at hand, they will almost always conduct a successful extrication operation.

Review Questions

1. How are buses classified?
2. What are distinguishing features of each type of school bus?
3. How are passenger seats arranged in transit and commercial buses?
4. What are the hazards associated with bus fuel systems?
5. What specific size-up concerns should an incident commander consider during a bus extrication operation?
6. What hazard control procedures should be employed during a bus extrication operation?
7. What methods can be used to gain access to the interior of a bus?

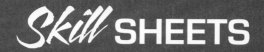
REMINDER: Not all agencies advocate the following procedures and practices. The following skill sheets present a snapshot of various procedures utilized during extrication operations. As always, local agency procedures and protocols must be followed.

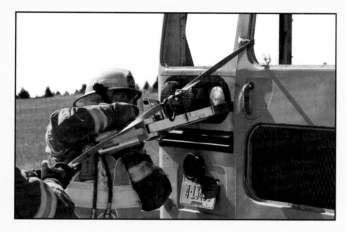

Forcing the rear door:

Step 1: Insert a prying or spreading tool between the door and the frame.

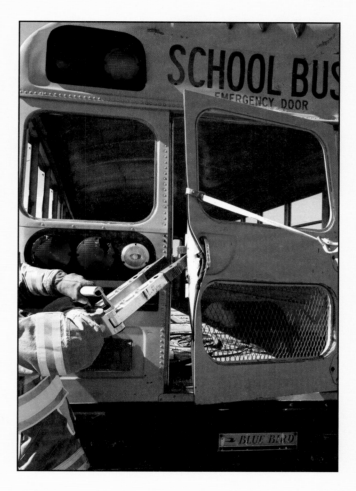

Step 2: Pry or separate the door and frame.

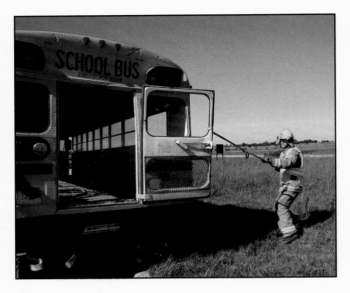

Step 3: Open and secure the door in the open position.

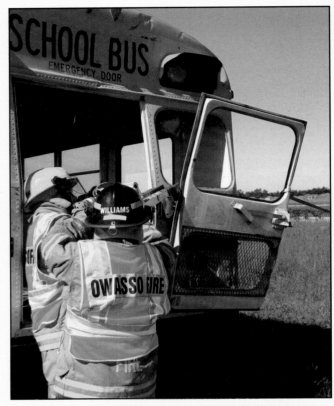

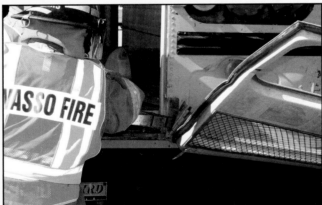

Removing the rear door:

Step 1: Insert a prying or spreading tool between the door and the frame.

Step 2: Pry or separate the door and frame.

Step 3: Open the door.

Step 4: With the door in the open position, remove, cut, or displace the door hinges.

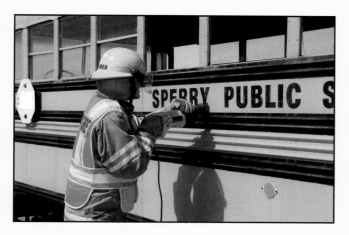

Step 1: Cut away the window frame.

Step 2: Make vertical cuts straight down from two window posts. The cuts should extend down only as far as the floor level.

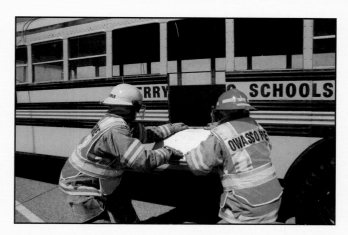

Step 4: When these cuts have been made, the wall section can be pushed/pulled down to create an opening in the side wall.

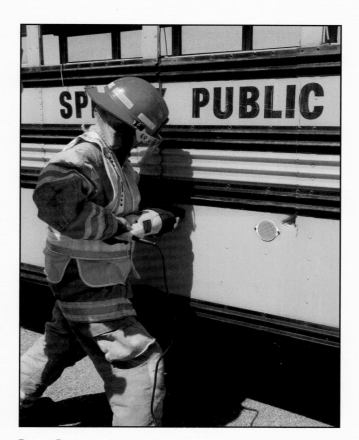

Step 3: At the floor level, make short horizontal relief cuts, 1 to 2 inches (25 mm to 50 mm) long, toward the center of the portion to be laid down.

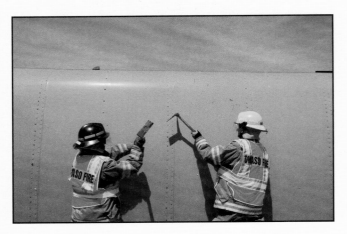

Step 1: Create an access hole near a row of rivets with either a pick-head axe or the point of a Halligan tool.

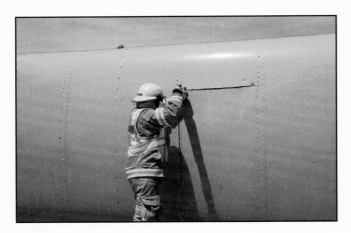

Step 2: Insert the saw blade into the hole and make a horizontal cut across one row of rivets, but stopping short of the second row.

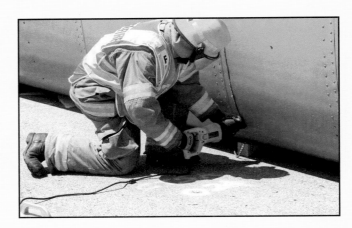

Step 3: Make vertical cuts from the ends of the horizontal cut down to ground level.

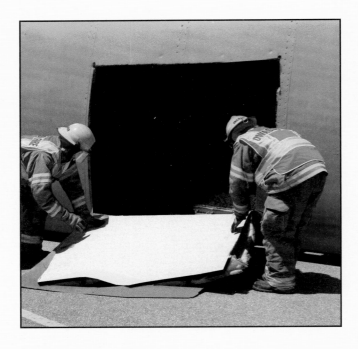

Step 4: Fold the flap of roof down to the ground.

Note: This procedure is specifically for cutting an access opening in the roof of a school bus. The same procedure can be used with transit and commercial buses except that commercial buses have overhead storage bins along each outside wall. To avoid these bins, rescuers must cut access openings as near the centerline of the roof as possible.

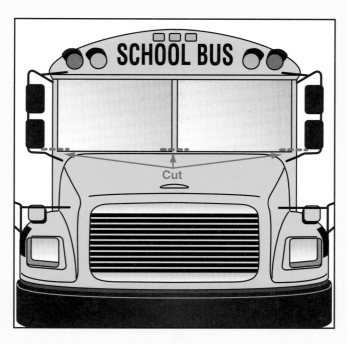

Step 1: After removing the windshield, cut the three front window/roof posts.

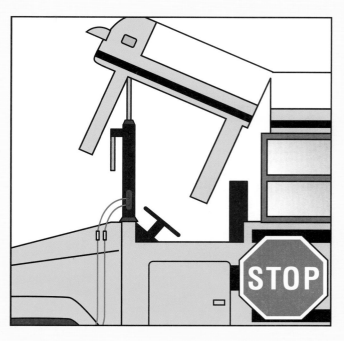

Step 4: Position an extension ram in the middle of the windshield opening and push the roof up.

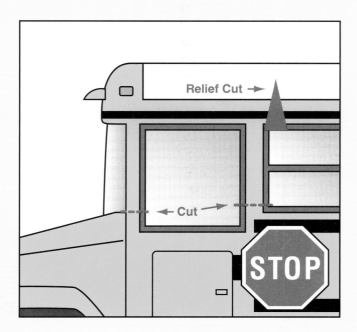

Step 2: Cut the B-posts on each side.

Step 3: Make relief cuts into the roof slightly aft of the B-posts.

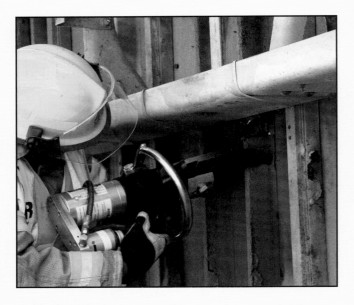

Step 1: Identify the two adjacent main supporting beams between which the opening will be made.

Step 2: Using an air chisel or power shears, make two cuts in the end of each of the nonsupporting beams that lie between the main supporting beams. The first cut should be at the end of each beam, and a second cut should be at least 3 inches (75 mm) inside the first cut.

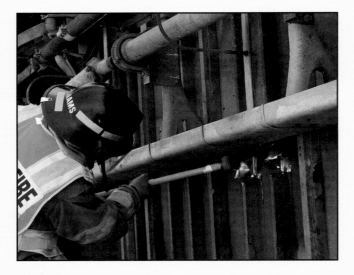

Step 3: Using a sledgehammer or similar tool, knock out the small section of beam between the cuts.

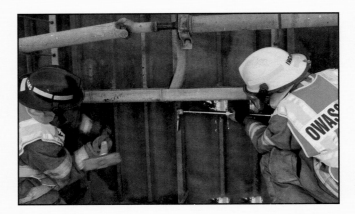

Step 4: Using an air chisel or other tool, cut an access hole in the floor of the bus.

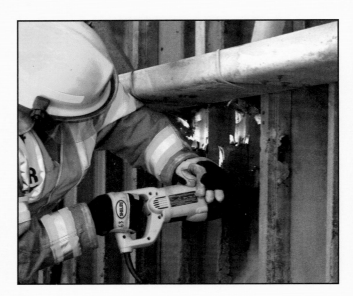

Step 5: Insert the blade of the reciprocating saw into the access hole and cut the floor.

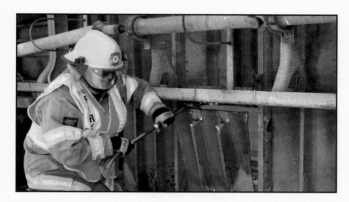

Step 6: When three sides of a square or rectangular opening have been cut, fold back the flap of flooring to create the access opening.

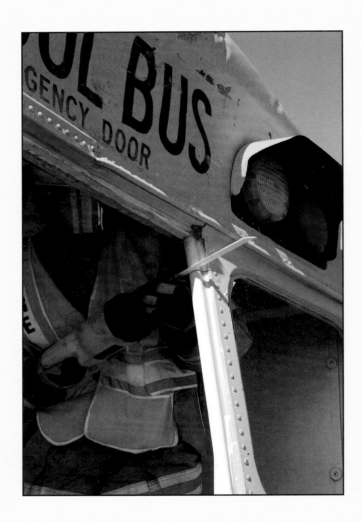
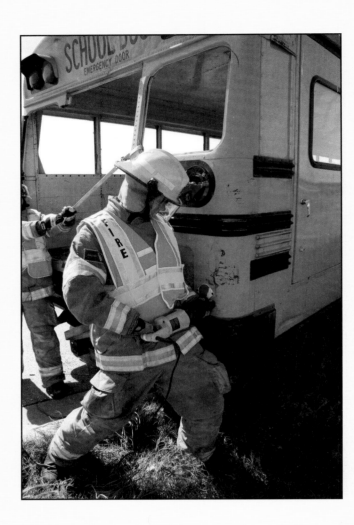

Step 1: Using a cutting tool, make cuts to the top of the window post nearest the door and along the floor level of the rear wall.

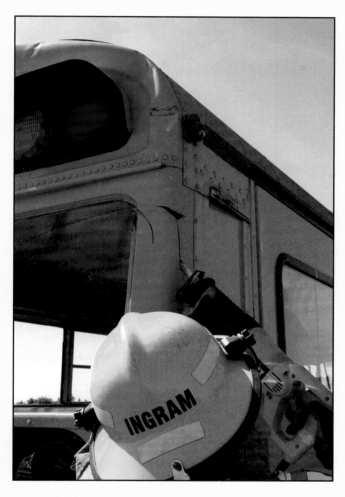

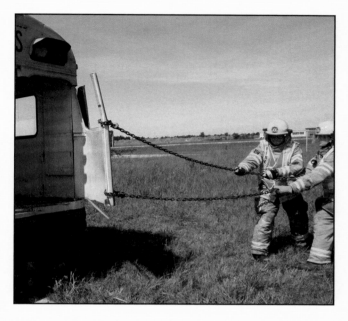

Step 3: Once these cuts are made, the end wall can be folded to the side to increase the opening size.

Note: It may be necessary to remove the last few rows of seats to take full advantage of this wide opening.

Step 2: Make vertical relief cuts just inside the corner post of the bus.

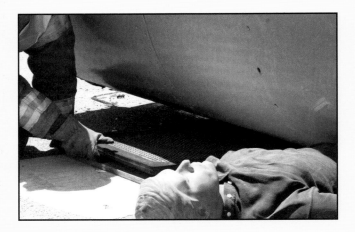

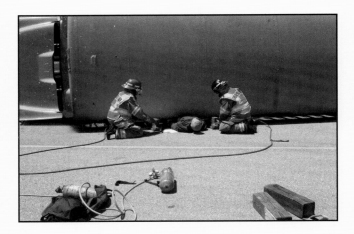

Step 1: Insert at least one pneumatic lifting bag beneath the bus on each side of the patient. Center the middle of each bag beneath a roof truss support. These supports are clearly marked by rows of rivets across the roof structure. If more air bags are available, a small one can be stacked on top of a larger one when they are put into place. This increases the height, but not the lifting capacity, that can be achieved.

WARNING: Stack pneumatic lifting bags only if the manufacturer of the bags approves of this practice.

RECOMMENDATION: When using air bags, place a solid piece of plywood, as large or larger than the air bag, below the air bag to prevent sharp objects from puncturing the air bags.

Step 2: While the bags are being pushed into place, assemble cribbing or place step chocks on either side of the patient. The cribbing or chocks are used to shore up the bus as the bag(s) are inflated.

Step 3: Once everything is in place, begin lifting. Build up the box cribs or adjust the chocks as the lift progresses. This will minimize the risk to the rescuers and patient if the lifting bag fails. Because the roof of a bus is curved where it meets the side wall, it may be necessary to use wedges to maximize the contact between the cribbing and the bus, or invert the step chocks and use them as large wedges.

Step 4: Evaluate and maintain the integrity of the cribbing.

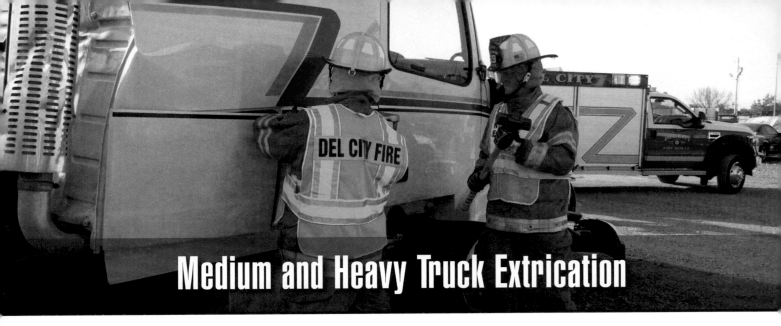

Medium and Heavy Truck Extrication

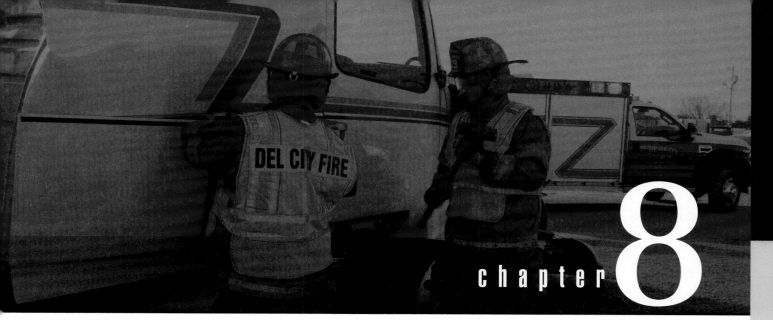

chapter 8

Key Terms

Job Performance Requirements

This chapter provides information that addresses the following job performance requirements (JPRs) of NFPA® 1001, *Standard for Fire Fighter Professional Qualifications* (2008), NFPA® 1006, *Standard for Technical Rescuer Professional Qualifications* (2008), and NFPA® 1670, *Standard on Operations and Training for Technical Search and Rescue Incidents* (2009).

NFPA® 1001 JPRs
6.4.1
6.4.2

NFPA® 1006 JPRs

5.2.2	**10.2**	**10.2.4**
5.2.3	**10.2.1**	**10.2.5**
5.3.2	**10.2.2**	
5.5.1	**10.2.3**	

NFPA® 1670 JPRs

8.2.2	**8.3.3**
8.2.3	**8.3.4**
8.3.2	**8.4.2**

Learning Objectives

1. Describe each class of medium and heavy truck.

2. Describe anatomical features of medium and heavy trucks.

3. Identify anatomical features of trailers associated with medium and heavy trucks.

4. Identify specific size-up concerns associated with medium and heavy truck extrication operations.

5. Explain methods for stabilizing medium and heavy trucks.

6. Describe methods for gaining access into medium and heavy trucks during extrication operations.

7. Identify medium and heavy truck extrication tactics.

Chapter 8
Medium and Heavy Truck Extrication

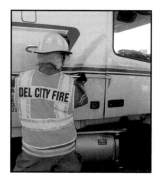

Case History

Fire and rescue units were dispatched from two neighboring departments to an accident involving an SUV and a tractor trailer truck pulling two trailers. As a result of the collision, the truck and trailers overturned. The SUV driver was shaken but otherwise uninjured. Rescuers found the driver of the truck trapped inside the wreckage of the vehicle's cab. Because of the size of the truck and its condition following the accident, rescuers first stabilized the wreckage, then began efforts to gain access to the driver. Once rescuers accessed the driver, EMS personnel began patient stabilization efforts. Structural components of the cab were spread or cut away to free the patient who was then packaged and transported in critical condition to a nearby trauma center by helicopter.

Medium and heavy trucks include a broad range of vehicles including, but certainly not limited to, the following:

- Delivery vans
- Highway tractors pulling multiple trailers
- Tanker trucks carrying a variety of hazardous and nonhazardous liquids
- Cement mixers
- Refuse Haulers
- Fire apparatus

There are laws that limit the number of hours a driver can operate a commercial truck without a break, and vehicle safety inspections are conducted at weigh stations along major highways. However, considering the number and variety of trucks on the road, it is not surprising that some become involved in collisions with other vehicles, bridge abutments, or a host of other objects. Because of their size and weight, medium and heavy trucks fare better in collisions with smaller vehicles, so there are fewer times when truck drivers are trapped in their vehicles. For these same reasons, air bags are not required in long-haul trucks that fall under federal safety regulations, but seat belts have been required in trucks manufactured in the U.S. since September of 1989.

This chapter discusses:

- The different classifications of medium and heavy trucks and their anatomy

- The elements needed to properly size up an extrication incident involving a medium or heavy truck

- The steps on how to stabilize collision-damaged trucks in a variety of positions

- The steps involved in gaining access into them and extricating patients from collision-damaged trucks

Classification of Medium and Heavy Trucks

There are several different classifications of medium and heavy trucks. The most common are straight trucks and tractor/trailer combinations, including tankers, grain transports, and auto transports. There are also a number of specialty trucks within this size range, including cement mixers, refuse haulers, ambulances, and fire apparatus **(Table 8.1)**.

Type	Class(es)	Gross Vehicle Weight Rating (GVWR)	Examples:
Medium	3, 4, or 5	10,001 pounds (4 536 kg) and 19,500 pounds (8 845 kg)	Straight trucks and vans
Light Heavy	6	19,501 pounds (8 845.5 kg) to 26,000 pounds (11 793 kg)	Beverage trucks and two-axle vans
Heavy-heavy	7	26,001 pounds (11 794 kg) to 33,000 pounds (14 968.8 kg)	Fuel trucks, refuse haulers and two-axle highway tractors
Heavy-heavy	8	33,001 pounds (14 969kg) or more	Three-axle dump trucks, cement mixers, and three-axle highway tractors

Table 8.1 Medium and Heavy Truck Classifications*

Based on the U.S. Department of Transportation Vehicle Inventory and Use Survey (VIUS).

Straight Trucks

The straight truck is perhaps the most common of all the truck types — those built on a rigid frame and not intended to pull a trailer. Most have either two or three axles and a gross vehicle weight rating (GVWR) between 10,000 pounds (4 540 kg) and 40,000 pounds (18 160 kg). Some have large, rather boxy bodies, and are used as local delivery vans. Others have either flatbeds or large box bodies mounted on their frames **(Figure 8.1)**.

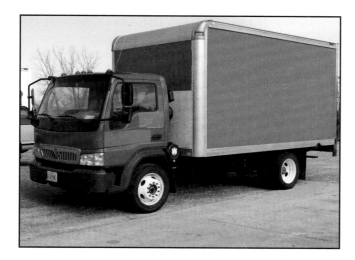

Figure 8.1 This delivery vehicle is an example of a straight truck. *Courtesy of Alan Braun, University of Missouri Fire and Rescue Training Institute.*

Truck/Semitrailer Combinations

Truck/Semitrailer combinations consist of a highway tractor and one or more separate trailers. The tractors may have either two or three axles and may weigh up to 18,000 pounds (8 172 kg) by themselves. The entire truck/trailer combination may weigh up to 140,000 pounds (63 560 kg). The trailers may be flatbeds, enclosed box trailers, tankers (in any of a variety of shapes), or any of a number of specialized types such as grain transports and vehicle transports **(Figure 8.2)**. While some of these vehicles will be labeled or placarded to indicate the nature of their cargo, others will not — and they may be carrying almost any commodity, including up to 440 pounds (200 kg) of hazardous materials. The load can be made up of combinations of these without being placarded for each.

Trailer — Highway or industrial-plant vehicle designed to be hauled/pulled by a tractor or truck.

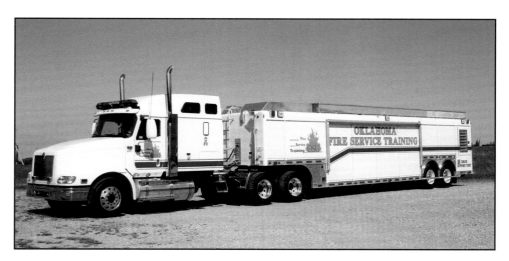

Figure 8.2 A tractor/semitrailer combination.

Specialty Trucks

Specialty trucks are differentiated only by their unique purposes. Otherwise, they may have the same configuration as any of those already described, and they are likely to weigh as much as any other truck of the same type and size.

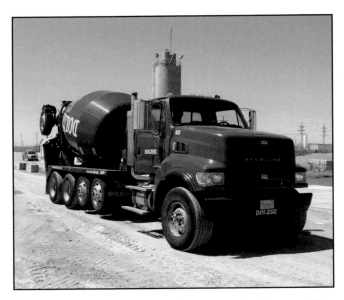

Figure 8.3 This cement mixer is an example of a specialty truck.

As mentioned earlier, specialty trucks can include everything from cement mixers, refuse haulers, tow trucks, and grain transports, to ambulances, fire apparatus and countless others **(Figure 8.3)**.

Truck Anatomy

As with automobiles, light trucks, and buses, medium and heavy trucks all have certain characteristics in common and others that are unique. The most distinguishing characteristic of all types of medium and heavy trucks is that they are relatively big and often extremely heavy. Their sheer size and weight can complicate an otherwise routine extrication problem and necessitate the use of specialized resources such as booms, cranes, or other massive lifting devices.

Cabs

Except for delivery vans, all medium and heavy trucks have a cab of some sort. In delivery vans, the cab is merely the front portion of the vehicle's body, separated from the cargo area only by a bulkhead on either side of the center aisle. The two most common types of cabs are conventional and cab-over units **(Figures 8.4a and b)**. The sections that follow not only describe these two types of cabs, but also describe other aspects of cab anatomy.

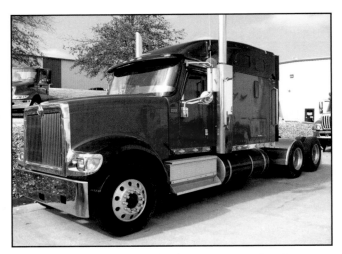

Figure 8.4a A conventional cab on a tractor. *Courtesy of Alan Braun, University of Missouri Fire and Rescue Training Institute.*

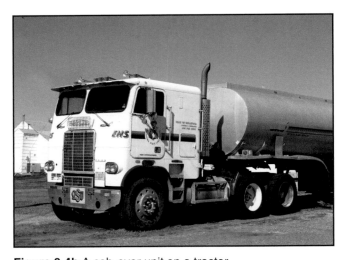

Figure 8.4b A cab-over unit on a tractor.

Conventional Cabs

In a conventional cab, the passenger compartment is located aft of the engine compartment. A conventional cab is longer from front to back than is a cab-over model, and the cab does not tilt forward to provide access to the engine. The engine is accessed by raising the sides of a hood that is hinged down its midline, or the hood and front fenders may be a molded fiberglass unit that tilts forward. The remainder of a conventional cab is usually made of steel, aluminum, or a combination of fiberglass panels over a steel framework.

Cab-Over Units

In this design, the engine is located directly under the midline of the passenger compartment, roughly between the seats. The cab-over unit is designed to tilt forward to allow access to the engine. Generally, the cab is attached to the chassis at three points — in the center behind the cab (latch point) and by a hinge at the forward end of each frame rail. As with conventional cabs, cab-over units may be made of steel, aluminum, fiberglass, or a combination of these materials.

Sleepers

Because many long-haul trucks drive great distances and the law limits the number of hours a driver can operate a commercial vehicle without a rest period, many heavy trucks are equipped with a sleeping compartment in or behind the cab **(Figure 8.5)**.

Sleeper — A compartment built into or behind the cab of a large truck to be used by the driver for rest and relaxation.

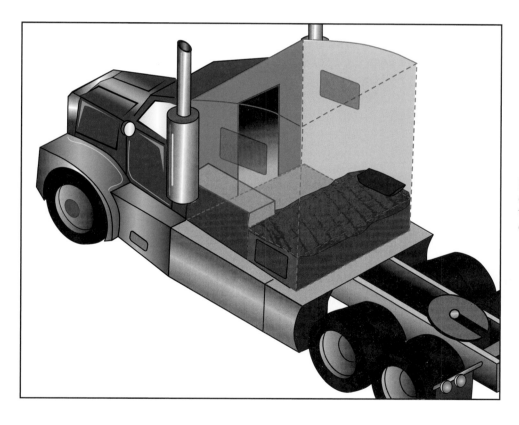

Figure 8.5 A sleeping compartment attached to the rear of a conventional cab.

The vast majority of sleepers are merely an extension of the cab and not a separate unit, so access into these units is through the cab or by forcing entry through the required exterior door. In those units that are separate compartments, they must have an intercom between the sleeper and the cab. The access door to the sleeper may be on either side of the unit.

The fact that a truck has a sleeper attached to the cab should alert rescue personnel to check there for another possible occupant during the size-up of an incident involving one of these rigs. Often, team drivers will have a sign indicating the driving team on the driver's door area. Since the occupant of a sleeper is not required to be restrained, rescuers should expect to find an injured patient in the sleeper following a collision.

Cab Doors

The forward doors on most delivery vans are pocket doors that slide rearward into the vehicle's side wall to open. These doors have a single latch point at the center of the front edge of the door. Newer delivery vans have conventionally front hinged doors.

The doors on both conventional and cab-over units are much heavier and stronger than those on automobiles and light trucks. They are equipped with either conventional or piano-type hinges. Most have a single latch with a two-step locking action. Because of the height of the doors above the ground, the door latch handle is usually located in the lower rear corner of the door.

Cab Windows

The windshields and rear windows of medium and heavy trucks are made of laminated safety glass, and they are set in center-bead rubber gaskets. The cab side windows are made of tempered glass that is heavier than that used in automobiles and light trucks.

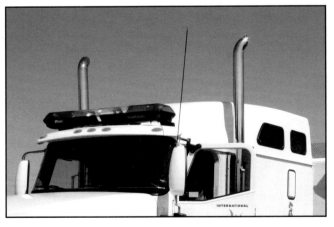

Figure 8.6 The roof configuration of a conventional cab.

Fairing — An auxiliary structure or the external surface attached to or part of the roof of a large truck that serves to reduce drag.

Cab Roofs

The cab roofs of most medium and heavy trucks are usually covered with the lightest gauge metal or fiberglass on the vehicle, and the skin is supported by two or more ribs running from front to rear. Many heavy trucks have a large fiberglass fairing (wind deflector) mounted on the roof, behind which are often an air horn and an air-conditioning unit **(Figure 8.6)**.

Seat Belts and Supplemental Restraint Systems

Like passenger vehicles, medium and heavy trucks are equipped with seat belts and supplemental restraint systems to protect the driver and any passengers riding in the vehicle. These systems operate in much the same manner as those found in passenger vehicles and present the same types of concerns as discussed in Chapter 6, *Passenger Vehicle Extrication*.

Batteries

Medium and heavy trucks have either a 12-volt or 24-volt electrical system supplied by one or more banks of batteries. The battery banks may be in more than one location on the vehicle. Those with 24-volt systems normally have four 6-volt batteries in series, with a negative ground.

Fuel Systems

Most medium and heavy trucks operate on diesel fuel, rather than gasoline. Use of diesel fuel reduces, but does not eliminate, the danger of a flash fire following a collision. While the flashpoint of diesel fuel varies from 126° to 204° F (52° C to 95° C) it can easily be heated to that point if it leaks onto exhaust system components or even very hot pavement. The diesel fuel is usually contained in large external saddle tanks attached to either side of the frame **(Figure 8.7)**. The capacity of these saddle tanks may vary from 50 to 300 gallons (200 L to 1 200 L) each. Many vehicle saddle tanks are interconnected by a small tube that equalizes the volume of fuel in both tanks. At one or both ends of this tube is a small valve that can be used to isolate the tanks from each other if one tank is leaking. This will limit the amount of fuel that can escape.

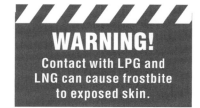

Figure 8.7 This truck is equipped with large saddle tanks to carry the truck's fuel supply.

Just as with buses and some light trucks, some medium and heavy trucks operate on alternative fuels — either liquefied petroleum gas (LPG) or compressed natural gas (CNG). A small number of trucks now operate on liquefied natural gas (LNG) or hydrogen. Decals or other signs should be visible to alert rescue personnel that a particular vehicle uses an alternative fuel. The locations of the fuel tanks vary considerably. Leaking fuel may present more than fire and explosion hazards.

WARNING!
Contact with LPG and LNG can cause frostbite to exposed skin.

Auxiliary Power and Hydraulics Systems

Some larger trucks are equipped with auxiliary power systems. These may include generators and inverters. Other vehicles are equipped with separate hydraulic systems used to operate specialized equipment on the vehicles. Two such systems are described as follows:

1. *Generators and Inverters* — Some vehicles have a generator or battery powered inverter to provide 110-220 volt power. This power may be used to operate climate control and other electrically power equipment while the vehicle is traveling or parked overnight.

2. *Hydraulics* — Some vehicles are equipped with a separate hydraulic system. That system may power vehicle components such as a concrete trucks drum, crane, or a dump trailers lift. These systems may be running continually or when needed by the operator.

Brake Systems

Medium and heavy trucks are equipped with either hydraulic brakes, air brakes, or a combination of the two. The hydraulic brake systems are similar to those in automobiles and light trucks, but they are heavy-duty. The most common type of breaking system is drum type, however disc brake systems are becoming more popular. Some trucks have hydraulic brakes that are assisted by air pressure. In the air brake systems, compressed air is used to apply the brakes under normal operation. Under abnormal conditions, such as a complete loss of air pressure in the braking system, heavy-duty springs automatically apply the rear brakes.

Because the trailers on tractor/trailer rigs also have air brakes, the trailer's air system is connected to that of the tractor by a breakaway valve (commonly called "glad-hand connections") at the rear of the cab. The flexible air line connecting the tractor and trailer is often supported on a vertical stand (sometimes called a "pogo stick") mounted on the rear of the tractor or by some other securing device.

Both trucks and tractor/trailer combinations with air brakes have air brake chambers mounted under each axle. The double chambers (called "piggyback chambers") under the rear axles contain large compressed springs that are designed to apply the brakes mechanically for parking or if there is a loss of air pressure. The parts of each double chamber are held together with a metal clamp **(Figure 8.8)**. Rescuers should never loosen the clamp on an air brake chamber. Loosening this clamp can release a spring that has sufficient force to cause serious injury. Also, rescuers should stay clear of the rear of air brake chambers when they are involved in fire. If the chamber melts, the compressed spring can break.

NOTE: The buses discussed in Chapter 7, *Bus Extrication*, include brakes identical or very similar to those described in this section.

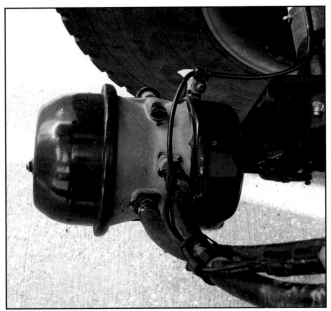

Figure 8.8 A double chamber air brake unit on a heavy truck. *Courtesy of Alan Braun, University of Missouri Fire and Rescue Training Institute.*

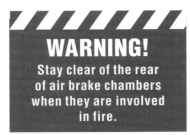

WARNING!
Never loosen the clamp on an air brake chamber.

WARNING!
Stay clear of the rear of air brake chambers when they are involved in fire.

Leaf Spring Suspension — A type of suspension system consisting of several long, narrow, layers of elastic metal bracketed together.

Suspension Systems

Most medium and heavy trucks have conventional heavy-duty suspension (leaf and/or coil springs). However, a growing number of heavy trucks are equipped with air suspension systems. In these systems, the conventional metal springs are replaced with compact rubber air bags that are somewhat similar to a bellows. At each wheel, there are air suspension bags — two on each axle. An on-board compressor maintains the air pressure within the bags as high as 120 psi (840 kPa). Depending upon the load of the vehicle and the condition of the road, the pressure within each bag is automatically increased or decreased to maintain the vehicle in a level state. If the pressure in an air suspension bag is lost because of damage to the bag or its associated piping, the truck chassis can suddenly drop several inches without warning.

Fifth Wheel

Mounted on the rear of every highway tractor is a heavy-duty circular steel plate called a fifth wheel. The fifth wheel allows the trailer to rotate more than 90 degrees from center in both directions. The fifth wheel turntable can pivot approximately 15 degrees front to rear and, on some vehicles, it can be adjusted fore and aft. The fifth wheel has a wedge-shaped slot in its rear aspect to receive the trailer's king pin. When the king pin reaches the center of the fifth wheel during coupling, the pin is locked into place by two spring-loaded jaws. A pull handle on the driver's side of the tractor opens the jaws to allow the trailer to be uncoupled from the tractor **(Figure 8.9)**. On some vehicles, the jaws can be opened by air from the cab.

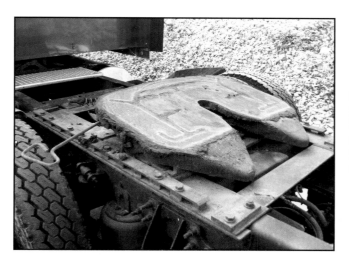

Figure 8.9 A fifth wheel mounted on rear of a highway tractor. *Courtesy of Alan Braun, University of Missouri Fire and Rescue Training Institute.*

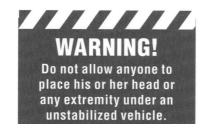

Coil Spring Suspension — A type of suspension system consisting of numerous elastic steel bodies wound spirally that recover their shape after being compressed, bent, or stretched.

WARNING!
Do not allow anyone to place his or her head or any extremity under an unstabilized vehicle.

Trailer Anatomy

Trailers are available in a wide variety of shapes and sizes — depending upon their intended use. There are flatbed trailers used for hauling virtually anything that can be lashed to the bed. There are trailers with bottom-dump capability used for hauling sand, gravel, grain, and other dry products. There are long cylindrical tankers in a variety of styles depending upon what they are intended to carry. There are trailers with spherical tanks for carrying cryogenic materials. Probably the most common trailers seen on the highways are the huge box trailers used for hauling almost anything that will fit inside the box. These box trailers may also be insulated.

Regardless of whether the trailer is a flatbed, box, or tanker, they are all designed in one of two basic styles: trailers or semitrailers **(Figure 8.10)**. A trailer is a freestanding unit with wheels front and rear. These trailers are usually shorter than semitrailers. The front axle on a trailer is connected to a turntable that can be turned from side to side for better tracking, and the rear axle is fixed. A trailer couples to a tractor or another trailer with a long tow bar, often called a dolly. Semitrailers only have wheels at or near the rear end, and the front end is supported by the tractor when locked into the fifth wheel described earlier. When a semitrailer is not coupled to a tractor, its front end is supported by a pair of small wheels or plates (sometimes called "landing gear") that are attached to the underside of the trailer by two struts. When not in use, the trailer's landing gear can be lowered with a hand crank. On many of these trailers, the hand crank has two speeds — push in and crank for slow raising or lowering, pull out and crank for fast raising or lowering. The landing gear can be used for additional temporary stabilization, but not for lifting the trailer.

Figure 8.10 An illustration showing the difference between a semitrailer and a trailer.

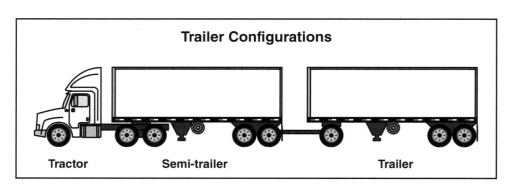

Trailer Configurations

Tractor   Semi-trailer   Trailer

Many trailers and semitrailers are equipped with air suspension systems as described earlier in the section on truck anatomy. The same precautions apply to working under these trailers as apply to working under trucks with similar suspension systems. The sections that follow provide rescuers with more detailed information about various types of trailers they will encounter at accident scenes.

Box Trailers

With the exception of refrigerated trailers that have heavily insulated walls and roofs, most box trailers have a relatively lightweight metal frame that is covered by thin metal or fiberglass or a combination of the two. There may be rub rails along the inside walls of the box to protect it and add shear strength. The roof of the box is the area most easily penetrated because the covering material is thinnest and there are the fewest structural members. While there are many exceptions, most box trailers have 110 inches (2.8 m) of vertical clearance inside, from front to rear. The sections that follow familiarize rescuers with the various doors common to box trailers.

Rear Cargo Doors

The rear cargo doors on box trailers may be one of two types: swinging or roll-up. Trailers with swinging doors usually have two single-leaf doors that latch near the middle and swing outward on conventional or piano-type hinges. Most roll-up doors on trailers are constructed in sections similar to a garage door. Most types of roll-up doors latch in the center at the bottom of the door.

Side Cargo Doors

Some box trailers have one or two side cargo doors, usually located at the mid-point of the trailer's length on either one or both sides. These doors are generally swinging doors on conventional or piano-type hinges. These doors may consist of a single-leaf door or two single-leaf doors that latch near the middle.

Livestock Trailers

Livestock — Cattle, horses, sheep, and other useful animals raised or kept on a ranch or farm.

While not as numerous as other types of trailers, livestock trailers bear mentioning because unlike most other trailers on the highway, they often contain a significant life hazard. Horses or other livestock that are already frightened and upset because of the collision can be further agitated by the sounds of power tools being used in the extrication operation. In their panic, they can seriously injure themselves, other animals, or rescue personnel. It may be possible to calm the animal by blindfolding it and/or restricting its hearing. If this is not successful, it may be best to free the animal as quickly and as quietly as possible. However, be aware that a frightened animal that is freed from the confines of a wrecked trailer may bolt and attempt to flee. Fleeing animals can create a traffic hazard for other motorists and may result in harm to the animal. It is sometimes advisable to call a veterinarian to the scene to tranquilize any animal that cannot be extricated quickly.

Tanker Trailers

Tanker trailers are made of steel, aluminum, stainless steel, and other materials and have capacities that range from 200 to 14000 gallons (757 to 55 996 L). There are many different types and styles of trailer on the roads today, responders should be concerned with the contents of the tank during the response and upon arrival. Another concern is the ability of the contents to shift during extrication efforts.

Lowboys

Lowboy trailers make up a small part of road traffic, however their load capacity makes them worth mentioning. These trailers feature a low center deck area designed to carry large heavy loads up to several hundred tons. Trailers may also have a heavy steel beam framework that the load is mounted to for transportation. Lowboy trailers commonly have two or three rear axels with two wheels per side; trailers that carry heavier loads may also have additional sections with multiple axels to support the heavy loads. These loads may be over 175ft (53 m) long and/or over width (greater than 8 feet [2.4 m] wide). The loads that lowboy trailers carry are of special concern to rescuers because of the difficulty in stabilizing the large size and heavy weight. These types of loads may overwhelm our resources due to the large volume of material needed to stabilize them.

Lowboys are made with most of the same equipment as other standard over-the-road trailers. They have air brakes supplied by the tractor. Most heavy-duty trailers are hydraulically operated. Some operate from the cab of the tractor while others are operated by generators and electric hydraulic pumps. These methods are used to split them apart to unload equipment.

Dump Trailers

Dump trailers are a common sight on highways and the interstate system. In the United States, their gross vehicle weight is limited to 80,000 pounds (36 287 kg) by the DOT. These trailers may have a frame structure or the trailer body may be used as the frame. Trailers can be constructed of steel, aluminum, or stainless steel. Dump trailers can carry many different loads including rock, dirt, scrap metal and hazardous materials. Care should be taken when assessing dump trailers due to the many different load possibilities, weights, and potential load shifting during extrication.

These trailers are equipped with most of the same equipment as standard over-the-road trailers. They have air brakes supplied by the tractor. Most heavy duty trailers are hydraulically operated from the cab of the tractor. Some of the smaller ones are operated by generators or battery powered electric hydraulic pumps.

Specific Size-Up Concerns for Medium and Heavy Truck Extrication

One of the potentially most important parts of assessing the scene of an incident involving a medium or heavy truck is identifying the cargo that the truck is carrying. In addition to the other hazards that may be present — fuel leaks, downed wires, incipient fires, etc. — the cargo itself may be hazardous. *49 CFR*

172 allows up to 440 lbs [200 kg] of hazardous cargo without placarding. The load can be made up of combinations of materials without being placarded for each. Before approaching a crashed medium or heavy truck, stop a safe distance away and use binoculars to look for hazardous materials labels or placards.

If any labels or placards are seen, follow agency protocols for the material indicated **(Figure 8.11)**. These protocols will usually follow the recommendations contained in the Emergency Response Guidebook.

Pedestrians fleeing the scene may be the first indication of the need to stop and assess the scene before approaching. If people are running from the scene with a look of panic on their faces or if pedestrians have collapsed in the area of the crashed vehicles, it would be imprudent to jeopardize rescue personnel by approaching the scene without taking the necessary precautions.

If it appears that an airborne contaminant has been released in the collision, use public address systems or bull horns to instruct those near the scene to vacate immediately. A hazardous materials response team should be called, and all incoming units informed of the situation. They should be instructed to stage uphill and upwind of the incident scene. If SCBA and full PPE will protect the wearer from the chemical involved, rescue personnel should cordon off the scene and deny entry until the haz mat team arrives. If this level of protective equipment will not protect rescuers from the chemical involved, rescuers should stay out of the area.

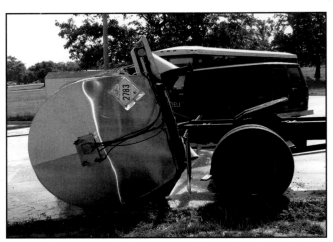

Figure 8.11 This trailer is placarded as carrying a Class 6, Poison.

Even if the cargo is labeled as hazardous, it may be contained and represent no immediate threat. The cargo area should still be cordoned off until a hazardous materials specialist can assess the situation, but the extrication operation can proceed. All nonessential personnel and spectators should be kept upwind of the scene in case of a subsequent release. The adjacent highway should be closed to all but emergency vehicle traffic. Emergency vehicles should stage uphill and upwind.

When responding to a motor collision with trucks, one of the most critical size-up factors is locating the driver/operator of the truck. If the truck driver/operator is conscious, he may be able to tell rescue personnel what the cargo is and if it needs any special handling to maintain safety. If not, rescuers should attempt to locate the bill of lading (cargo manifest) which is usually carried in a pocket on the driver's door.

Other concerns regarding cargo include its weight, location, and configuration. Additionally, these factors can affect the stability of the vehicle during extrication operations. Extremely heavy cargo adds weight to the vehicle, and this weight could exceed the lifting capability of the available tools and equipment. More powerful lifting equipment may be needed and may take time to arrive on the scene. Where the cargo is located and how the cargo is configured could affect the stability of the vehicle as it is being lifted or as vehicle components are removed. The cargo could shift in its location causing the vehicle's center of gravity to shift. Shifting can cause negative energy (potentially harmful movement) to be released into the in the passenger compartment or cause the vehicle to move off of any stabilizing devices.

Perhaps the best thing that can be said about incidents involving medium or heavy trucks is that there is usually a small number of occupants who can become trapped in the wreckage. Most medium and heavy trucks are occupied by the driver only, the driver and a helper, or two drivers.

Medium and Heavy Truck Stabilization

Before rescue personnel can enter the cab or sleeper of a crashed truck, it is imperative that the truck be stabilized. When the truck has been stabilized, rescuers can conduct a more thorough assessment of the patients inside and properly package them for extrication. Stabilization may be accomplished by creating a sufficient number of points of contact between the truck and a stable surface — the ground or the pavement. While the equipment used remains the same as described in earlier chapters, the techniques employed to stabilize a medium or heavy truck will vary depending upon the position in which the vehicle is found. As always, stabilization includes preventing the vehicle from moving in any direction, shutting off the engine, and disconnecting the batteries. The sections that follow discuss the stabilization techniques used for a medium or heavy truck that is upright, on its side, on its roof, and in other positions.

Truck Upright/On Wheels: Stabilization

Even though some medium and heavy trucks have a relatively high center of gravity, the majority of trucks involved in collisions will be found upright. However, because a truck is resting on its wheels does not mean that it is stable. The inflated tires allow a certain amount of movement, especially laterally. Also, the vehicle's suspension system is designed to allow the vehicle's chassis to move in various directions. Even these small amounts of bounce and sway are enough to aggravate a trapped patient's injuries. Therefore, the truck must be stabilized as quickly as reasonably possible.

There are major differences between stabilizing an automobile or pickup truck and a medium or heavy truck. First, the vertical distance between the road surface and the bottom of the chassis is significantly greater in medium or heavy trucks than in other vehicles. As a result, the truck's center of gravity is significantly higher. And second, medium and heavy trucks generally weigh much more than the smaller vehicles.

In some cases, a four-point box crib installed under the front portion of the vehicle's frame and both sides of the truck frame is needed **(Figure 8.12, p. 372)**. Large wheel chocks, such as those carried on fire apparatus, should be used to prevent the vehicle from rolling forward or backward. On cab-over units, the cab should be secured with rope, webbing, or chains to prevent it from tilting forward unexpectedly during extrication operations. Other truck cabs are mounted on air suspension systems that allow movement of the cab independent of the chassis. Rescuers should attempt to minimize this movement by "marrying" the two components together. Once these measures have

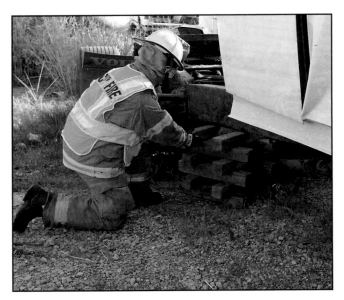

Figure 8.12 A rescuer constructing a box crib under a heavy truck frame.

been taken, the truck should be stable enough for rescuers to start the patient assessment phase of the operation. Rescue personnel should secure and stabilize anything attached to the truck.

Truck on its Side: Stabilization

A medium or heavy truck on its side can sometimes be easier to stabilize than other smaller vehicles because the weight and shape of these trucks often make them relatively stable when they come to rest. However, a truck on its side may behave differently if it is fully loaded than it would if it were empty. In the case of a tractor/trailer, the tractor's center of gravity is different than the trailer's. Therefore, if someone uncouples the tractor from the trailer, the tractor may suddenly shift back toward the upright position while the trailer remains on its side. As with automobiles and other vehicles, chocks or other supports should be installed at the cab's door posts. Because of the roundness of the cab's roof edge, it may be advisable to invert the step chocks before sliding them under the vehicle. Depending upon how stable the truck is after the cribbing is installed, it may be advisable to shore the underside of the truck to prevent any possibility of it rolling back onto its wheels **(Figure 8.13)**. Securing the truck with rope, chain, or webbing can also be used to prevent it from rolling back onto its wheels. However, if rapid extrication is needed, removing the cab's windshield may be the best course of action.

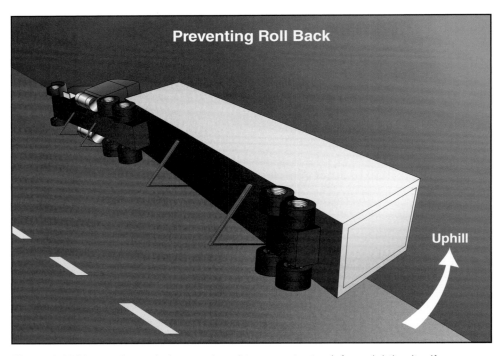

Figure 8.13 Heavy shores being employed to prevent a truck from righting itself.

Truck on its Roof: Stabilization

A truck on its roof can be even more of a challenge to stabilize than one on its side. The roofs of most truck cabs are rounded and offer few if any positive purchase points. However, inverted step chocks installed at the door posts and box cribbing or Hi-Lift® jacks installed under the front will often suffice. In some cases, it may be necessary to crib the truck's bed to prevent the truck from rocking fore and aft. Again, depending upon the situation, it may be practical to stabilize these trucks with ropes, chains, or webbing.

Trucks in Other Positions: Stabilization

Stabilizing trucks found in positions other than those already described will test the ingenuity of rescue personnel assigned to perform this task. However, regardless of what technique is used to stabilize a truck, the emphasis must be on safety. While speed and efficiency are highly desirable, the security and effectiveness of the stabilization measures are far more important. A rapidly installed crib that fails is far worse than one that takes longer to install but does the job.

When deciding how to stabilize a truck that has come to rest in an unusual position, rescue personnel should remember the discussions in Chapter 3 regarding center of gravity, mass, and vehicle integrity. These basic physical principles will dictate how a truck is likely to move when its components are manipulated or removed during extrication operations. If a truck is on a steep slope or hanging over the edge of a bridge or cliff, shoring and/or rigging can be used to offset the forces of gravity and secure the vehicle in place. If the vehicle is wedged under another vehicle or other object, the goal is to limit if not eliminate the vehicle's reaction when the overlying object is removed. Sometimes it is best to attach two vehicles or objects together, often called "marrying the two together," to make extrication safer. Exactly how this is done will be dictated by the specific situation. Given the size of these trucks, extrication personnel may have to call for secondary or outside sources to secure and stabilize these trucks such as tow rigs, commercial riggers, and even cranes.

Secondary Vehicles, Overrides and Underrides

Medium and heavy trucks are frequently involved in accidents with smaller vehicles. The amount of damage these vehicles receive in such accidents will depend upon size of the smaller vehicle or vehicles and the type of impact that occurred. Rescuers must search each vehicle involved in the accident as well as the area surrounding the accident scene to locate any potential patients. Medium and heavy duty trucks usually require more time and personnel to perform extrication tasks due to the size and structural components of the vehicles.

Medium and heavy trucks can become involved in over-rides and under-rides. Truck overrides often result in extreme damage and injury to other, smaller vehicles and their passengers. It is extremely difficult to gain access to the patients in the smaller vehicle because of the size and weight of the truck. Underride situations, while rare, can cause severe damage and injury to the truck and its occupants.

Gaining Access into Trucks

Once a truck has been stabilized, the next step is to gain access to the interior of the cab. Attempting to open the doors as normal is the first step in gaining access: rescuers should try before they pry. However, in many cases, the doors are either locked or jammed, or both. Rescuers should also consider the additional height that rescue operations will take place. This height issue can be resolved by building a platform from cribbing material, working from ladders, or working from another vehicle such as a pickup truck or flat bed wrecker.

NOTE: Unless otherwise stated in this section, the equipment and techniques for gaining access to medium and heavy trucks are the same as those described in Chapter 4, *Extrication Equipment*, and Chapter 5, *Extrication Techniques*.

Windows and Doors

If the cab doors are either locked or jammed, removing the side windows to allow access to the door locks/handles is often necessary. Once the windows have been removed, the door lock/handle can be reached through the window opening.

When the cab door has been unlocked, the door handle should be tried. If that allows the door to be opened, the door handle can be held in the open position by inserting a short piece of angle-iron, cut specifically for this purpose, between the handle and the door handle recess. Holding the door handle in the open position prevents the door from latching again if it closes when released. If operating the exterior or interior door handle does not open the door, it sometimes helps to operate both of these handles simultaneously. Whether the doors need to be removed or merely opened will be dictated by the specific situation. **Skill Sheet 8-1** describes the procedures for removing truck doors.

Roof Removal

When patients are trapped inside a truck that has come to rest on its side, one of the fastest and most efficient ways of gaining access is by opening the door that is on the top side of the vehicle. However, removing all or part of the vehicle's roof is a preferable and much better route for extricating patients.

Shears, reciprocating saws, or other suitable cutters can be used to cut through those door/roof posts that are accessible, depending upon how the vehicle is lying. If the vehicle is lying on its side, but the door/roof posts are accessible, all of the posts can be cut and the entire roof removed. If the vehicle is lying on the door/roof posts on one side of the vehicle, the other posts can be cut and the roof flapped down to the ground. Or, depending upon the situation and the tools and equipment available, it may be best to cut around the edge of the roof and remove the sheet metal and any cross members, leaving the door/roof posts and the roof frame intact. **Skill Sheet 8-2** describes the procedures for gaining access through truck roofs.

Floors

While it is possible to make access through the floor, such access should be considered a last resort. The cab floor and underlying structures are usually made of heavy gauge material. There are also multiple components bolted to the floor such as seats, cabinets, and other cab components. These components may limit the amount of room rescuers have to work in. Tool selection will be critical in this type of extrication due to the heavy floor structure and patient location.

Cab/Sleeper Wall Access

This technique involves using cutting tools to flap or remove the sides or rear panel of a vehicle. To gain access in these locations, rescuers should cut the outer skin away, cut the inner support structures, and then pull or cut away any interior cladding, insulation, cabinets, and other components to allow access to patients. Rescuers should not remove more material than necessary because doing so could jeopardize the vehicle's structural integrity. **Skill Sheet 8-3** describes the procedures for removing truck cab and sleeper walls.

Third Door Conversion

This technique involves using cutting tools to flap the side panel of a vehicle. This technique may be needed in a truck collision only if the sleeper area is an extension of the cab and not a separate compartment. In this case, the side wall of the cab aft of the door is flapped rearward.

Medium and Heavy Truck Extrication Tactics

Once the truck has been stabilized and access to the cab's interior has been gained, the trapped patients must be disentangled and removed from the vehicle. As mentioned earlier, the techniques and procedures involved in medically stabilizing and properly packaging an injured patient for extrication are beyond the scope of this manual. Therefore, in the extrication techniques that follow, it is assumed that medical stabilization and packaging have been or are being done. As with the other phases of the process, the extrication techniques used will vary depending upon the position of the truck. A well organized plan that all personnel can understand and implement is a key to an effective extrication operation.

Truck Upright/On Wheels: Extrication

Regardless of where the trapped patients are located within the cab, rescuers must focus their efforts on disentangling the patients — that is, removing the vehicle from the patients. And, they must do so in a way that will not aggravate the patients' injuries. This means that the extrication team must closely coordinate their efforts with those who are stabilizing and packaging the patients.

Disentanglement may involve cutting the brake and/or clutch pedals or bending them out of the way to free the driver's feet. It may involve removing the seat backs or the entire seats. Or, it may involve removing or flapping the roof.

Once the vehicle has been removed from the patients and they have been properly packaged, the extrication team should work with the medical team to secure each patient to the appropriate-sized backboard. Then, working together, the team members carefully lift each patient and remove them from the wreckage. Once clear of the wreckage, the patients can be transferred to those responsible for transporting them to a medical facility.

Truck on its Side: Extrication

Disentangling and extricating patients from a truck on its side can sometimes be very challenging. However, because the patients may be piled on top of each other at the bottom of the wreckage, the greatest challenge may be for the medical team responsible for stabilizing and packaging the trapped patients. Roof removal is probably the best option for creating a clear opening through which the patients can be extricated — provided that it can be done without compromising the vehicle's stability. Given a well-trained and equipped extrication team, the roof of a truck's cab can be flapped down or removed in less than a minute.

If the truck's stability cannot be maintained if the roof is flapped down or removed, then cutting through the roof and leaving the roof frame intact is another option. Using a cutting tool, rescuers should cut around the edge of the roof and remove the sheet metal and any cross members to create a relatively large opening through which patients can be extricated. However, compared to roof removal, cutting through the roof takes considerably longer.

Truck on its Roof: Extrication

When a truck has come to rest on its roof, the occupants may be in dire need of extrication — and as quickly as safely possible. The possibility of the vehicle catching fire is greater than when in other positions because of the fuel and other flammable fluids that are almost surely to be leaking from the vehicle. Therefore, time is of the essence.

Depending upon the structural condition of the vehicle, members of the extrication team may be available to assist the medical team in freeing patients and with packaging them for extrication. As in all extrication operations, rescue personnel must work together cooperatively for the good of those in need of their help.

Disentanglement and extrication from a truck on its roof may be complicated by the fact that removing door posts or other components may weaken the cab's structural integrity. Weakened cabs are more likely to move suddenly and unexpectedly, perhaps aggravating the patient's injuries. Therefore, rescue personnel must anticipate the consequences of each action before it is taken. If removing a structural component will weaken or destabilize the vehicle, steps must be taken to counteract those effects, or another option must be considered. Otherwise, disentangling and extricating patients from a truck on its roof are no different than from vehicles in the positions already discussed.

Trucks in Other Positions: Extrication

When a truck has come to rest in a position other than those already discussed, rescue personnel may have to use all of their ingenuity and skill to safely and efficiently disentangle and extricate the patients trapped inside. For example, if the patients are trapped in the cab of a truck that is wedged under a collapsed bridge or other structure, the working room inside the cab may be extremely limited. The space limitation may render the most reliable extrication techniques impractical if not impossible to perform. Members of the medical and extrication teams may have to work in either the prone or supine position inside the cab. They may also have to take turns working inside. However, regardless of how innovative the situation forces rescuers to be, they must never forget that the techniques employed must be safe for them to apply and as safe as possible for the patients. While the goal of extricating all patients without doing further injury still applies, these unusual situations may not allow that to happen. In some extremely rare instances, it may be medically necessary to sacrifice a limb to save a life. Such a decision must be made according to local protocols and through consultation between the incident commander (IC) and a physician at the scene. Stabilizing a collapsed bridge or other structure may be necessary prior to rescue operations to insure safer operations.

Summary

Extrication incidents involving medium or heavy trucks can be extremely challenging for rescue personnel. Therefore, if they are to function safely and efficiently at these incidents, personnel must be familiar with the nomenclature and anatomy of these sometimes massive vehicles. Regardless of the size of truck involved, rescue personnel must keep in mind that their role is to protect themselves and others from harm, to protect the trapped patients from further harm, and to free those patients as safely and as quickly as possible.

Review Questions

1. What are distinguishing features of each type of medium and heavy truck?

2. What are the hazards associated with medium and heavy trucks?

3. What types of trailers are commonly associated with medium and heavy trucks?

4. What specific size-up concerns should an incident commander consider during medium and heavy truck extrication operations?

5. What methods can be used to stabilize medium and heavy trucks during extrication operations?

6. What methods can be used to gain access to the interior of medium and heavy trucks?

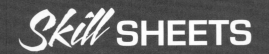
REMINDER: Not all agencies advocate the following procedures and practices. The following skill sheets present a snapshot of various procedures utilized during extrication operations. As always, local agency procedures and protocols must be followed.

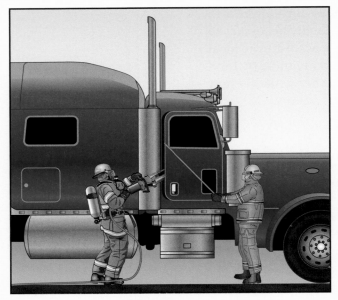

Step 1: Create a purchase point using any of the various methods used in your area.

Step 2: Insert the tips of the spreader at or slightly above the exterior door handle. Place the tips in such a position that they push the door outward and toward the ground.

Step 3: One person should maintain control of the door using a strap to prevent the door from striking anyone. Never use personnel and the door butt method to maintain control in close proximity when prying the door. Instead, a rope, chain, strap, or tubular webbing should be used to tether the door.

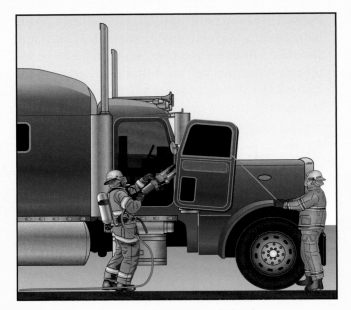

Step 4: Open the spreader arms until the door opens.

Step 5: With automotive style hinges, insert the spreader slightly above the first hinge. It is important to aim the tips of the spreader so the door is being pushed down and away from the vehicle.

Step 6: Open the spreader until the first hinge fails or can be cut.

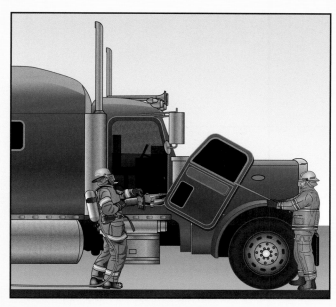

Step 7: If the top hinge was addressed first and the tool has a large enough spreading distance and is properly positioned, it may be possible to continue on and break the second hinge without repositioning. This will depend on the integrity of the doors components. If this is not possible, reposition the tool and repeat the spreading process to break the bottom hinge.

Step 8: If the bottom hinge was addressed first, reposition the spreaders above the top hinge and open the spreaders until the top hinge fails or can be cut.

Step 9: If the door has a piano style hinge, it is often necessary to remove the retaining bolts instead of attempting to cut/pry the hinge off.

NOTE: Freeing a door from a "Nader pin" is not always this easy and may require repositioning the tool or the angle of the tool several times to get the best purchase to overcome the "Nader pin" or other latching mechanism. Parts of the door may tear away without releasing the door from the retaining point.

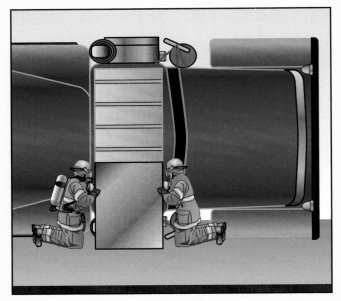

Step 1. Select the area to be opened.

Step 2. Cut the outer skin away.

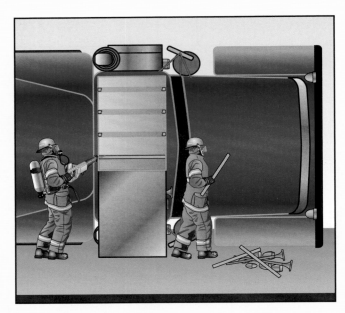

Step 3. Cut inner support structures to create an opening big enough to remove the patient. Do not remove more material than necessary.

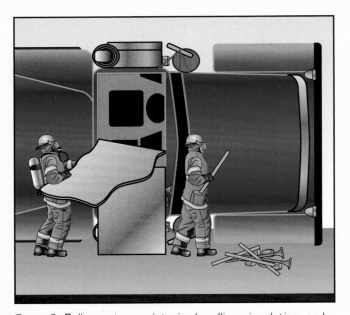

Step 4. Pull or cut away interior headliner, insulation, and other components to allow access to patient.

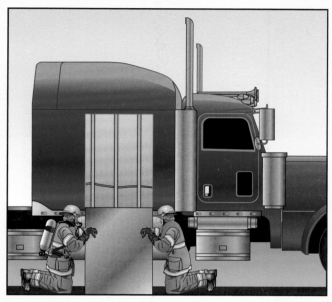

Step 1. Select the area to be opened.

Step 2. Cut the outer skin away.

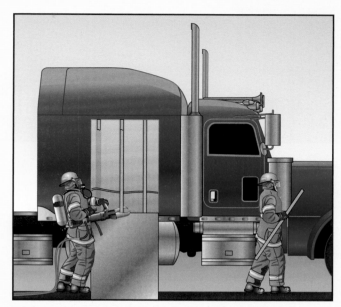

Step 3. Cut inner support structures to create an opening big enough to remove the patient. Do not remove more material than necessary.

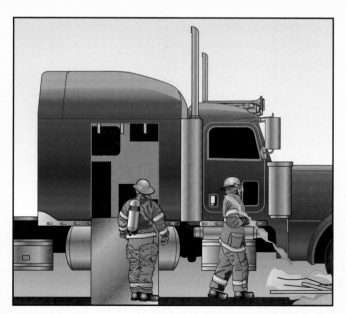

Step 4. Pull or cut away interior cladding, insulation, cabinets, and other components to allow access to patient.

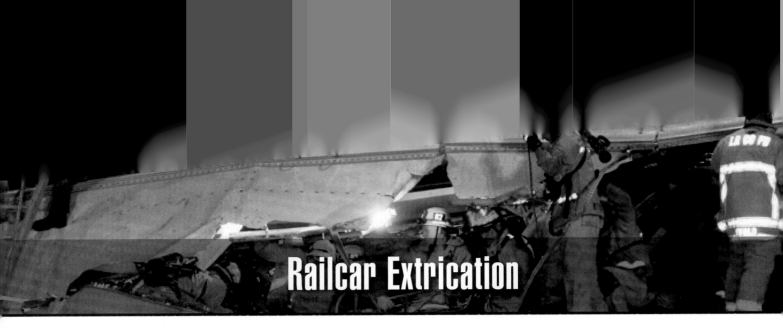

Railcar Extrication

Chapter Contents

Photo Courtesy of Los Angeles Fire Department (LAFD).

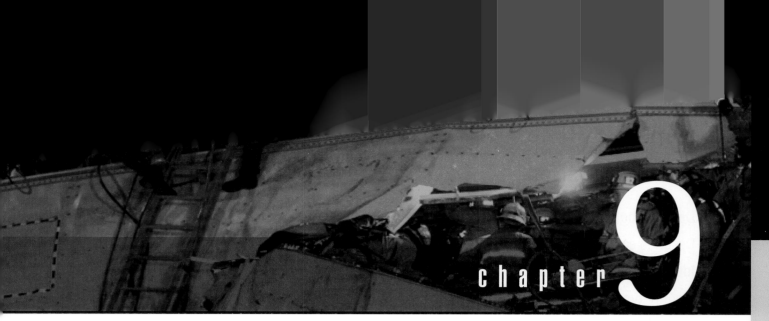

chapter 9

Key Terms

Job Performance Requirements

This chapter provides information that addresses the following job performance requirements (JPRs) of NFPA® 1001, *Standard for Fire Fighter Professional Qualifications* (2008), NFPA® 1006, *Standard for Technical Rescuer Professional Qualifications* (2008), and NFPA® 1670, *Standard on Operations and Training for Technical Search and Rescue Incidents* (2009).

NFPA® 1001 JPRs
6.4.1
6.4.2

NFPA® 1006 JPRs

5.2.2	5.3.2	10.2.1	10.2.4
5.2.3	5.5.1	10.2.2	10.2.5
5.3.1	10.2	10.2.3	

NFPA® 1670 JPRs

8.2.2	8.3.3
8.2.3	8.3.4
8.3.2	8.4.2

Railcar Extrication

Learning Objectives

1. Describe both classes of trains.

2. Describe each type of railcar.

3. Identify anatomical features of railcars.

4. Identify types of rails and roadbeds.

5. Identify specific size-up concerns associated with train incident extrication operations.

6. Explain methods for stabilizing railcars.

7. Describe methods for gaining access into railcars during extrication operations.

8. Identify railcar extrication situations rescuers must be prepared to handle.

Chapter 9
Railcar
Extrication

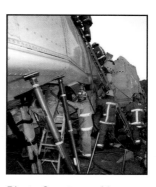

Photo Courtesy of Los Angeles Fire Department (LAFD).

Case History

The collision of a passenger train and a cargo train resulted in a large scale response by the local fire department. In all, a deputy district chief, four battalions chiefs, two EMS chief officers, an EMS assistant deputy chief paramedic, a mobile command and communications unit, four truck companies, four engine companies, a heavy rescue squad, and seven ambulances were initially dispatched to the accident.

An incident command post was established, and hose lines were laid to provide fire protection should diesel fuel from the locomotive's tanks ignite. A nearby school was used as a treatment/transport area and a shelter for the passengers. Triage was conducted once patient injuries were assessed. Rapid transport moved the critically injured to local hospitals.

Additional rescue units and personnel arrived and continued to arrive throughout the incident. Other triage and treatment sites were setup. All passengers were removed from the train and either transported to area hospitals for treatment or received treatment at one of the on-scene treatment locations.

The locomotive of the passenger train was sufficiently damaged to entrap the two engineers inside. While the engineers were not pinned inside the cab, doors into the cab were too heavily damaged to open normally. The locomotive did not have roof access panels or structural weak points that could be exploited to gain access into the cab. Rescuers were finally able to breach one door on the locomotives right side only to find an interior door jammed by the raised floor of the cab. This door was removed as was part of the right-side cab window allowing one engineer to exit the cab through the window and the other through the door.

Of all forms of land-based transportation, passenger trains have the greatest potential for large-scale extrication operations. Large passenger trains may carry hundreds of people at a time. When in motion, the size and weight of a railcar can produce tremendous inertial forces. These forces tend to create an accordion effect in collisions and derailments. The cars often come to rest in a characteristic zigzag pattern with the forward cars stacked upon each other. Added to this scene are the cries for help from trapped and injured passengers and the hysterical screams of horrified onlookers. An incident involving a loaded passenger train can challenge the resources and abilities of even the most capable emergency response organizations because of the potential for mass casualties and the difficulty involved in accessing the trapped victims.

Unlike automobiles, trucks, and buses, which can be found in virtually every area, a jurisdiction either has rail lines or it does not. If the jurisdiction has no rail lines, there is no need to be prepared for incidents involving trains, unless responding to rail incidents on mutual aid is anticipated. On the other hand, if passenger trains regularly travel through the district, rescue personnel should be familiar with them and the techniques required for removing people from the railcars should a collision or derailment occur. The importance of thorough pre-incident planning, followed by realistic training exercises, cannot be overemphasized.

While the information in this chapter is based primarily on Amtrak passenger trains, it is applicable to most rail transportation systems and vehicles. The information on locomotives applies to all locomotives regardless of what type of cars make up the train. The information on passenger cars, all-electric units, and electrical systems also applies to equipment used in local commuter transportation systems. For the most part, this information will also apply to subway systems, although the construction of some subway cars may differ slightly.

Fires and other emergency incidents that occur in railway tunnels, on elevated tracks, or in trams suspended high above the ground are among the most hazardous that rescuers may encounter. Because of these hazardous environments, such incidents are considered to be technical rescue incidents and are beyond the scope of this manual. NFPA 1670, *Standard on Operations and Training for Technical Rescue Incidents* requires fire and rescue organizations having such exposures within their jurisdictions to make provisions for handling these emergencies. The standard allows agencies to train and equip their own personnel to perform these tasks, to enter into automatic aid agreements with other agencies that are trained and equipped to handle these incidents, or to contract with another public or private entity for these services.

This chapter describes:

- Classification of trains and train anatomy
- Make-up of rails and roadbeds
- Steps to size-up of train incidents including:
  — train car stabilization
  — height considerations
  — gaining access
  — extrication situations and techniques
- Considerations taken in special situations involving trains

Train Classifications

In general, trains can be classified into two broad categories — passenger trains and freight trains. Within each of these classifications, many different types of cars may be used. In passenger trains, there may be baggage cars and various types of passenger cars in addition to the locomotives (engines) **(Figure 9.1)**. In freight trains, there may be any of a variety of cars such as flatcars, boxcars, tank cars, and others. In the United States, the word *consist* is used to identify a group of railroad vehicles that make up a train.

Passenger Trains

Whether long or short, main line or local, all passenger trains consist of one or more locomotives or self-propelled cars and a number of passenger cars. Passenger trains vary from relatively slow-moving local commuter trains (light rail) to high-speed express trains that travel up to 150 mph (240 km/h) **(Figure 9.2)**.

Also in this classification are trams and cable cars **(Figures 9.3)**. These small vehicles are designed to carry a few passengers (rarely more than two dozen) a relatively short distance (usually less than a mile [1.6 km]). The motive power for trams may be all-electric, diesel, or hoist cable.

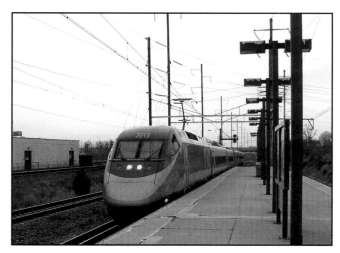

Figure 9.2 A high-speed express passenger train. *Courtesy of Rich Mahaney.*

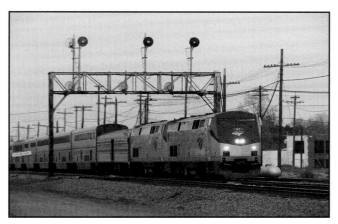

Figure 9.1 A common passenger train. *Courtesy of Rich Mahaney.*

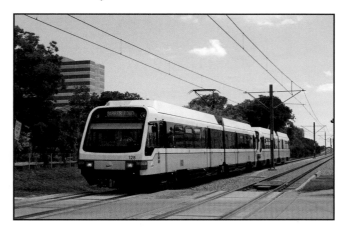

Figure 9.3 A larger tram. *Courtesy of Ed Chapman.*

Freight Trains

Like passenger trains, freight trains are composed of one or more locomotives and a string of cars. Freight cars include flatcars, boxcars, hopper cars, tank cars, and a number of other specialized cars **(Figure 9.4)**. In addition to hauling lumber and similar products, flatcars are also used to carry semitrailers and huge intermodal shipping containers. With the exception of the locomotive, extrication is likely to be needed only if a freight car has come to rest on top of a railroad passenger car or an occupied highway vehicle.

The contents of freight cars and shipping containers can greatly complicate any incident in which they are involved. A derailed tank car that is leaking a flammable, corrosive, or toxic liquid is a threat to rescue personnel, trapped victims, and the environment. Even if the load is not hazardous in itself, if tons of lumber

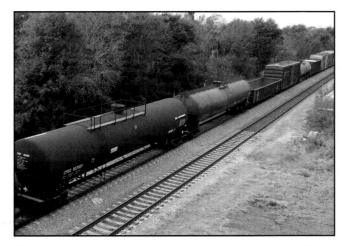

Figure 9.4 An example of a freight train. *Courtesy of Rich Mahaney.*

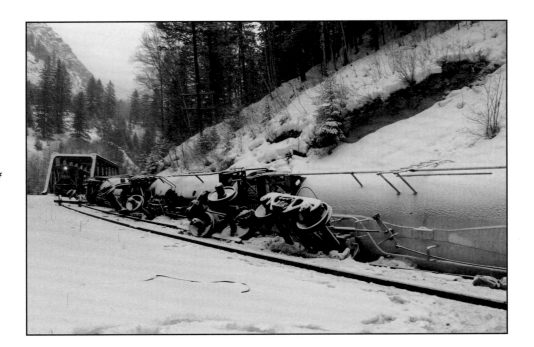

Figure 9.5 A freight train accident scene. *Courtesy of Phil Linder.*

or thousands of boxes or other containers are strewn about the scene, it can make all phases of the operation much more difficult, dangerous, and time consuming **(Figure 9.5)**.

Types of Railcars

In the United States, Amtrak operates a wide variety of railcars. There are several different types of locomotives, passenger coaches, dining cars, and lounge cars as well as specialized cars such as auto carriers. These cars are organized in different fleets that have common characteristics and styling. These fleets are named Heritage, Superliner I and II, Amfleet (Amcans) I and II, Viewliner, Horizon, Turboliner, Talgo, and Acela. Rescue personnel who serve in areas where rail travel is common should familiarize themselves with the various types of railroad equipment common to their area. However, most rescue personnel cannot be expected to know and remember the intricacies and variations of all these various types of cars — especially under emergency conditions. Therefore, only general information about railcars and railcar anatomy is presented here.

On freight trains, the only cars likely to contain a life hazard are the locomotives; therefore, the locomotives are the only freight cars to be discussed in the balance of this chapter. Instead, the chapter focuses primarily on railroad passenger cars and those other types of railroad cars that may involve extrication or body recovery.

Locomotives

Locomotives differ in how they are powered and how they are employed. The most common types of locomotives are:

- Diesel only
- Diesel/electric
- Electric only
- Steam

Some locomotives are powered by diesel engines only. Others are dual-mode units — that is, they have diesel engines but can also be powered by electricity from a 600-volt DC third rail. A few steam locomotives are still in service but only as part of local tourist attractions. As mentioned earlier, trams may be all-electric, diesel powered, or cable operated.

Diesel and Diesel/Electric Locomotive Hazards

Most of the locomotives in both passenger and freight service in North America are diesel/electric — that is, diesel engines operate onboard generators that power electric motors on each axle to drive the wheels. In addition to those used in main line operations, many of these locomotives are used as switching engines in terminals and shop areas.

Diesel/electric locomotives can weigh from 130 tons (118 tonnes) up to 175,000 tons (158 757 tonnes), develop as much as 4,250 horsepower, and carry between 1800 to 2,200 gallons (6 814 to 8 800 L) of diesel fuel inside or under the locomotive **(Figure 9.6)**. Locomotives have a top speed of up to 125 mph (201 km/h). The volume of combustible diesel fuel carried by such locomotives present one type of hazard found during train incidents/accidents. While running, diesel/electric locomotives generate both high- and low-voltage AC and DC electrical current for train operation. There are two electric drive motors in each locomotive truck.

Electric Locomotive Hazards

The primary hazards associated with electric locomotives is the high voltage involved in such systems and the danger of electrocution. Most operate with power from a 12,000 volt AC to 25,000 volt AC catenary system of wires suspended above the tracks. A roof-mounted pantograph maintains contact with the overhead wires to provide power to the locomotive **(Figure 9.7)**.

NOTE: Both catenary systems and pantographs are discussed in greater detail later in this chapter. These locomotives weigh as much as 100 tons (91 tonnes), develop as much as 7,000 horsepower, and have a top speed of up to 150 mph (240 km/h).

Some Amtrak trains as well as local commuter trains have all-electric locomotives operated by power from an electrically charged third rail between or adjacent to the regular rails **(Figure 9.8, p. 390)**. As mentioned earlier, this enclosed third rail carries 600 volts DC and must be avoided by all but trained Amtrak personnel.

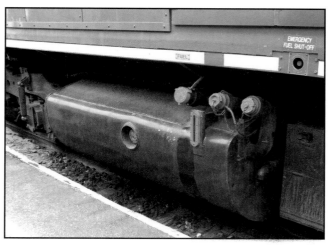

Figure 9.6 The fuel tanks on a diesel/electric locomotive. *Courtesy of Rich Mahaney.*

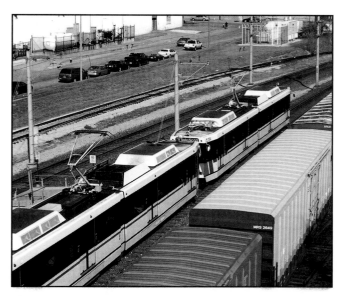

Figure 9.7 A catenary wire system and roof mounted pantographs on an electric powered rail sys tem. *Courtesy of Bill Accord.*

Pantograph — A mechanical linkage device which maintains electrical contact with a contact wire and transfers power from the wire to the traction unit of electric buses, locomotives, and trams.

Caternary wire system — A series of overhead wires used to transmit electrical power to buses, locomotives, and trams at a distance from the energy supply point.

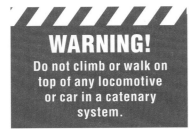
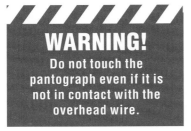
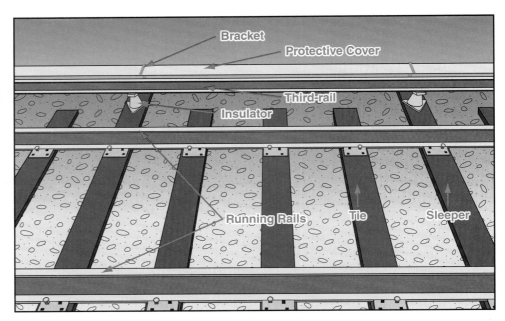

Figure 9.8 A third-rail electrical system.

Steam Locomotive Hazards

While extremely rare, some steam locomotives are still in use. These locomotives are used for tourist and sightseeing excursions, particularly in Colorado, California, and Arizona. Hazards associated with steam locomotives include the potential for extremely hot steam that may escape from damaged piping or boiler as well as the risk of fire from the unit used to heat the boiler **(Figure 9.9)**.

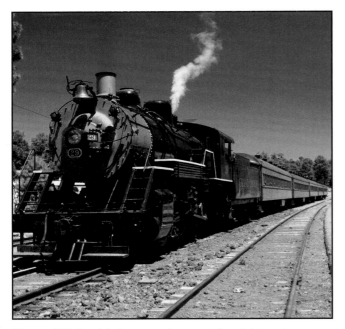

Figure 9.9 An old steam engine used for sight seeing excursions. *Courtesy of Bill Accord.*

Passenger Cars

Amtrak operates a variety of passenger cars, and they are representative of those operated by other rail systems. The construction of railroad passenger coaches is similar to that described in Chapter 7, *Bus Extrication,* for commercial buses. The primary difference is that railcars are constructed much more substantially, with heavier materials than those used in buses.

Coach cars and coach dome cars provide passenger seating space. High-level cars provide two levels of coach space for passengers. Some coach cars also provide crew sleeping space. Depending on the layout of the cars, they can seat anywhere from 44 to 85 passengers. Both passengers and crew members may be present during train operation. The 85-passenger coaches have seating facilities for passengers with disabilities. These coaches are usually the last in the consist, and some contain secondary controls that allow the train to be operated in reverse from the last car without turning the train around.

Sleeper cars provide passengers with seating room and sleeping accommodations. Some sleepers also provide daytime private rooms for first-class passengers. These cars are normally located either toward the front or rear of the train. Passengers and crew members may be present in these areas during train operation. All sleeping/bedroom, seating, and toilet areas should be checked for victims during size-up and search and rescue.

Lounge/Food Service Cars

Also known as "club cars," lounge/food service cars provide food/beverage service and entertainment to passengers aboard Amtrak trains. Some dining cars include an upper level dining area for passengers as well as a food preparation area in the lower level of the same car. Some variant configurations also provide limited passenger coach space. Full-dome lounge cars provide food and beverage service for passengers and crew members, as well as a panoramic view. These cars are normally located in the center of the consist. Passengers and crew members may be present in these areas during train operation. All dining, bar, and food storage areas should be checked for passengers and crew members during size-up and search and rescue.

Baggage Cars

With the exceptions of commuter trains and trams, all passenger trains will have one or more baggage cars in the consist. The purpose of the baggage car is to transport passenger baggage. Some coach/baggage cars provide upper level coach space for passengers and space on a lower level for transporting baggage. These cars are normally located directly behind the locomotive at the front of the consist. An assistant conductor may be present in the car during train operation. Therefore, it is essential that all areas of the car, including the toilet room, be checked for crew members during size-up and search and rescue.

Material Handling Cars

These are essentially standard boxcars used for carrying baggage and mail. They are usually located directly behind the locomotive or at the end of the consist. In addition to having side doors only, these cars have plug doors that must be pulled outward before sliding laterally. Material handling cars are usually unoccupied during train operation but rescuers must check these cars to ensure there are no patients in them.

Railcar Anatomy

Regardless of what type of railroad passenger cars are involved in an incident, they all have certain features and characteristics in common. The most common features are discussed in the following sections to help explain those features that either help or hinder them in an extrication operation.

Electrical Hazards

All Amtrak cars are equipped with 480-volt electrical circuits charged by power from the locomotive, commonly called "head-end power." The power may be supplied to the locomotive by an overhead catenary system or a third rail (both discussed later in this chapter) or from diesel generators aboard the

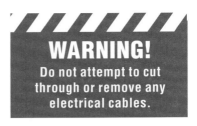

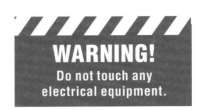

locomotive. Power is supplied to the individual cars by jumper cables connected between each car **(Figure 9.10)**. Rescue personnel should not remove or attempt to remove these cables. Only trained Amtrak crew members can safely perform the following actions:

- De-energize head-end power
- Lower locomotive pantographs
- Disengage third-rail shoes
- Ground electrical equipment when required
- Remove or install power cables

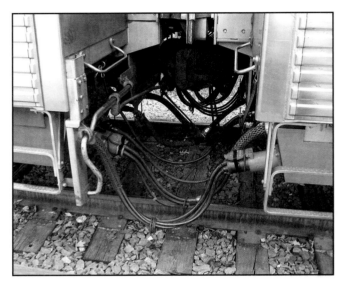

Figure 9.10 Electrical power "jumper" cables between rail cars. *Courtesy of Rich Mahaney.*

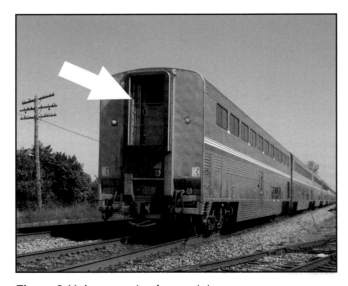

Figure 9.11 An example of an end door on a passenger railcar. *Courtesy of Rich Mahaney.*

Windows

Railroad passenger cars have windows along the full length of both sides of the car. Some have an upper and lower row, and they may be any of several different styles. Two different window pane materials are used: Lexan® plastic and tempered glass. The type of pane used will vary on different types of cars.

All Amtrak passenger coaches are equipped with emergency window exits. Each car will have at least four of these window exits — two on each side — and some have more. These windows have double panes — the outer pane is either Lexan® or tempered glass, but the inner pane is always Lexan®.

Doors

All railroad passenger cars have end doors. These doors either swing inward or slide sideways to open. Most sliding doors are power assisted — either electrically or electro-pneumatically. In case of power failure, they easily slide open manually. Car end doors are not locked during train operation and function normally while the train is in motion **(Figure 9.11)**.

Some passenger cars also have side-entry doors located at both ends of each car. These are pocket doors that slide sideways into the car body to open. Other passenger cars have inward-swinging side-entry doors located in the center of the car. Because these doors are closed and automatically locked during train operation **(Figures 9.12)**, rescuers may have to force entry through these doors following a collision and/or derailment.

Floors

Gaining entry through passenger car floors may be necessary if a car comes to rest on its side or roof. The floor framing is usually constructed of tubular steel or aluminum attached to the railcar frame. Most passenger railcar floors are composed of plymetal (plywood and metal, usually aluminum) panels that are attached to the

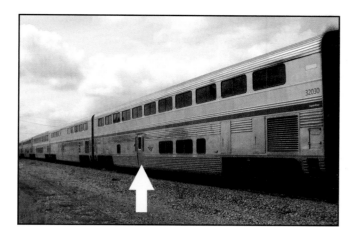

Figure 9.12 The location of a side entry door on a passenger railcar. *Courtesy of Rich Mahaney.*

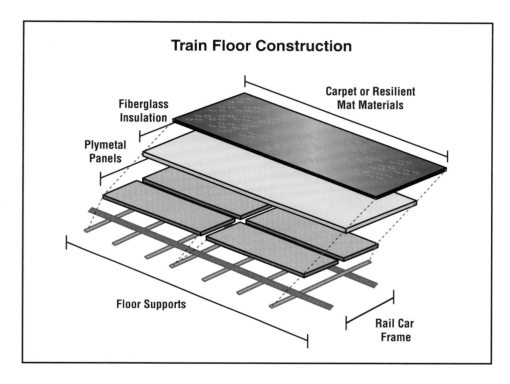

Figure 9.13 Examples of the components used to construct railcar floors.

framework. Floors are usually insulated with fiberglass insulation and covered with carpet and resilient matting materials **(Figure 9.13)**. It may be difficult to gain access through a car floor because of the following obstructions:

- Utility lines (gas, water, sewage, and electrical power)
- Train brake system air lines
- Heating, ventilation, and air conditioning (HVAC) units
- Water and waste water storage tanks
- Electrical generators attached to the underside of a car

Plymetal Panels – Railcar floor panels constructed of plywood sheets covered by sheets of metal, usually aluminum.

Walls/Roofs

Most Amtrak cars have exterior skins made of 3/32-inch (2.5 mm) stainless steel. Other cars have an aluminum skin. In many cases, the wall construction consists of steel framing members and plywood sandwiched between two sheets of stainless steel or aluminum. Heavy-duty framing members are placed 12 to 24 inches (300 mm to 600 mm) on center in the walls, floors, and roof structure. Roofs can also be covered with a thin fiberglass skin. Locomotive walls are made from 3/8 inch (3 mm) thick steel, the roof is made from 1/8 inch (10 mm) steel **(Figure 9.14)**.

Trucks

Trucks (also called railroad trucks) are the assemblies to which a railcar's wheel axles are attached. Trucks are constructed of cast steel and can weigh up to 7 tons. These assemblies are made up of the wheels, suspension and braking system **(Figure 9.15)**.

Brakes

Firefighters and other rescue personnel need to be familiar with the operation of the hand brakes on freight cars. On level tracks, applying the hand brake may be all that is needed to stabilize a car. Braking systems are operated by air pressure up to 140 psi (965 kPa). Responders should not attempt to disconnect the airlines prior to shutting off the air supply at the knuckle on the end of the car as serious injury or death may result **(Figure 9.16)**.

> **WARNING!**
> Do not attempt to disconnect airlines prior to shutting off the air supply at the knuckle end of a car.

Rails/Roadbeds

Most trains run on standard-gauge twin-rail beds. Some trams and tourist trains operate on narrow-gauge rail beds. However, from an extrication standpoint, the width of the rail bed is far less important than the electrical hazards associated with some systems. Some Amtrak locomotives and many local commuter trains obtain their motive power from wires suspended above the tracks (catenary systems), while other commuter trains and trams obtain motive power from an energized third rail between or adjacent to the regular rails.

Catenary Systems

The overhead catenary system consists of longitudinal wires and cables suspended from poles that hold an electrically charged trolley wire in a firm position above the track. The pantograph mounted on top of the locomotive maintains contact with the trolley wires to conduct 12,000 volts to 25,000 volts AC, 25 Hz, to the locomotive motors.

Catenary poles are 14-inch (350 mm) square steel H-sections weighing 84 pounds per foot (125 kg/m). They range in height from 70 to 170 feet (21 m to 52 m). At the top of each pole is a ground wire located approximately 9 feet (3 m) above the transmission conductors. The ground wire is a return for the propulsion current and protects the transmission line from lightning strikes. Approximately 3 feet (1 m) down from the ground wire are the transmission cross arms, 18 feet (6 m) across, held level by sag rods. Below these cross arms are two transmission lines energized at 138,000 volts **(Figure 9.17, p. 396)**.

On one side of the pole is a signal power line energized at 6,900 volts, 100 Hz. The signal line is a transmission line between substations to locations along the right-of-way. There, it is transformed into various voltages to feed signals, track circuits, and other equipment.

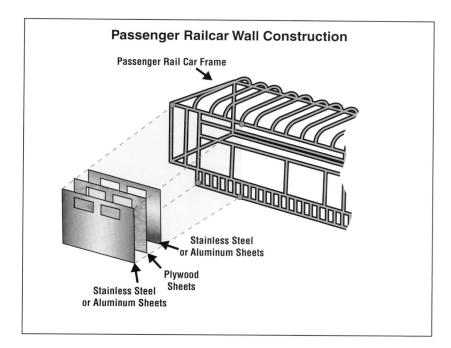

Passenger Railcar Wall Construction

Passenger Rail Car Frame

Stainless Steel
or Aluminum Sheets

Plywood
Sheets

Stainless Steel
or Aluminum Sheets

Figure 9.14 A cutaway view of passenger railcar wall construction.

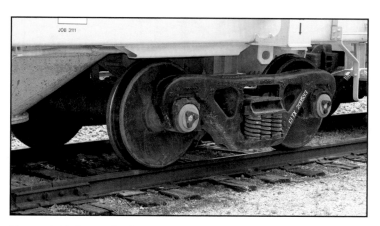

Figure 9.15 A standard railcar truck.

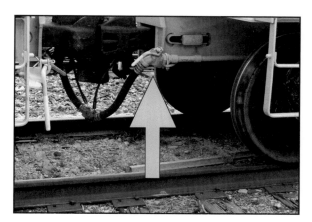

Figure 9.16 An air supply shut off valve handle.

The trolley wires above the tracks are supported between the body span by three units of 10-inch (250 mm) disk-type insulators. Immediately below the insulators is a longitudinal messenger wire. Below this is an auxiliary messenger wire supported by bronze hanger rods. Below the auxiliary wire is the contact or trolley wire, supported from the auxiliary messenger by clips spaced 15 feet (5 m) apart. All wires and hardware of the catenary system are energized at 12,000 volts.

Substations on the system are spaced 8 to 10 miles (13 km to 18 km) apart. These substations contain power control apparatus for the 12,000 volt, 25 Hz, catenary system; the 6,900 volt, 100 Hz, signal power line; and the 138,000 volt, 25 Hz, transmission line. Firefighters and other rescue personnel should not enter these facilities unless accompanied by qualified Amtrak employees.

Under no circumstances should any object be allowed to contact these wires. Materials such as wood, rope, and clothing that might be considered nonconductive at low voltages are not safe for use in close proximity to high-voltage wires.

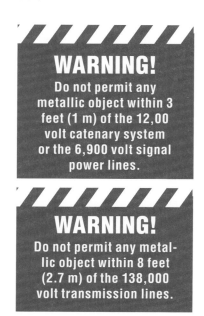

WARNING!
Do not permit any metallic object within 3 feet (1 m) of the 12,00 volt catenary system or the 6,900 volt signal power lines.

WARNING!
Do not permit any metallic object within 8 feet (2.7 m) of the 138,000 volt transmission lines.

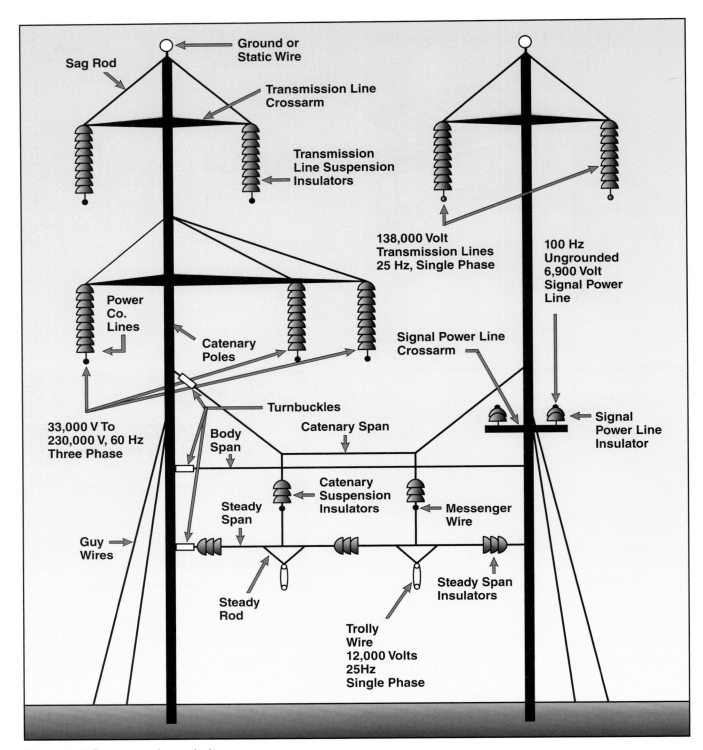

Figure 9.17 Catenary poles and wires.

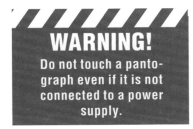

WARNING!
Do not touch a pantograph even if it is not connected to a power supply.

The pantograph on top of each car conducts electrical power from the overhead wires to the car. If there is no obvious electrical hazard following a collision and/or derailment on a catenary line, the overhead power should not be disconnected. Electrical power will provide for lighting and electric door operation. When an electrical hazard does exist, the overhead power supply can be disconnected by pressing the "Pantograph Down" button in the locomotive control cab and then grounding the locomotive. This is usually done by Amtrak crew members before emergency responders arrive. If it has not been done, rescuers should see that it is done by properly qualified personnel. Rescue personnel should not get on the roof of these type of locomotives as the roof area may be energized.

Third-rail Systems

Third-rail electrical-power distribution systems generally distribute 600-volt DC current. The third rail is usually located slightly above and to the side of the two regular rails on which the train's wheels run. No one should be allowed to touch a third rail or its protective cover. Third-rail power may be de-energized by contacting the appropriate power director/dispatcher or by using emergency switch boxes where installed along the right-of-way **(Figure 9.18)**. Only personnel from those agencies having direct authority from Amtrak or the local train authority should use these emergency switch boxes.

Roadbeds

Although some percentage of all roadbeds are at grade level, especially in switching yards and loading/unloading areas, much of their length is not. The rails and cross ties are set atop a berm that allows the roadbed to be more-or-less level throughout its length. To discourage the growth of vegetation along the roadbed, and thereby reduce the risk of fires, the spaces between the cross ties and down both sides of the berm are covered with coarse gravel **(Figure 9.19)**.

The steeply sloped sides of the roadbed embankment and the loose gravel make traction and footing difficult. Therefore, gaining access and stabilizing the crashed vehicles may be far more difficult than would be the case in other locations. The slope of the embankment and the lack of traction may make it difficult to position rescue vehicles close to the scene. It may be necessary to lay ground ladders on the slopes of the berm to provide secure footing for rescue personnel.

Specific Size-Up Concerns for Train Incident Extrication

As with any other type of extrication incident, those involving trains should be assessed (sized up) in a systematic way. First, the scene is assessed, followed by an assessment of the vehicles involved. Then, the victims are assessed as are the extrication requirements for that particular incident. As always, size-up continues throughout the incident.

Once on scene, the first responding officer must determine if a legitimate emergency exists. If so, he should assume command of the incident and begin a more thorough assessment of the vehicles involved. As with other types of extrication incidents, the incident commander (IC) must try to determine how many vehicles are involved and their conditions. In the derailment of a long passenger train, scene assessment can be a daunting task. With railcars resting at various angles and in various positions

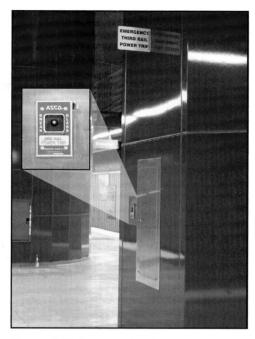

Figure 9.18 An example of an emergency power shut off switch for a third-rail electrical system. *Courtesy of Robert J. Tremberth.*

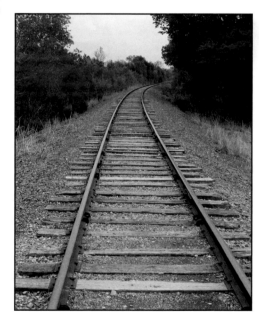

Figure 9.19 A common railroad bed.

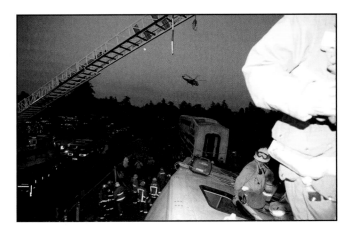

Figure 9.20 An example of just a small part of a railroad accident. *Courtesy of Los Angeles Fire Department (LAFD).*

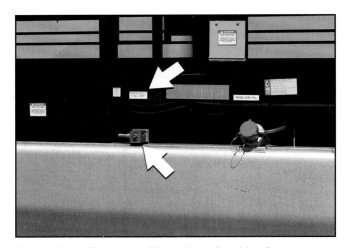

Figure 9.21a Fuel shut off switch on the side of a locomotive. *Courtesy of Rich Mahaney.*

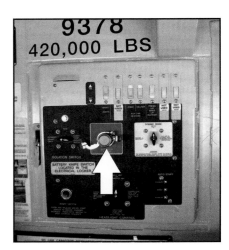

Figure 9.21b Fuel shut off switch inside the cab of a locomotive. *Courtesy of Rich Mahaney.*

along both sides of the track, it can be very difficult to see the entire scene from one location **(Figure 9.20)**. How the cars came to rest — upright, on their sides, upside down — will dictate how much and what types of shoring and cribbing materials will be needed.

Diesel/electric locomotives can carry up to 2,200 gallons (8 800 L) of diesel fuel in tanks located inside the locomotive or underneath it. Fuel shutoff devices (clearly marked FUEL SHUT OFF) are located on each side of the locomotive body side rails and also on the firewall of the cab behind the engineer **(Figure 9.21a and b)**. To shut off the fuel supply to the engine, push and hold the emergency fuel shutoff device for 8 to 10 seconds. The engine will stop running within about one minute.

In situations where there is a high likelihood of mass casualties, one of the highest operational priorities is setting up for triage, treatment, and transportation. Prior to the train cars being stabilized, any passengers who have escaped the wreckage should be questioned about the location and condition of others still trapped inside. After the cars are stabilized, rescue personnel should be assigned to quickly but thoroughly search all cars and triage the passengers trapped inside. The number and condition of the victims may indicate a need for additional ambulances or medevac helicopters.

Based on the specifics of the crash — the number of cars involved and their conditions and the number of trapped victims and their conditions — a determination must be made regarding how much and what types of extrication resources will be needed. Questions to assess are as follows:

- Are there a sufficient number of power spreaders, cutters, and similar equipment available on scene, or do more need to be requested?

- Is there a need for oxyacetylene cutting torches, plasma cutters, or burning bars?

- Is there a need for additional personnel to allow more tasks to be performed at the same time or for crew relief if the incident becomes protracted?

- Is there a need for a full Rehab Unit if the incident becomes protracted?

For incidents involving passenger trains, rescuers will need to triage patients carefully to determine who requires immediate medical treatment and who can wait for treatment at a later time. These triage efforts will assist in determining medical transportation requirements. The rescue agency should establish a standard operating procedure (SOP) for train incident triage procedures.

The IC should consider contacting the railroad company dispatcher to stop other rail traffic from entering the area. In areas not controlled with signals or dispatchers, the IC should place flare flaggers up to two miles away on either side of the incident. These flaggers should swing the flare from side-to-side in an arc at arms length. Engineers are trained to stop the train upon seeing this signal.

Railcar Stabilization

Because of the size and weight of most railroad cars, they are generally very stable. However, following a collision and/or derailment, some of the cars may have come to rest in unstable positions. They may need to be stabilized to protect trapped and injured victims and to provide a safe working environment for rescue personnel. Considering that much of the equipment used to stabilize highway vehicles will be of limited value when trying to stabilize these massive vehicles, determining how to stabilize railcars can be a tremendous challenge. Simply deciding where to start can be difficult. However, the survival of both the trapped victims and rescue personnel depend upon this critical step being performed quickly and effectively. Normal cribbing will not be sufficient in size or strength to handle railroad emergencies. If railroad ties are available at the scene, they can be used as cribbing for stabilization **(Figure 9.22, p. 400)**.

Railcar Upright

Because the majority of the weight of most railcars is concentrated in the lower third of their structure, railcars that are upright and still on the tracks are relatively stable. If a car is still upright but off the tracks and subject to sliding or rolling down the side of the roadbed embankment, then extensive stabilization may be required. Responders should apply the railcar's brake to limit movement of the car.

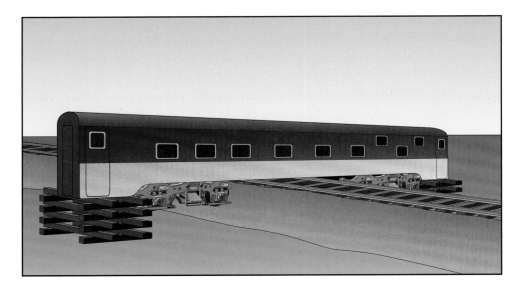

Figure 9.22 Railroad ties can be used by rescuers to construct cribbing to stabilize railcars.

Railcar on Its Side

Unless affected by slope or similar environmental influences, a railcar on its side is very stable. The shape, size, and weight of most railcars make it unlikely that they will move suddenly or unexpectedly when resting on their sides on a stable and level surface.

However, if the car is resting on mud, snow, or unstable soil, rescue personnel must be extremely cautious. Under these conditions, the biggest danger is that the car will suddenly roll back upright without warning. To reduce this possibility, the car should be stabilized with shoring from the underside.

Railcar on Its Roof

Because a railcar is top heavy when resting on its roof, this position can be very unstable. Unless its movement is limited by an adjacent embankment and/or leaning against other railcars, a car on its roof may suddenly roll to one side or the other. The car should be secured with webbing, chains, or heavy ropes, before personnel are allowed close enough to install shoring along both sides.

Railcars in Other Positions

The inertial forces involved in many train derailments leave railcars accordioned into a characteristic zigzag pattern, with the forward cars stacked upon each other. Stabilizing several cars at the same time can be very difficult. Only the specific situation can dictate which car should be stabilized first and how stabilization should be accomplished. As mentioned earlier, cars may need to be stabilized to prevent them from sliding or rolling down a steep embankment or into a body of water. Cars that have overridden other cars may need to be stabilized to prevent them from sliding or falling off the cars beneath them. Unlike highway vehicle extrication incidents, the time that would be needed to install a sufficient amount of rigging and heavy shoring to stabilize these railcars may eliminate this as an option. Instead, if heavy construction vehicles are available, they can be used to temporarily stabilize the railcars by placing their bucket, blade, or articulating arm against the sides of the cars.

Gaining Access into Railcars

Once the railcars have been stabilized, rescue personnel can enter the cars for search and rescue. Because of the relative ease of access and egress, using a railcar's doors is better than using the windows for extricating victims. Even if a railcar is on its side or on its roof, the door openings will still allow the easiest passage into and out of the car. If all doorways are blocked, then victims will have to be removed through the windows. In the most extreme cases, they can be removed through openings cut in the walls or roof of the car — but this should be attempted only as a last resort. The sections that follow describe these entry points in some detail.

Height Considerations

The height of the roadbed above grade, the steepness of the sides of the berm, and the poor footing afforded by the loose gravel covering the berm, may force rescue personnel to lay ground ladders on the sides of the berm just to be able to reach the roadbed. Where a paved road parallels the railroad, it may be possible to position an aerial device on the roadway to allow the use of the main ladder or articulating boom to reach the roadbed. Once on the roadbed, rescuers may need ladders to reach the doors and windows of the railcars.

Even when the roadbed is at grade, the height of the railcar doors and windows may make it necessary for rescue personnel to use their ingenuity to create stable working platforms for extrication operations. If immediately available, conventional aluminum scaffolding can be erected beside a railcar and moved along from car to car as needed. Wooden planks between two stepladders can be used as a makeshift scaffold. A flatbed truck or a fire engine positioned beside a railcar can provide a relatively large, stable platform from which to work, and it can be moved from car to car as needed. If railcars are stacked one upon the other, ground ladders and/or aerial devices may be needed to reach the necessary access points.

Locomotive Entry

Most locomotive cabs can be entered through either of two doors on each side or on some models, through an additional door in the nose. Almost all locomotive cab doors open by turning the door latch and pushing inward. These doors are not locked during train operation, so rescue personnel should not need to force entry following a collision and/or derailment.

Because the cab doors on most locomotives are too narrow to accommodate many standard litters, the best option for extricating injured crew members may be to remove the locomotive windshield or side windows and pass them out through the opening. Side door and sliding cab windows are single panes of either Lexan® or tempered glass that slide sideways to open and are not usually locked. Some locomotive windshields are single-pane, laminated safety glass; others are Lexan®. The windshield is over one half an inch thick and is held in by a heavy frame system. It is very time consuming and labor intensive to remove. If access is not possible through the side windows, remove the windshield protector, if the unit has one, and then remove the windshield. If entry cannot be made through the windows or doors, the roof is the next option as it is made from 1/8 inch (10 mm) steel.

Passenger Car Door Entry

All railroad passenger cars have end doors, and some have side-entry vestibule doors. These doors are the first points where rescue personnel should attempt entry into these cars. The sections that follow provide more detailed information about exterior entry doors on passenger cars.

Passenger Coach End Doors

Passenger coach end doors normally remain unlocked during train operation and are likely to be unlocked following a collision or derailment. If not, the majority have latches that are manually operated. Some end doors are power assisted and have push plates or bars marked "PUSH TO OPEN" or "PRESS." These push plates activate an electric or electro-pneumatic power assist opening device. If this device is not operable, the door can be opened manually by either pushing it inward or sliding it sideways. Power-assisted end doors have power cut-out switches on both sides of the door permitting door operation during malfunctions and emergencies. Lockable end door latches may be unlocked with a standard Amtrak coach key obtainable from a crew member.

Passenger Car Side-Entry Doors

Some passenger coaches, sleepers, and lounge/food service cars also have side-entry vestibule doors. Some of these doors are manually operated and pneumatically locked. These doors are automatically locked by an inflatable weatherseal that releases automatically when the door handle is pulled, opening the latch. If the seals do not deflate, open the ceiling panel directly above the door on the public address system locker side, and open the door seal cut-out valve. This allows both doors in that vestibule to be opened manually.

Other side-entry doors are electrically actuated and locked. They can be opened by obtaining a standard Amtrak coach key from a crew member. If electrical power is still on to the door circuits, the door will slide open. If the power is off, open the door manually by grasping the outside door indentation and pushing it sideways. These doors may be opened from the inside by pulling down on the door lock handle located in a ceiling recess above the door. The door can then be opened manually by sliding it sideways.

Some side-entry doors may be opened from outside the car by opening the door seal cut-out valve located under the car adjacent to the door. Preferably, a trained Amtrak crew member should perform this function to ensure that nearby air brake lines remain operative.

While many side-entry vestibule doors slide sideways to open, the side-entry doors on some other cars swing inward to open. These doors are closed and latched during train operation. When unlatched, the door can be opened manually. If the door is jammed, open the door window using the latch handle in the frame.

Passenger Car Window Entry

While most passenger coaches have relatively small side windows measuring 29½ inches wide by 16½ inches high (737 mm by 412 mm), the Talgo coaches have larger side windows that measure 5 feet 3 inches wide by 39 inches high (1.6 m by 1 m). With the glass completely removed, these windows offer adequate clearance for most backboards and litters.

As discussed earlier in this chapter, railcar window openings are covered with either tempered glass or Lexan®, or both. Since tempered glass is designed to fracture into many small pieces when broken, rescuers and victims may suffer minor scratches and small cuts from contact with these small pieces of glass. Tempered glass is easily broken by striking a bottom corner of the pane with a pointed object, such as the pick end of an axe. Smaller panes can be broken by pressing a spring-loaded center punch into the bottom corner of the window pane.

Lexan® is a polycarbonate plastic 250 times stronger than glass and 30 times stronger than Plexiglas®. It will not break when struck with a forcible entry tool. In fact, the tool will bounce off the Lexan®, and that could injure the rescuer or others nearby. The only successful methods of dealing with Lexan® are to remove the entire pane or to cut through it with a power saw.

Window panes are removable from the outside in a manner similar to those used for over-the-road trucks. Emergency exit windows can be removed from the outside of the car. The emergency windows can be identified by a plate with the removal instructions located next to each emergency exit window. These plates are also located at the ends of each car. **Skill Sheet 9-1** describes how to remove tempered glass windows.

Passenger Car Roof/Wall Entry

As described earlier in the section on railcar anatomy, the construction of railroad passenger cars is similar to but much heavier than that used in the construction of buses. The exterior walls are generally reinforced stainless steel designed to resist impact forces. This type of construction resists forcible entry, and it should be attempted only if other means of access are unavailable. Breaching the walls of a railroad passenger car will almost certainly require the use of oxyacetylene cutting torches and/or other exothermic cutting devices.

Unlike buses and heavy trucks, the roof of a railroad passenger car is made of the same gauge material as the walls. Therefore, forcible entry through this area is unlikely to produce positive results.

Interior Door Locks/Latches

Once inside a rail passenger car, rescue personnel will find a variety of locking and latching mechanisms on interior doors. Most are similar to those found in industrial settings and their operation is obvious from their construction. Mechanical locks may require a standard Amtrak coach key obtainable from a train crew member. This section covers only those locks and latches unique to trains or those whose functions may not be immediately apparent.

Toilet Door Latches

The toilet room latch is similar on most models of cars. When the "Occupied" display is showing, rescuers should assume that someone is inside. To open the door, rescuers should insert a screwdriver or similar object into the oval opening in the slide bolt and move the bolt to the left. The door will unlock and open inward. The toilet doors on other models may be unlocked using standard Amtrak coach keys.

Sleeping Car Bedroom Door Latches

Some sleeping car bedroom doors can be opened by removing the two Phillips head cover plate screws exposing the keyway. The lock may now be opened using a standard coach key.

Sleeping Car Intercommunicating Door Latches

These doors are generally locked and unlocked by one of three different slide bar devices. Rescuers should use the following instructions to open each different type of slide bar latch:

- Slide bar #1 is opened by using the standard Amtrak coach key
- Slide bar #2 is opened by the slide mechanism on one side of the bedroom divider
- Slide bar #3 is opened by the slide mechanism on the other side of the bedroom divider.

Sleeping Car Room Door Latches

All sleeping car rooms are designed to be locked from the inside. To open locked doors from the outside, remove the two slotted screws on the outside door handle. The pin inside the door is attached to the outside cover plate. When the plate is removed, the latch drops allowing the door to slide open.

Lounge/Food Service Car Entry

Entry into lounge cars should be attempted through their side-entry vestibule doors and if that is not successful, through the end doors. Diner and buffet cars do not have side-entry doors, so the end doors should be used. The kitchen and bar loading doors are locked during train operation, so entry should be made through other doors or windows. If door entry is unsuccessful, entry should be made through the emergency exit windows.

Baggage Car Entry

Entry into baggage cars can be made through the sliding side doors or through the end doors. The side doors are usually locked during train operation. They feature a slide-type lock a few inches above the floor of the car. The end doors will usually not be locked if a crew member is inside the car. If entry through the end doors is not possible and the side doors are locked, the quickest method of entry is through the windows in the side doors. The door window panes consist of a single pane of Lexan® that can be removed using the procedure described earlier.

Material Handling Car Entry

Material handling cars have plug doors that must extend clear of the door opening before sliding sideways. The door automatically extends outward when the lever handle or wheel is operated. These doors are normally closed and locked during train operation, so forcible entry will be required following a collision and/or derailment. If it is necessary to enter one of these cars, the best way to do so is through the side doors. If the doors are jammed, they will have to be forcibly opened using a rescue saw or power-spreading equipment.

Railcar Extrication Situations

As mentioned earlier, extrication incidents that occur in tunnels, on elevated railways, on railroad bridges, and in similar high-hazard environments are considered to be technical rescue problems that are beyond the scope of this manual. However, there are still numerous special situations with which firefighters and other first responders must be prepared to deal, some of them are explained in the sections that follow.

Disentanglement/Tunneling

Even though railroad cars are substantially built, the tremendous inertial forces involved in many train wrecks can cause significant damage to the cars. These forces can rearrange the cars' interior configurations and thereby entrap passengers and crew members **(Figure 9.23)**. The heavy gauge material of which these vehicles are constructed makes the entrapment that much more complete. The same problems involved in disentangling victims trapped in buses are involved in freeing those in railcars, but made more difficult by the heavy construction.

Because of the mass of railroad passenger cars, when they are stacked one upon the other, it may be necessary for rescue personnel to tunnel through the wreckage in much the same way that rescuers tunnel through rubble and debris following structural collapse. And, many of the same tunneling techniques can be used. Before rescue personnel are allowed to work beneath heavy overhanging objects — heavily damaged railcars or parts thereof — these objects must be supported with appropriate shoring. Box cribbing may be sufficient in some cases, but heavy timber shoring or hydraulic/pneumatic shoring is more likely to be needed.

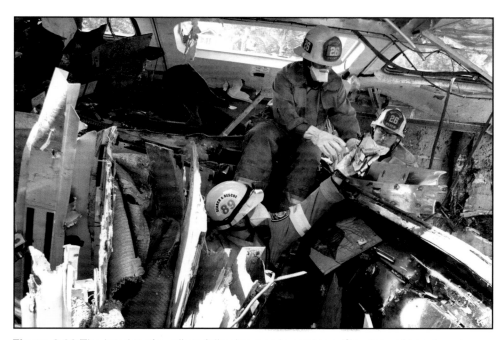

Figure 9.23 The interior of a railcar following a train collision. *Courtesy of Los Angeles Fire Department (LAFD).*

Loading Platform Incidents

These incidents most often involve one or more individuals who, in one way or another, have left the platform and are on the roadbed. They may be in close proximity to a third rail, lying on tracks used by high-speed commuter trains, or under a standing railcar. In most cases, railway personnel will be on the scene when rescue personnel arrive — in fact, they may have initiated the 9-1-1 call. In these cases, a unified command made up of the first arriving officer and a railway representative is most appropriate. In this way, the incident action plan (IAP) can accurately reflect the expertise, capabilities, and limitations of both agencies and is most likely to be a realistic, safe, and effective plan.

If rescue personnel are on the scene before railway personnel, the railway operator should be notified of the situation and asked to send emergency response personnel. Rescue personnel should avoid the third rail (if present), cordon off the area, and deny entry to all but authorized personnel. Depending upon the specifics of the situation, rescue personnel may be able to take effective action to rescue the victim prior to the arrival of railway personnel. However, these actions should only be initiated if they have a reasonable expectation of success and they do not involve unnecessary risk for rescue personnel.

Train/Highway Vehicle Collisions

Unfortunately, this type of incident is all too common. Motorists who have their car windows rolled up, the stereo system at high volume, and are perhaps distracted by interaction with others in the vehicle may not hear a train approaching an ungated crossing. Or, as is too often the case, a motorist misjudges the speed of a train approaching a gated or ungated crossing and attempts to cross the tracks before the train arrives. These and other similar scenarios can produce tragic results. It should be noted that trains have the right of way, not automobile vehicle traffic.

There are two basic types of train/highway vehicle collision incidents: those where the train is derailed and those where it is not. Obviously, those that involve train derailment can be very complex incidents, especially if there are victims trapped in both the highway vehicle and the railcars. This type of incident lends itself to a command structure with two divisions or sectors: one for each mode of transportation and group of victims.

Just because an incident does not involve a train derailment does not mean that it may not be complex. A collision between a train and a highway vehicle carrying hazardous materials can create a very complex incident — especially if it occurs in a densely populated area. A locomotive colliding with a loaded bus or with a truck loaded with farm workers can create mass casualty incidents that will severely tax the resources of many small agencies. Also, these incidents may occur at relatively remote rural crossings that may be many miles from the nearest trauma center or fully staffed emergency medical facility. Fast and efficient on-scene triage, treatment, and transportation — perhaps by medevac helicopter — may be critical to the victims' survival.

Train/Pedestrian Collisions

These incidents occur in every locality that has one or more active rail lines. Pedestrians put themselves in the path of an oncoming train for a wide variety of reasons. Some, like foolhardy motorists, attempt to dash across the tracks before the train arrives. Others, under the influence of alcohol or other drugs, may fall asleep on the tracks or fall and knock themselves unconscious. And others do so consciously in an attempt to do away with themselves.

Regardless of why a person is hit by a train, unless all or part of the victim is in or under the railcar somehow, it is technically not an extrication incident but merely a medical trauma call that occurred on railroad property. However, if it is an extrication incident involving a train, the goal as always is to use whatever resources are available to save the victim's life and remove him from further harm. Again, working closely with on-scene railway personnel is likely to produce the best result and will increase the victim's chances of survival.

Trams

Like other classes of transportation vehicles, trams come in a wide variety of sizes and configurations. They range from individual railcars powered by diesel engines or electric motors to cable-drawn vehicles such as the famous San Francisco cable cars. There are also cable-drawn trams that travel at a very steep angle on rails set against a mountainside and those that are suspended from a cable high above the ground. How incidents involving these vehicles are handled, and who handles them, will vary depending upon the specific situation and on local protocols.

Many trams are like buses or street cars that travel on rails, and extrication operations in them can be handled much the same way as extrication from buses as described in Chapter 7, *Bus Extrication*. When dealing with trams that are powered by electricity, either from a third rail or an overhead catenary system, rescue personnel should follow the same safety precautions as those described earlier in this chapter. Extrication incidents involving trams that travel either on elevated tracks or are suspended by an overhead cable — essentially those that are beyond the reach of fire department ground ladders or aerial devices — operate in a hazardous environment. Subject to the dictates of local protocols, these incidents should be handled by technical rescue teams trained and equipped to operate in these environments.

Summary

Extrication incidents involving fully loaded railway passenger cars can be some of the most challenging that rescue personnel may ever face. The potential for large numbers of trapped and injured victims, the often remote incident locations, the size and weight of the railcars themselves, and the difficulty of gaining access into them combine to make these incidents very difficult to handle. Personnel in jurisdictions that have rail lines running through them should familiarize themselves with the various types of railcars that travel through their areas. In areas where trains operate on electrical power, personnel should be especially diligent in their pursuit of knowledge about those systems and the vehicles that operate in them. Also of critical importance is that agencies with the potential for this type of incident follow NFPA® 1670 and develop pre-incident plans before the need arises.

Review Questions

1. What are distinguishing features of each class of train?

2. What are distinguishing features of each type of railcar?

3. What are the hazards associated with railcars?

4. What are the hazards associated with rails and roadbeds?

5. What specific size-up concerns should an incident commander consider during train incident extrication operations?

6. What methods can be used to stabilize railcars during extrication operations?

7. What methods can be used to gain access to the interior of railcars?

8. Which railcar extrication situations must rescuers be prepared to mitigate?

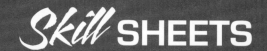

REMINDER: Not all agencies advocate the following procedures and practices. The following skill sheets present a snapshot of various procedures utilized during extrication operations. As always, local agency procedures and protocols must be followed.

Removing Tempered Glass Windows

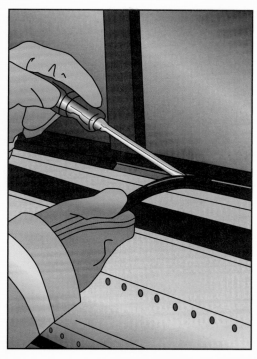

Step 1: Use a small screwdriver or key to pry the zipper strip from the center of the rubber seal surrounding the window unit. This zipper strip may be a different color from the seal itself.

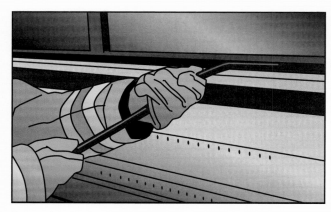

Step 2: Pull the rubber strip from around the window.

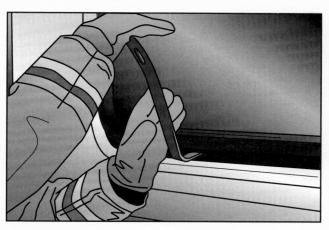

Step 3: Insert a large screwdriver or small pry bar under the corner of the window between the window seal and the car body. Pry down, pulling the window out.

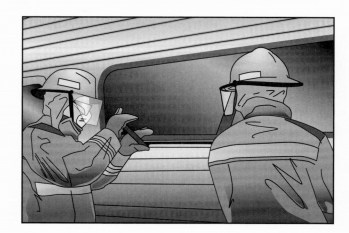

Step 4: Continue pushing down on the prying tool, pulling the window outward from the lower edge. The window will fall free outside the car.

CAUTION: Set removed windows out of the way of the rescue area to prevent a tripping hazard.

Removing Lexon® Windows

These window panes are removable from the outside by using the following procedure:

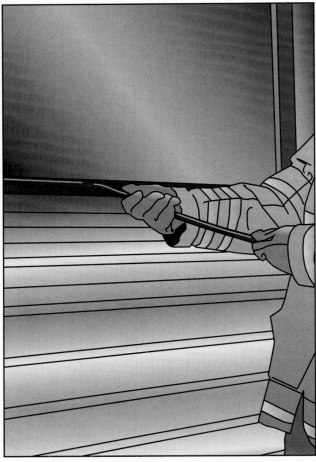

Step 1: Grasp the split end of the window rubber molding and pull straight out until all the molding is completely removed.

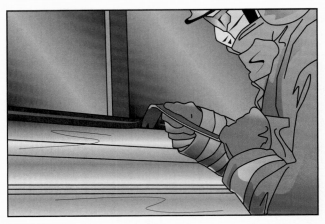

Step 2: Insert a pry bar between the Lexan® pane and the window frame at the pry point, and pry out the frame. The Lexan® pane will fall inside of the car.

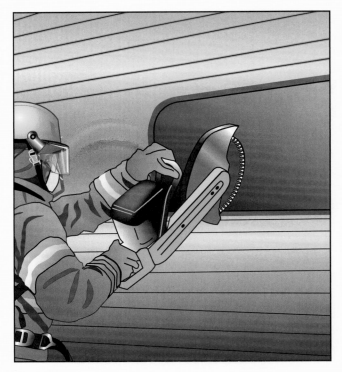

Step 3: If prying is not successful, cut out the pane with a power saw, but be prepared for the Lexan® to melt onto the saw blade.

Removing Emergency Exit Windows (Outside)

The following procedure should be used to remove these windows from outside the car:

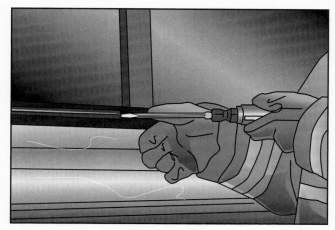

Step 1: Use a small screwdriver or key to pry the zipper strip from the center of the rubber seal surrounding the window unit. This zipper strip may be a different color from the seal itself.

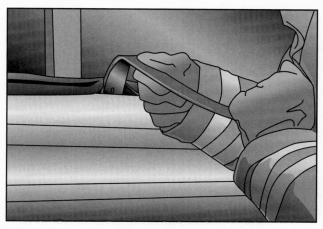

Step 3: Insert a large screwdriver or small pry bar under the corner of the window between the window seal and the car body. Lift upward and inward.

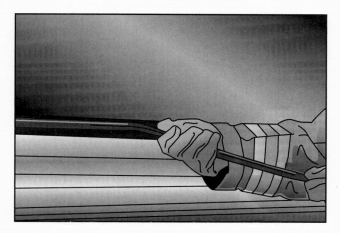

Step 2: Pull the rubber strip from around the window.

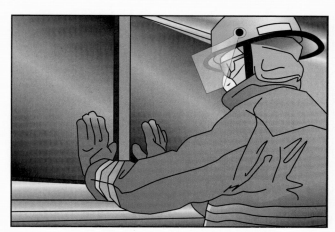

Step 4: Warn passengers inside to stand clear. Push the lower edge of the window firmly to break it loose from the car body. Continue to pry until the window falls free to the inside of the car. Cover any sharp edges before making entry.

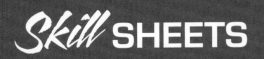
Removing Emergency Exit Windows (Inside)

Emergency exit windows can also be removed from inside the car. To remove these windows from inside the car, use the following procedure:

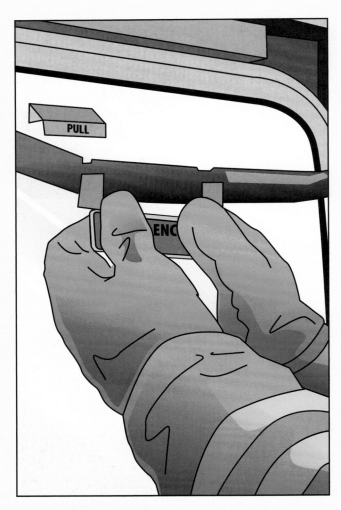

Step 1: Pull the red emergency handle in, and remove the rubber molding.

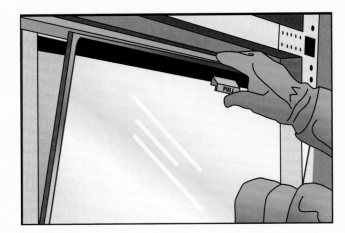

Step 2: Use the newly-exposed metal handle attached to the pane to pull the window toward the inside of the car. Only one-half of the window is designed to be removed.

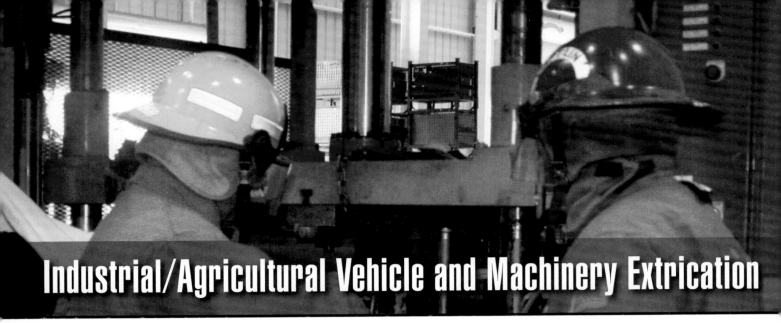

Industrial/Agricultural Vehicle and Machinery Extrication

Chapter Contents

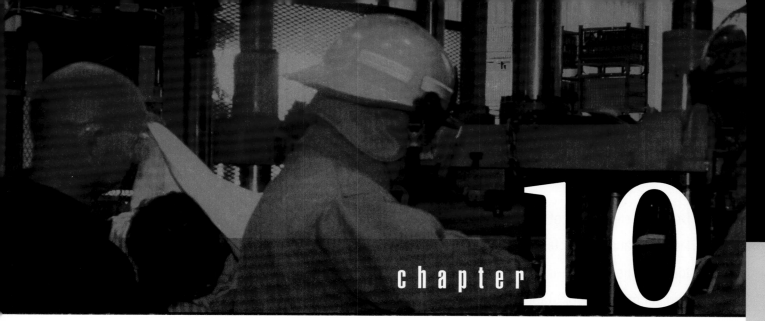

chapter 10

Key Terms

Job Performance Requirements

This chapter provides information that addresses the following job performance requirements (JPRs) of NFPA® 1001, *Standard for Fire Fighter Professional Qualifications* (2008), NFPA® 1006, *Standard for Technical Rescuer Professional Qualifications* (2008), and NFPA® 1670, *Standard on Operations and Training for Technical Search and Rescue Incidents* (2009).

NFPA® 1001 JPRs

6.4.1

6.4.2

NFPA® 1006 JPRs

5.2.2	5.5.1	10.1.2	10.1.5	10.1.8	10.2	10.2.3
5.2.3	10.1	10.1.3	10.1.6	10.1.9	10.2.1	10.2.4
5.2.7	10.1.1	10.1.4	10.1.7	10.1.10	10.2.2	10.2.5

NFPA® 1670 JPRs

8.2.2	8.3.3	12.1	12.2.3	12.3.3	12.4.2
8.2.3	8.3.4	12.2.1	12.3.1	12.3.4	
8.3.2	8.4.2	12.2.2	12.3.2	12.4.1	

Industrial/Agricultural Vehicle and Machinery Extrication

Learning Objectives

1. Describe each class of industrial and agricultural vehicle.

2. Describe anatomical features of industrial and agricultural vehicles.

3. Identify specific size-up concerns associated with industrial and agricultural vehicles.

4. Explain methods for stabilizing industrial and agricultural vehicles.

5. Describe methods for gaining access into industrial and agricultural vehicles during extrication operations.

6. Identify tactics used in industrial and agricultural vehicle extrication operations.

7. Describe industrial and agricultural machinery extrication procedures.

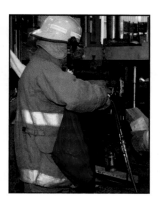

Chapter 10
Industrial/Agricultural Vehicle and Machinery Extrication

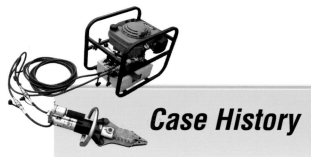

Case History

Rescue personnel were dispatched to a report of a man entrapped by a conveyor belt at a paper recycling plant. Arriving personnel established command and conducted a scene and patient size-up. They found the patient's left arm wedged between a conveyor belt roller and the frame of a paper shredding machine. The patient's left hand was also impaled by metal parts of the conveyor belt itself. EMS personnel began treating the patient with an IV and oxygen.

The decision was made to disassemble the conveyor belt to extricate the patient's arm. Because of the large amount of shredded paper littering the area, a charged handline was setup to protect the patient and the rescuers. Lacking lockout/tagout devices, rescuers and plant personnel ensured the power to the paper shredding unit was off and a guard was positioned to ensure it remained off.

Rescuers removed the bolts of a heavy cover, raised the cover to expose the roller bearing mount, and used cribbing to keep the cover out of the way. A heavy duty come-along anchored to a beam overhead was employed to stabilize the roller. Rescuers then unbolted the roller bearing assembly and used a Halligan tool and pry bar to raise the assembly. Wedges were inserted as needed to prevent the roller from falling. The cover and bearing mount on the opposite end of the roller had to be raised to provide sufficient space to free the patient's hand. With this done, the patient received medication from EMS personnel to prevent Crush Syndrome effects and the hand was freed. EMS personnel then packaged the patient for transport to a hospital.

The variety of shapes and sizes of industrial and agricultural vehicles is almost endless. These vehicles are as varied as the tasks that they are designed to perform. They range from small farm tractors to huge earthmovers used in construction and mining. New types of vehicles and improved models of existing vehicles are continually being introduced. Some of them are modern versions of vehicles that have existed for many decades. Others may have never been seen in our society before because the tasks that they have been designed to perform did not exist before.

To add to the challenge of extrication involving these vehicles, the incident scene may be on a construction site, in an enormous open-pit mine, inside a vast industrial complex, or on a huge corporate farm. In these types of incidents, there is usually only one patient to extricate unless one vehicle collides with or rolls over onto another.

This chapter discusses the following information about industrial, agricultural, and mechanical extrication:

- The classification and descriptions of the most common of the myriad types of industrial and agricultural vehicles in use

- The sizing up of an incident involving one or more of these vehicles, including stabilizing and gaining access into them

- The process for terminating an incident involving an industrial or agricultural vehicle

Classification of Industrial and Agricultural Vehicles

But, like automobiles and other types of vehicles, industrial and agricultural also have many characteristics in common. Some of these vehicles have enclosed cabs, others do not. Some of them are two-wheel drive while others are all-wheel drive. Some have no wheels at all because they are tracked vehicles.

Commercial Vehicles

As discussed in chapters 6, *Passenger Vehicle Extrication,* and 8, *Medium-Heavy Truck Extrication,* pickup and medium trucks are commercial vehicles but will not be explored here. Instead small utility vehicles and four-wheel all terrain vehicles (ATVs) that are commonly used at industrial and agricultural sites for moving personnel and small amounts of materials **(Figure 10.1)** will be explored.

Tractors

Tractors are used in a variety of industrial and agricultural settings that range from airports and construction sites to farms, ranches, and highways. Like other types of vehicles, tractors come in many different sizes and configurations. There are two broad classes of off-road tractors: wheeled tractors and tracked vehicles. The tracked vehicles are commonly called "crawlers" or "tracklayers."

Wheel Tractors

Typical wheel tractors have very large rear wheels (normally up to 50-inch [120 cm]) and smaller front wheels (normally up to 38-inch [95 cm]), with rubber tires. Depending upon the specific use for a tractor, the front wheels may be set the same distance apart as the rear wheels or they may be very close together **(Figure 10.2)**. Some wheel tractors are two-wheel drive and others are all-wheel drive, often referred to as manual front wheel drive (MFWD). On some two-wheel drive tractors, the rear tires have traction treads and the front tires are grooved for lateral purchase, however some may be found with turf or industrial type tires. The front and rear tires on all-wheel drive trac-

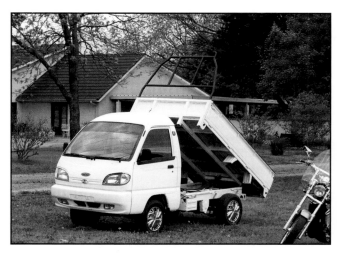

Figure 10.1 Utility vehicles, such as this small utility truck with a dump bed, are useful in agricultural applications.

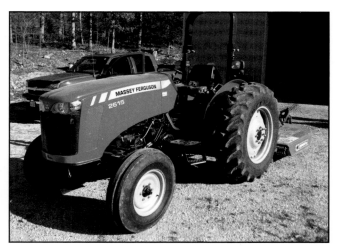

Figure 10.2 A wheel-based agricultural tractor. *Courtesy of Alan Braun, University of Missouri Fire and Rescue Training Institute.*

tors have heavy traction treads. Because these tractors are relatively light in weight and are often used to pull very heavy loads, large cast-iron weights are sometimes bolted to the wheels, and/or the tires are filled to approximately 90 percent with a solution of calcium chloride or ethylene glycol and water to improve traction. In other cases, tractors are equipped with multiple front and/or rear wheels for the same purpose.

Regardless of how individual wheel tractors are configured, they all tend to have a rather high profile and are more prone to rolling over than other types of vehicles. Their relatively narrow track (horizontal distance from 60 to 100 inches [144 cm to 240 cm] between wheels on the same axle) and their high ground clearance make them susceptible to lateral rollovers. The Occupational Safety and Health Administration (OSHA) requires that all wheel tractors manufactured after October of 1976 be equipped with seat belts and roll bars — officially known as roll-over protection systems (ROPS).

On flat, level ground, the center of gravity of these tractors is along their centerline roughly halfway between their front and rear axles. When a wheel tractor is traveling on a hillside, its center of gravity shifts toward the downhill wheels. If the downhill wheels drop into a depression or the uphill wheels hit a slight bump, or both, it may cause the tractor to roll over laterally. Likewise, if a wheel tractor is climbing a steep slope, its center of gravity shifts to the rear axle. If the front wheels hit a large enough bump while the rear wheels are in a depression, it can cause the front wheels to leave the ground and the front end to rotate around the rear axle, with the unit coming to rest upside down — perhaps pinning the operator beneath it. To reduce this possibility, some wheel tractors are equipped with up to 1,400 pounds (635 kg) of cast iron weights attached to the front of their chassis.

Crawlers

Steel or rubber tracks, rather than wheels, provide the locomotion for some tractors. These tractors are generally larger and heavier than most wheeled tractors, have a wider track, and a lower profile **(Figure 10.3, p. 420)**. Therefore, crawlers are less susceptible to rollover than are wheel tractors.

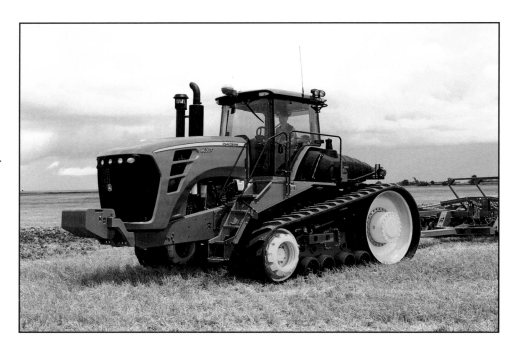

Figure 10.3 A crawler-type tractor with rubber tracks. *Courtesy of John Deere.*

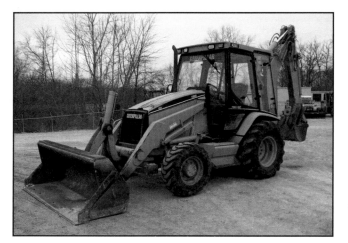

Figure 10.4 This tractor is equipped with a front-end loader and backhoe attachments. *Courtesy of Alan Braun, University of Missouri Fire and Rescue Training Institute.*

Attachments/Implements

In addition to pulling heavy loads, tractors are designed to accommodate a wide variety of attachments and implements. Attachments are those auxiliary appliances, such as front-end loaders, backhoes, and scraper blades that are more or less permanently attached to the chassis of the tractor **(Figure 10.4)**. Attachments are important to rescue personnel because these devices can affect a tractor's stability and sometimes result in tractor rollovers. Implements are those appliances that are temporarily attached to and usually towed or carried by the tractor. Typical farm implements are planters, manure spreaders, chemical spraying rigs, hay rakes, and balers.

While some wheel tractors are equipped with a scraper blade on the front or rear for snow removal and light-duty grading, heavy-duty grading and excavation is done by crawlers equipped with massive steel blades on their front ends. Some crawlers also have trenching attachments, huge rippers, or other attachments on the rear of the vehicle. Crawlers are sometimes used at airports, especially during inclement weather, to tow aircraft from one point to another. These vehicles are often equipped with rubber tracks or rubber pads on steel tracks to avoid damaging the taxiway surface. As with wheel tractors, the number and variety of attachments and implements for crawlers is virtually endless.

Forklifts

While the OSHA regulations in 29 CFR 1910.178 refer to forklifts as powered industrial trucks, they are also known as lift trucks or fork trucks. Forklifts are found in a variety of working environments such as warehouses, lumberyards, construction sites, and many other locations where relatively heavy objects need to be lifted and transported over relatively short distances **(Figure 10.5)**. They are also used by urban search and rescue (US&R) teams in structural collapse incidents. While lifting capacity varies with the manufacturer and the model of the vehicle, most forklifts are capable of lifting from 2,000 to 80,000 pounds (4 400 kg to 176 200 kg). Some forklifts operate on rechargeable lead-acid batteries of either 24, 36, or 48 volts. Others have internal combustion engines that operate on gasoline, diesel, or liquefied petroleum gas (LPG). Some have dual fuel systems that can operate on both gasoline and LPG.

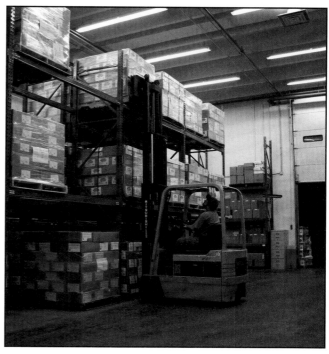

Figure 10.5 Forklifts are useful in lifting and moving products and materials.

Most forklifts are equipped with two broad lifting forks, approximately 4 feet (1.2 m) long. The forks can be moved laterally to adjust to the width of a particular load. Some forklifts are equipped with more special-ized lifting devices for lifting unique loads. Regardless of what type of lifting device is used on the front of the vehicle, the device is attached to a horizontal cross beam that can be elevated or lowered on rollers that travel in a pair of vertical tracks called the mast. These masts can be deflected from five to seven degrees from vertical to increase control of the load. Some masts are designed to also telescope to increase vertical lift range and may have a side shift feature to move the load laterally. Forklifts equipped with a four-stage telescoping mast have a vertical lift range of up to 30 feet (10 m). However, the higher the lift, the greater the chance of the unit falling over because of the increase in leverage at the top of the lift mechanism. As with fire department aerial devices, when these high-lift units are extended in close proximity to power lines, there is the additional danger of the mast or the load coming into contact with the power lines.

The design of each forklift chassis varies with the manufacturer and the intended purpose of the vehicle, but all have a relatively low profile and are made of very heavy materials such as cast iron and steel. Some forklifts weigh as little as 2,000 pounds (907 kg) while others weigh as much as 36,000 pounds (16 329 kg). The bulk of the weight of a forklift chassis is concentrated at the end opposite the lift mechanism to act as a counterweight. Some forklifts have additional counterweights added to the end of the chassis. Many fork-lifts, especially those operated in warehouses and other areas with concrete floors, have small solid rubber tires mounted on 12-inch (300 mm) to 21-inch (525 mm) wheels. Forklifts intended for outdoor use generally have either pneumatic tires or "cushion" tires. All of these design features are intended to increase the stability of these vehicles and decrease the chances of them turning over.

All forklifts have some form of overhead operator protection system de-signed to deflect falling objects. Most are heavy-gauge wire screen or a steel grille over a steel frame. Forklifts that routinely operate outdoors are some-times equipped with a fully enclosed cab. The enclosure usually consists of the standard operator protection system enclosed with Plexiglass® panels or window panes and a laminated safety glass windshield.

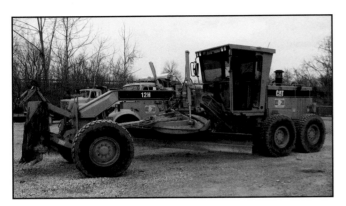
Graders/Maintainers

These road maintenance vehicles may be found anywhere that unsurfaced roads are common or where highway construction is being done. Despite the ability to laterally tilt their front wheels, given a sufficiently steep slope and enough lateral force, these vehicles can roll over. Their enclosed cabs are similar to those on tractors and other industrial or agricultural vehicles **(Figure 10.6)**. These vehicles are very heavy and may have movable scraper blade mid-mounted and ripper teeth on the blade or rear end.

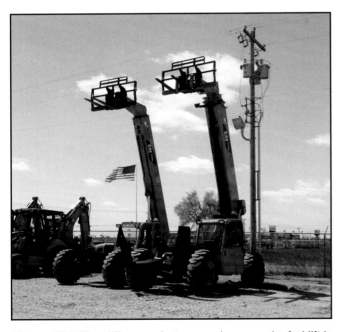

Figure 10.6 A standard grader or maintainer. *Courtesy of Alan Braun, University of Missouri Fire and Rescue Training Institute.*

Booms

These are some of the most versatile single purpose vehicles. They consist of a vehicle-mounted boom that can telescope more than 40 feet (12 m) and lift from 7,000 to 10,000 pounds (3 200 kg to 4 500 kg). The end of the boom may be fitted with forks for lifting material on pallets, a platform or basket similar to those on fire service aerial devices, or a bucket as is used on front-end loaders **(Figure 10.7)**. Many of these vehicles not only have all-wheel drive but also have all-wheel steering. Some have fully enclosed cabs similar to those described in the section on forklifts.

Like fire department aerial devices, when booms are operated in close proximity to power lines, there is a danger of them coming into contact with the power lines. These vehicles often operate on unsurfaced construction sites where the soil may be uneven and/or unstable. When the boom is fully extended vertically, these conditions make the boom vulnerable to turning over — especially if there is a strong crosswind.

Cranes

These massive vehicles may have large pneumatic tires and can be driven from site to site, or they may be crawlers that must be transported from site to site on lowboy trailers. Regardless of their means of locomotion, these vehicles are subject to the same hazards as the booms just described **(Figure 10.8)**.

Harvesters

Sometimes called "combines," these vehicles are wide, have a relatively low center of gravity, and are usually very stable. However, like crawler tractors, given a sufficiently steep slope and enough lateral force, these vehicles can roll over. Many harvesters are designed to discharge grain into a truck or trailer following the harvester **(Figure 10.9)**. Farm workers that enter the truck bed or trailer to manipulate the material inside, can become trapped in the grain and suffocate if not extricated in time. In addition, some harvesters discharge the grain into a following vehicle by means of an enclosed auger. Many farm workers

Figure 10.7 The difference between a boom and a forklift is that a boom can lift materials higher.

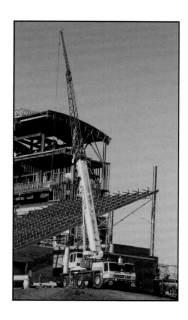

Figure 10.8 A wheel-based crane at a construction site.

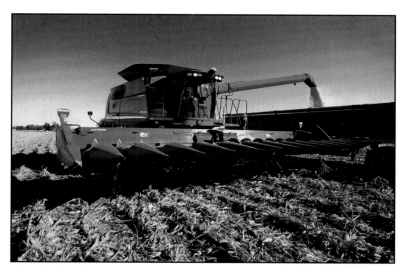

Figure 10.9 A harvester or combine. *Courtesy of John Deere.*

have had an extremity pulled into these augers when their clothing became entangled in the mechanism. Disentanglement in these cases most often involves disassembly of the drive chains, gears, or belts before entry. Some units are operated by flowing hydraulics. Where hydraulic lines are concerned, the end that is farthest from the patient should be addressed first.

Auger – A screw-like shaft that is turned to move grain or other commodities through a farm implement.

Anatomy of Industrial and Agricultural Vehicles

These vehicles can be differentiated by:

- Their means of locomotion
  - two-wheel drive
  - all-wheel drive
  - tracklayers
- Their configuration
  - articulating
  - telescoping
- Their sheer size

The sections that follow describe these differentiations and also discuss various of industrial and agricultural vehicle anatomy that are common to all such vehicles.

Two-Wheel Drive Vehicles

Many wheel tractors and similar vehicles have two-wheel drive. In most of these vehicles, the driving wheels are at the rear of the vehicle and the steering wheels are at the front. However, most forklifts are configured the other way around — the front wheels are the driving wheels and the rear wheels do the steering. Regardless of which wheels provide locomotion, poor traction makes two-wheel drive vehicles prone to rollovers on hillsides and other slopes. A two-wheel drive vehicle attempting to move diagonally up and across a slope may begin to slide sideways and then down slope. If it hits an obstruction while moving in this way, the vehicle may roll over **(Figure 10.10, p. 424)**.

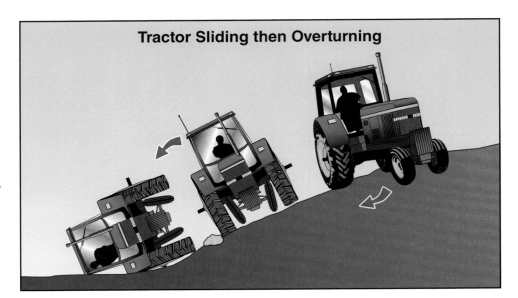

Figure 10.10 Two-wheel drive tractors can slide sideways and roll over if they strike an obstacle while trying to travel over a slope.

All-Wheel Drive Vehicles

Four-wheel or all-wheel drive vehicles are much better equipped to handle situations involving poor traction and steep slopes. Some of these vehicles have all-wheel steering as well. These are especially agile vehicles that are capable of some extraordinary maneuvers. However, because all-wheel drive vehicles are so capable and maneuverable, their drivers can be lulled into a false sense of invulnerability. This cavalier attitude can cause the operator to take imprudent risks — sometimes resulting in a rollover.

Tracked Vehicles

The direction of travel for tracked vehicles is often controlled by manually operated levers or joysticks that apply or release a separate brake for each track. However, because the tracks spread the weight of the vehicle, some crawlers exert a ground pressure of as little as 2.5 psi (35 kg/cm ^{2}). The same physical laws apply to crawlers as to wheel tractors. Considering the extreme environments in which they are often used, if the angles involved are steep enough, tracked vehicles are vulnerable to rollovers. Once rolled over, their size and weight can make extrication much more difficult than with most wheeled tractors.

Articulating Telescoping Vehicles

The most common articulating vehicles are large earthmovers and large tractors **(Figure 10.11)**. Other examples of articulating vehicles are all-wheel drive farm tractors, log skidders, large front-end loaders, rough-terrain forklifts, and large dump trucks. Normally quite stable because of their huge wheels and low center of gravity, earthmovers can be rolled over if all the necessary elements are present — steep slope, unstable soil, and sufficient lateral force. Telescoping vehicles include booms and cranes that are capable of lifting heavy loads.

Oversized Vehicles

Perhaps the most common of the oversized vehicles are massive dump trucks used in strip mining and similar activities. Similar types of vehicles are used in heavy construction. Some other examples of oversized vehicles would be drilling rigs, tunnel boring machines, and steam shovels **(Figure 10.12)**. Given

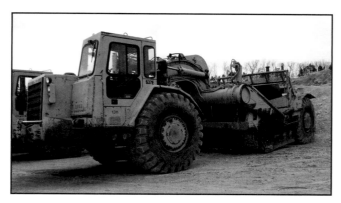

Figure 10.11 An example of an articulating earthmover. *Courtesy of Alan Braun, University of Missouri Fire and Rescue Training Institute.*

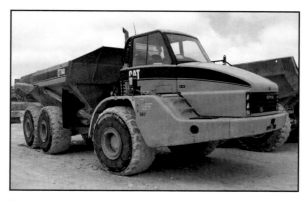

Figure 10.12 Oversize dump trucks are frequently used in strip mining operations. *Courtesy of Alan Braun, University of Missouri Fire and Rescue Training Institute.*

the environments in which these vehicles operate, rock slides, cave-ins, and similar events can cause these vehicles to overturn.

Operational Controls

Industrial and agricultural vehicles employ a variety of control devices. While some vehicles use a steering wheel, others may be maneuvered by hydraulics or a "clutch-brake" system. Many modern tracked vehicles uses a joystick control to steer the vehicle **(Figure 10.13)**. Some of these are steering devices, some are used to increase a vehicle's stability, and still others are used to power or control auxiliary devices. On some equipment, a global positioning satellite (GPS) system may be used to guide the equipment without input from the operator.

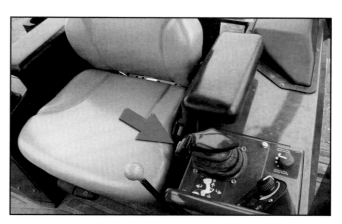

Figure 10.13 The joystick controls on a tractor.

Auxiliary Power Sources

To increase versatility, some tractors and similar vehicles are equipped with one or more auxiliary power sources. They may have power take-offs (PTOs) that can be used to operate implements such as portable grain augers or conveyor belts or chains. They may have hydraulic pumps that can be used to raise or lower any number of farm implements such as plows or mowers. As with any power source, if the proper guards are not in place or if the operators fail to exercise appropriate caution when using the devices, parts of their clothing can become entangled in the mechanism and this can pull the operator into the machinery.

Rollover Protection Systems (ROPS)

OSHA requires a ROPS on every industrial and agricultural vehicle except those in which the operator stands **(Figure 10.14, p. 426)**. Even in vehicles not covered by the OSHA regulations, ROPS are often installed by the manufacturer for liability reasons. Sometimes ROPS are required by the operator's insurance carrier, however, these systems are often removed or altered by owner to reduce the height of the vehicle.

> **CAUTION**
> Rescuers should ensure that they do not accidentally re-engage "live" PTO systems.

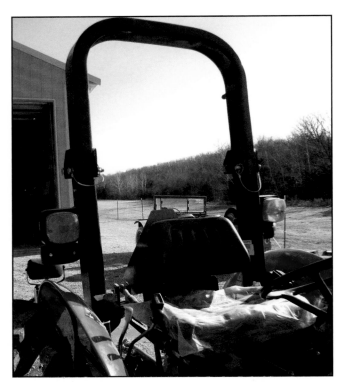

Figure 10.14 The rollover protection system (ROPS) on a tractor. *Courtesy of Alan Braun, University of Missouri Fire and Rescue Training Institute.*

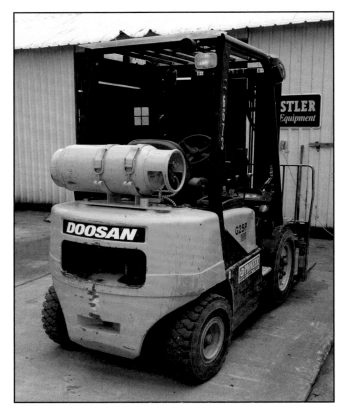

Figure 10.15 The compressed gas fuel tank on a forklift.

Fuels

Industrial and agricultural vehicles operate on a variety of fuels. Many of the largest and heaviest vehicles operate on diesel fuel and carry up to 100 gallons (378.5 L) in their tanks. Other industrial and agricultural vehicles operate on gasoline and/or LPG, usually propane. Still others operate on compressed natural gas (CNG) **(Figure 10.15)**. Some forklifts and other vehicles are powered by electricity from banks of rechargeable wet-cell batteries.

Vehicles that operate on liquid or gaseous fuels add the danger of fire to the other hazards associated with collisions, rollovers, and other extrication incidents. Part of the size-up process must be to assess the need for Class B foam to suppress flammable vapors and/ or flammable or combustible liquid fires. Flammable gases must be shut off at the source or allowed to burn out. Careful attention should be given to the possibility of fuel tank failure due to the lightweight material that make up some tanks. Sudden failure of these tanks or fuel lines could release large amounts of fuels that would potentially surround the firefighter.

Brakes

Brakes on agricultural equipment are typically mounted inside the rear axel and can be wet or dry systems; most do not have front brakes. The rear brakes can be operated independently or locked together with a bar mounted to the pedals, using them independently allows the operator to turn the tractor in a very short distance. Crawler tractors and other tracked vehicles use brakes for changing direction — steering. When the operator of one of these vehicles wants to turn left, he pulls a lever or steps on a pedal that applies a brake to the left track, slowing or stopping it. Since the left track is at least momentarily moving slower that the right track, the vehicle veers to the left. The greater the difference in the speed of the right and left tracks, the faster and more abrupt the turn will be. A fully applied brake to one track or the other will cause the vehicle to spin around a fixed point.

Tires

Industrial and agricultural vehicles may be equipped with pneumatic or solid rubber tires, with tread designs that are selected depending upon the vehicle's use and the environment in which it works. Pneumatic tires can be found on vehicles as small as converted golf carts, used as runabouts in warehouses and industrial complexes, and as massive as the huge earthmoving vehicles used in mining and heavy construction. To improve the traction of drive wheels with large pneumatic tires, it is common practice to fill the tires to about 90 percent with water or some other inert fluid such as anti-freeze, and then inflate the tires to their normal operating pressure with air.

Some forklifts and similar vehicles have what are called "cushion" tires. These are solid rubber tires that look like the pneumatic tires used on auto-mobiles and light trucks. One obvious difference between a cushion tire and a pneumatic tire is the absence of a valve stem on the cushion tire. Other solid rubber tires on forklifts are quite obvious for what they are. They generally are smaller in diameter than either cushion or pneumatic tires, and they usually have no traction treads.

Jacks

Also called "stabilizers" or "outriggers," these hydrauli-cally-operated devices, similar to the stabilizing jacks on a fire department aerial device, extend from both sides of a vehicle so equipped. As the name implies, these de-vices are intended to stabilize a tractor or other vehicle that is operating an attachment such as a backhoe or a boom **(Figure 10.16)**. When applied, stabilizing jacks normally lift the vehicle's wheels off the ground, and the jacks bear the full weight of the vehicle. These jacks make the vehicle quite stable — unless something goes wrong. If one or more of the jacks suddenly loses hy-draulic pressure, the vehicle can lurch to one side. If the vehicle were positioned across a slope and the downslope jacks failed, the vehicle could easily topple over. Also, if the ground under the jacks on one side of the vehicle collapsed into an excavation, the vehicle may roll over.

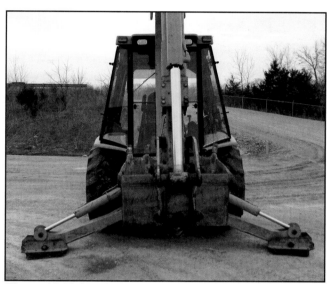

Figure 10.16 A stabilizing systems of jacks on a backhoe. *Courtesy of Alan Braun, University of Missouri Fire and Rescue Training Institute.*

Specific Size-Up Concerns for Industrial and Agricultural Incident Extrication

The size-up of an extrication incident involving an industrial or agricultural vehicle should be done systematically including assessments of the follow-ing:

1. Overall scene

2. Vehicles involved

3. Trapped patients

4. Extrication requirements of the particular incident

    NOTE: As always, size-up continues throughout the incident.

    Initial size-up should answer the following questions:

- Is the incident location clearly known and readily accessible, or will rescue personnel have to search for the scene?

- Is the trapped operator the only person at the scene who is familiar with the operation of the machine, and will a farm advisor or other expert be needed?

- Is a medevac helicopter required due to remoteness of the scene?

As the responder nears the scene, consideration of the following questions may identify the presence of other collateral problems:

- Is smoke (especially that with an unusual color) or steam rising from the scene?
- Will fire protection be a higher than normal priority because of a known flammability hazard?
- Will large-scale foam-making capability be needed?
- Will a hazardous materials team be needed because of a known release or a high potential for the release of a pesticide or other IDLH (immediately dangerous to life or health) substance?
- What additional resources will be needed to control and mitigate the known and potential hazards in this incident? Whatever those resources are, they should be requested immediately.

The IC must identify what the vehicle may be carrying and how that material is configured or arranged. The IC must ask any of the following questions:

- What type of load is the vehicle carrying?
- What are the load's contents?
- How are these arranged?
- Are the materials (packages in a crate or liquid within a tank) visible?
- How will the load affect the vehicle during the rescue operation?
- Is the load stable or will it need to be secured or removed in order to perform the rescue safely?

In industrial and agricultural settings, the load the vehicle carries may contain hazardous materials. The load may have placards or other identification decals on them; however, in a farm setting the contents of tanks may not be readily apparent. Farmers and private individuals are not required to placard individual tank loads of product. Many of these products, such as anhydrous ammonia, fungicides, and pesticides, are hazardous to responders and patients. Many materials are safe until they come in contact with another material. Often these chemicals and/or materials are packaged separately, but transported together.

In most incidents involving industrial and agricultural vehicles, there will only be one occupant in each vehicle but rescuers must consider the possibility that several persons may have been riding the vehicle even if it was not designed for that use. However, the size and weight of these vehicles may make extricating one patient more challenging and time consuming than extricating several from more conventional vehicles. This phase of the size-up process involves looking for patients to determine how many there are, where they are, and what their medical conditions are. Even though an industrial or agricultural vehicle may seem very stable in its present position, rescuers must attempt to assess the trapped patients without jostling the vehicle — especially the cab.

Some industrial equipment will require specialized tools beyond what rescue vehicles normally carry. Rescuers should consider using plant resources or local dealers for the equipment that would be needed in such instances. Contact numbers, including after hours contacts, for these resources should be readily available

Key points to consider when attempting a tractor rollover rescue include the following:

- Fire is a threat in an overturn situation if there is spilled fuel present. Ideally, an 1½ hoseline should be available throughout the rescue however, at a minimum, ABC-type extinguishers should be present.

- Before using thermal cutting equipment to free a patient, consider using alternative methods.

- Shut off the tractor engine. Rescuers should always stop a running tractor engine. Even if it is not running, rear wheel movement could start it up.

- If the ground is soft, it may be possible to dig the patient out from under the tractor.

- The machine should be blocked or cribbed to prevent it from tipping and causing more injuries.

- Lifting the tractor is the best way to deal with rollovers of large, modern tractors. A second tractor or a tow truck may be needed to perform the lift. If a tractor must be rolled away from the patient, careful blocking is required to minimize settling of the lower side.

- As the tractor is raised, cribbing should be added for proper stability.

- Hydraulic jacks can be used to lift smaller tractors. Block the axle on both sides to prevent the tractor from rocking onto the patient.

- Air bags can be used to raise an overturned tractor. They are more stable if stacked alternately with the blocking **(Figure 10.17)**.

Industrial and Agricultural Vehicle Stabilization

Because of the size and weight of many of these vehicles, they are generally quite stable. However, following a collision or rollover, these vehicles must be assumed to be unstable. Like any other vehicle from which one or more patients must be extricated, an industrial or agricultural vehicle must be stabilized before rescue personnel can enter to assess, stabilize, package, and disentangle trapped patients. As with other types of vehicles, the techniques and equipment used to stabilize an industrial or agricultural vehicle may vary depending upon how the vehicle came to rest — upright, on its side, on its roof, or in some other position.

Vehicle Upright

Unlike automobiles and light trucks, when an industrial or agricultural vehicle is upright following a collision or other destructive event, it is likely to be very stable vertically because of the extremely heavy suspension, or absence of suspension, on many of these vehicles. However, because the destructive event may have damaged or destroyed the vehicle's suspension system (if

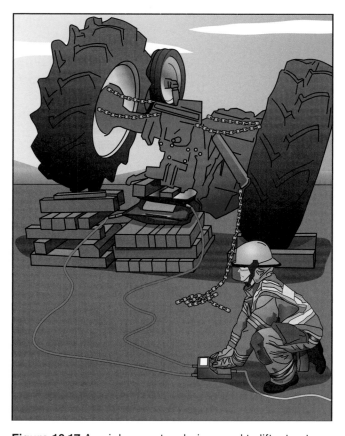

Figure 10.17 An air bag system being used to lift a tractor.

any), the same vertical stabilization measures described in earlier chapters should be applied. In addition, the vehicle should be stabilized horizontally using chocks, wedges, etc., to immobilize the wheels.

Both vertical and horizontal stabilization may involve the usual equipment and techniques — four-point or six-point cribbing, timber shores or pneumatic shores, installed at the appropriate points. In addition, wheel chocks, wedges, and/or webbing and chains may be needed to provide horizontal stability. How and where these techniques are applied will depend on the specifics of the situation.

Vehicle on Its Side

Just as with train cars and heavy trucks, once industrial or agricultural vehicles roll onto their sides they may appear to be very stable. However if the vehicle has come to rest on a slope or on unstable soil, there is the ever present danger of it suddenly and unexpectedly rolling back onto its wheels or tracks, or onto its top. To create a safe working environment for rescue personnel, it may be necessary to first secure the vehicle from the top with webbing and/or chains attached to a bombproof anchor point. Then, with that antiroll protection in place, shoring can be installed on the underside of the vehicle.

Vehicle Upside Down

Since many industrial and agricultural vehicles do not have roofs, the vehicle may be resting on a roll bar or on its fenders. Regardless of what part of the vehicle is supporting the rest of it, in this position it is likely to be very unstable. Because the vehicle's center of gravity is relatively high in this position, it is imperative that it be effectively stabilized as soon as possible.

Stabilizing an upside down industrial or agricultural vehicle may involve installing cribbing, shoring, and/or pneumatic struts at various points. Wheel tractors and similar vehicles may require box cribbing under the rear axle, one stack on each side between the differential and the wheel **(Figure 10.18)**. Other types of vehicles may require four-point or six-point cribbing depending upon the situation. Because of the unusually heavy weight of many of these vehicles, it may be necessary to build solid cribbing stacks to provide adequate support.

Vehicles in Other Positions

As described in earlier operational chapters, stabilizing vehicles that are in positions other than those already discussed can test the ingenuity and innovative thinking of the most skilled and experienced rescue personnel — and the same is true of industrial and agricultural vehicles. Very often, the vehicles come to rest at odd angles and in precarious positions. These unusual angles can dictate that extraordinarily long shoring be used or that the vehicle be stabilized from the top side with webbing and/or chains or cables. If timber shoring is used, a shoring system similar to those used to stabilize weakened building walls may have to be constructed. As always, the goal is to create as many points of contact between the vehicle and a stable surface as are necessary to stabilize the vehicle.

Machinery Incidents

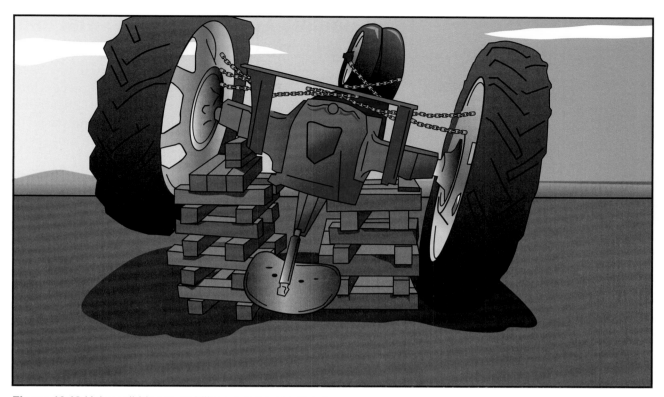

Figure 10.18 Using cribbing to stabilize an overturned tractor.

Industrial and agricultural workers often work in close proximity to moving conveyor chains or belts, augers, or gears. If the OSHA-required guards are not in place and if a worker wears loose clothing, when clothing becomes entangled in the operating machinery, that can pull the worker into the machine. In some cases, the worker can be freed simply by cutting the clothing free of the machine or having the worker slip out of the entangled clothing.

In most machinery entrapments, the machine will have been de-energized before rescuers arrive — either by an overload switch being triggered when the machine jams or by a coworker using an emergency shutoff. If not, power to the machinery may need to be left on until the machine is stabilized. If so, a guard should be posted at the control switch to prevent anyone from switching it off prematurely.

Leaving the power on may be necessary to protect the trapped worker by preventing the machine from completing its normal cycle when the power is shut off. Power may also be needed if the mechanism must be moved to extricate the patient. If the equipment can be de-energized, lock out/tag out procedures should be followed to ensure the machinery is not re-energized. The mechanism may have to be stabilized with rescue tools, wedges, cribbing, chocks, webbing, chains, or cables as necessary to prevent any movement or only allow for controlled movement **(Figure 10.19, p. 432)**. Rescuers may have to rely on the knowledge and expertise of the patient's coworkers or plant maintenance personnel to help them decide where and how to place the stabilization equipment if they are not familiar with the machinery in which the patient is trapped.

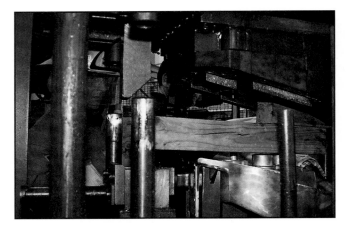

Figure 10.19 Cribbing can be used to limit or control the movement of machinery during an extrication operation.

Gaining Access into Industrial and Agricultural Vehicles

Once an industrial or agricultural vehicle has been stabilized, crews can safely work on gaining access into the vehicle's cab. Unless the cab is crushed beneath the upside down vehicle, the tools and techniques used to gain access into the cab are no different than those used to gain access into other vehicles.

NOTE: Unless otherwise stated in this section, the equipment and techniques for gaining access to industrial and agricultural vehicles are the same as those described in Chapter 4, *Extrication Equipment,* and Chapter 5, *Extrication Techniques.*

Window Entry

The tools and techniques used to remove the windshield and/or windows from the cab of an industrial or agricultural vehicle will vary depending upon the materials used in the windows. Some of these vehicles have Plexiglass in the side and rear windows, with tempered glass or laminated safety glass in the windshield. Others have tempered glass in the windshield as well as in the side and rear windows. Some of the windows are mounted in rubber frames. Others are held in place with industrial adhesive. Still others are bolted to steel hinges or brackets attached to the frame of the cab and have steel safety bars or screens mounted to them.

Door Entry

The cabs of most industrial and agricultural vehicles have outward swinging doors with a window that may or may not be designed to open. Those that open may be of the split-pane type that slide horizontally to open or of the type designed to swing open either partially or fully. Because the cabs of these vehicles are usually 4 feet (1.2 m) or more above the ground, the door latches are located near the bottom of the door panel (**Figure 10.20**).

If the door is jammed and must be removed, the hinge pins are exposed on the outside of the cab and can be cut off with a rotary saw equipped with a metal-cutting blade or with an oxyacetylene torch. Once the hinges are cut through, the door can be lifted or pried off manually or with a power spreader.

Roof Entry

If no other route of entry into the cab of an industrial or agricultural vehicle is accessible, then roof entry is feasible. However since the roof panel is part of the ROPS, it is made of rather substantial material — usually steel — so entry through the roof can be a slow process. There are exceptions, however. Some roof panels gain strength from stamped-in contours, so they can be made of metal

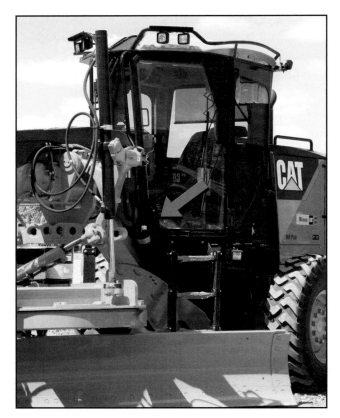

Figure 10.20 The door handle for this grader is located where the operator can reach it from the ground.

thin enough to be cut with most standard extrication tools. Some manufacturers are using fiberglass or plastic roof panels for access to equipment (such as heating, air conditioning and computer modules) housed under them. These roofs will be easier to gain access through. Depending upon the manufacturer, there may be one or more steel cross members under the panel. These cross members will have to be removed by cutting.

Floor Entry

Floor entry may be the option for removing the patient. Some vehicles may be equipped with a floor hatch for this purpose. However, due to the methods of construction, floor access is often virtually impossible.

Industrial and Agricultural Vehicle Extrication Tactics

As always, the goal during the process of extricating the operator of an industrial or agricultural vehicle is to remove the vehicle from the patient without causing further injury. Likewise, if a patient is caught in some piece of machinery, the machinery must be removed from the patient — not the other way around.

Disentanglement

Because the vehicle's cab is essentially the ROPS designed to protect the operator, the strength of the structure can make freeing the operator extremely challenging. If the vehicle's rollover protection system (ROPS) is intact, cutting or removing any part of it may cause the vehicle to fall injuring the patient and rescuers. Cutting any part of a ROPS should be done only when necessary. When sufficient force has been applied to these structural components to deform them enough to entrap the operator, rescuers may have to apply an equal amount of force to disentangle the patient. Otherwise, the cab or ROPS may have to be dismantled. To do this, power spreaders, shears, and extension rams are most often needed. These devices should be applied as described in Chapter 4, *Extrication Equipment.*

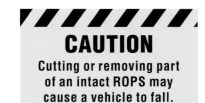

CAUTION
Cutting or removing part of an intact ROPS may cause a vehicle to fall.

If the patient is not in the cab of the vehicle but pinned under it or is caught in some piece of machinery, the tools and techniques used will be dictated by the specifics of the situation. Whether the patient is caught in a conveyor chain, an auger, or in some other piece of equipment, the equipment must be dismantled to the point that the patient is freed.

Patient Removal

Removing an injured patient from inside of the wrecked cab of an industrial or agricultural vehicle can be very difficult because of the limited working room within the cab. There may only be enough room for one rescuer to enter the cab of the vehicle to assess, treat, stabilize, and package the patient for removal. In this situation, it may be faster (and less traumatic for the patient) to simply dismantle the cab before attempting to extricate the patient.

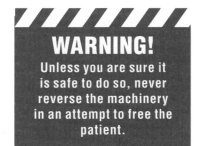

WARNING!
Unless you are sure it is safe to do so, never reverse the machinery in an attempt to free the patient.

Power Take Off (PTO) Incidents

PTO shafts are used to transmit power from a tractor or other source of power to an implement **(Figure 10.21)**. The two speeds commonly used with PTO shafts are 540 and 1000 rpm. PTO shafts can wrap 424 feet (138 m) of rope in one minute at 540 rpm while at 1000 rpm a shaft can wrap 785 feet (239 m) of rope in one minute. In terms of injury to patients, a 540 rpm shaft can wrap a patient's extremity 9 times a second, while a 1000 rpm shaft can wrap a patient's extremity 16 times a second. PTO shaft injuries range from minor lacerations to complete body dismemberment. PTO entanglement injuries can produce different injury patterns depending on the type of clothing the patient is wearing. Patients may be found with first and/or second degree burns, even if the PTO strips only the clothing from their body. Nylon and other synthetics tend to cut into skin and muscle tissue of a patient rather than rub across it. PTO shafts can grind away skin, muscles, tendons, and break bones starting in less than three-fourths of one second when a patient becomes entangled by an unshielded PTO shaft. Rescuers must also bear in mind that the tools required to rotate the PTO shaft backward may not be readily available and the patient may occupy the space you require to disassemble the shaft. **Skill Sheet 10-1** describes the procedures for freeing a patient entangled in a PTO.

Figure 10.21 A power take off (PTO) shaft that can provide power from a tractor to a mowing attachment.

Power Take-Off (PTO) — A rotating shaft that transfers power from the engine to auxiliary equipment. All farm tractors are designed to operate the PTO shaft at either 540 or 1,000 revolutions per minute.

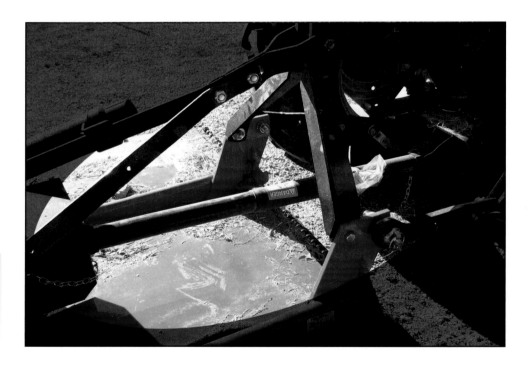

Industrial/Agricultural Machinery Extrication

When someone becomes entangled in a piece of machinery by clothing, jewelry, hair, or an extremity, the patient can be in danger of serious injury, loss of a digit or limb, or loss of life. If the entanglement did not stop the machine by tripping a circuit breaker or pressure limit switch, well meaning bystanders may turn off electrical power to the machine or switch off its hydraulic or pneumatic pressure. This loss of energy may cause the machine to automatically complete a revolution or cycle or return to its original position. Either way, this sudden and unexpected movement may make the original entrapment even worse by forcing an entangled body part to be pulled further into the mechanism — or back through the mechanism a second time.

To reduce the chances of inadvertently making a bad situation worse, rescue personnel must know how to safely and securely stabilize a machine in which a patient is entangled. To do this, they can sometimes enlist the aid of plant personnel who are intimately familiar with the involved machine. If technical assistance is unavailable, rescuers must have enough mechanical aptitude to recognize the mechanism of entrapment. They must also be able to use the tools, equipment, and techniques that will be needed to secure the machine and dismantle it sufficiently to perform the rescue.

The sections that follow cover a wide range of topics concerning extrications from machinery including the following:

- Pre-incident planning
- Tools and equipment
- Four phases of machinery extrication assessment and operations

Pre-Incident Planning

Pre-incident planning is essential to the timely and efficient handling of machinery rescue incidents. Rescue personnel need to be familiar with the locations and types of machinery installations found in their response district. It is critical that the emergency information be kept up to date and note any changes in the facility or machinery installations **(Figure 10.22)**. Unless the emergency response personnel have this information before an incident occurs, and an opportunity to study it and devise appropriate contingency plans, valuable time can be at the scene during an incident.

Machinery Extrication Tools and Equipment

Many of the tools and equipment used in machinery extrication incidents are the same as those used in other rescue disciplines but how those items are used can be different.

Examples of tools that can be used in a variety of situations are as follows:

- Cribbing
- Jacks
- Spreaders
- Mechanics tools

There are other tools that are more specific to machinery extrication that will be addressed in the sections the follow.

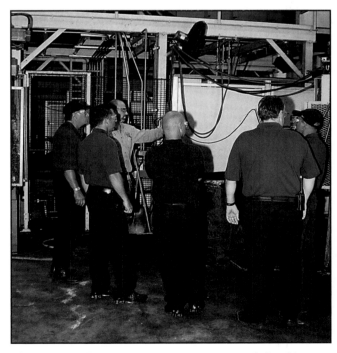

Figure 10.22 Emergency response personnel should receive familiarization training on industrial facilities within their communities.

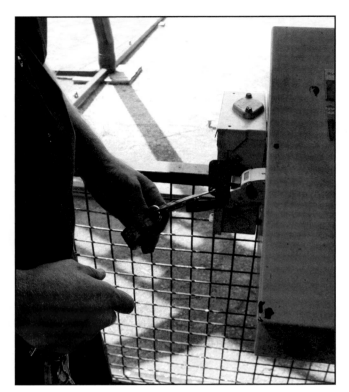

Figure 10.23 Lockout/tagout devices can prevent power from being restored to a machine during an extrication operation.

Lockout/Tagout Device — A device used to secure any power switches on a machine to prevent accidental or otherwise undesirable re-energization of the machine.

Blank — A thin piece of metal inserted between flanges in a pipe system to isolate part of the system.

Blank flange — A device that attaches to the end of a pipe in order to cap the end.

Lockout/Tagout Devices

Lockout/tagout devices are used to ensure that the position of certain valves and switches is not changed at a critical moment in the rescue operation **(Figure 10.23)**. Opening a valve or flipping a switch could re-energize the machine in which a patient is trapped. This could cause sudden and unexpected movement of the machine and place the patient and rescue personnel in serious jeopardy.

Flanges

When it is critical that the flow within a pipe be stopped —with absolute certainty—during a rescue operation, the time needed to dismantle and install a blank or a blank flange may be justified. A blank or a blank flange may be used to isolate the section within a system where a rescue is underway while allowing flow to the rest of the system.

Phase I: Assessment on Arrival

The assessment of the situation that must be made by the first-arriving rescuer can be subdivided into a primary and a secondary assessment.

Primary Assessment

During the size up of a machinery rescue incident, rescuers need to gather information about the number, condition, and location of patients:

- Is there more than one patient?
- If so, are they injured or merely entangled?
- How long have they been entangled?
- Are they conscious, and if so, are they coherent?
- What type of machinery is involved?
- Is the mechanism of entrapment the same in all cases?
- Has the machinery been stabilized?
- Is anyone on scene familiar with the machine?
- Is there an emergency call number for a machinery repair technician?

The answers to these questions will help the first-in rescuer make the first critical decision: Can the resources on scene or en route handle the situation, or do additional resources need to be called? If more resources are needed they must be requested immediately to get them on scene as quickly as possible. Size-up of the situation should be continued using the following checklist:

- Talk to patient (if possible).
- Interview witnesses.
- Identify hazards.

- Evaluate what has been and is being done.
- Weigh risk vs. benefits of available options.
- Contact expert assistance.

If the information gathered during the primary assessment confirms that this is a legitimate rescue emergency, then the area around the rescue site should be cordoned. Working zones (hot, warm, and cold) should be established.

Secondary Assessment

The secondary assessment involves some reconnaissance of the scene to gather information about the type of machine and its condition and status. All information gathered during both the primary and secondary assessments helps determine the mode of operation.

Type of machine. The rescuers only need to classify the machine in general terms — that is, by energy source and how it operates. The most common types of machines are as follows:

- Those driven by electricity, air pressure, hydraulic pressure, steam, or internal combustion engine.
- Those in which large rollers rotate in opposite directions to flatten, emboss, or imprint material that is fed through the rollers.
- Those in which enclosed or unenclosed augers rotate.
- Those in which conveyor belts or chains move materials horizontally or at low angles.
- Those that shape or form sheet metal by the impact of forging hammers.
- Those in which material is compacted by vertical or horizontal hydraulic rams or presses.
- Those in which materials are cut with spinning blades.
- Those in which materials are rotated at high speeds during shaping operations.
- Those in which materials are shaped or polished with spinning abrasive wheels.
- Those in which products are molded from molten material.

Condition. In this context, *condition* refers to the functionality of the machine. In other words, is it intact and fully operational, or was it damaged in the entrapment event? If it is was damaged, how seriously? This can help determine if the machine's own mechanism can be used to free the patient or if it will have to be dismantled.

Status. In this context, *status* refers to whether the machine is energized or not. If not, have the energy sources been secured?

Phase II: Pre-Extrication Operations

During this phase, which may last from a few minutes to an hour or more, all of the things that will make the rescue operation as safe and efficient as possible must be done. This phase includes:

- Monitoring patient status
- Finalizing the Incident Action Plan (IAP)
- Gathering the necessary resources
- Monitoring the atmosphere in the rescue area

Monitoring Patient Status

If the patient is accessible, his or her vital signs should be continuously monitored **(Figure 10.24)**. Any change in status (respirations, heart rate, level of consciousness) should be reported to the IC immediately. If the patient is out of reach, a continuous conversation should be maintained with him or her. Any needed medical treatment that can be started should be.

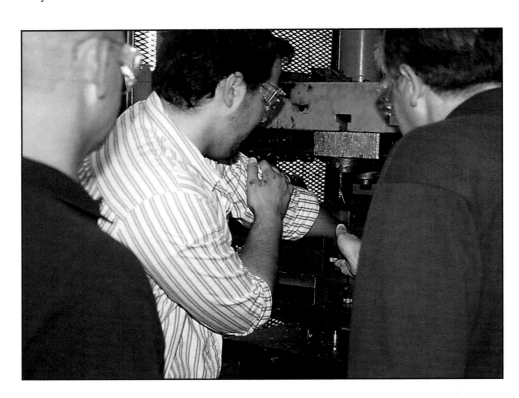

Figure 10.24 EMS personnel should monitor the medical condition of entrapped persons.

Finalizing the Incident Action Plan (IAP)

On small, relatively simple rescue operations the IAP need not be in writing, but *there must be a plan*. On larger, more complex operations the plan should be in writing and should reflect an incident management system. In either case, the plan must be finalized and communicated through channels to everyone involved in the operation. The plan should be structured enough to guide those involved in the operation, but flexible enough to deal with the unexpected. For example, if it should become necessary to rescue the rescuers, the plan should accommodate this contingency.

Gathering Resources

Resources consist of personnel and equipment, and both are critically important to the operation. The resources gathered at the scene should reflect the IAP. If either or both the personnel and equipment in the initial response are insufficient for the rescue problem at hand, additional resources should be requested as soon after arrival as possible.

Personnel. If there are too few rescue personnel, or if they are insufficiently trained to perform as needed, the best equipment in the world will not get the job done. Likewise, the most highly trained and motivated rescuers will not be able to do what is necessary if they do not have the tools and equipment they need. The number of extrication personnel needed will vary depending upon the nature and extent of the extrication problem.

Equipment. The amount and types of equipment needed will also vary with the nature and extent of the rescue problem. Highly specialized tools and equipment unique to the machine or industry involved may also be needed.

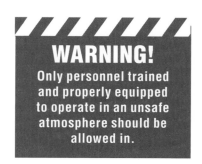

WARNING!
Only personnel trained and properly equipped to operate in an unsafe atmosphere should be allowed in.

Monitoring the Atmosphere

In many machinery entrapment incidents, the atmosphere in the immediate rescue area can be contaminated by escaping gases or vapors from fluids leaking from the damaged machine. It can also be become contaminated with the exhaust from gasoline-driven rescue equipment.

If the machinery entrapment also happens to be in a confined space, the atmosphere within the space should be monitored from *outside* the space. The atmosphere inside the space should be checked for oxygen concentration, flammability, and toxicity – in that order.

Whatever the source of contamination, personnel should be assigned to monitor the atmosphere in the immediate rescue area. These personnel should use single- or multi-gas detectors as dictated by the situation **(Figure 10.25)**.

Ventilation

Once the source of contamination has been found and controlled, it may be necessary to ventilate the area before attempting a rescue. If the atmosphere in the immediate area of the rescue is outside the acceptable range, the area must be ventilated with either positive pressure from a fan blowing fresh air into the area or an intrinsically safe fan exhausting air from within the area. Because many toxic gases and vapors are also flammable, the same precautions should be taken when ventilating areas with toxic atmospheres. If gasoline-powered fans are used, the engine exhaust must not be allowed to further contaminate the rescue area.

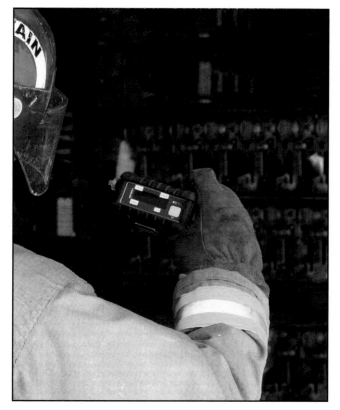

Figure 10.25 Atmospheric monitoring should be conducted in and around machinery extrication operations.

Lighting

In many cases, the rescue area will have sufficient natural illumination for the operation to be conducted without the need for additional lighting. In others, portable lighting will be needed. If there is any possibility of flammable gases or vapors being in the rescue area, only intrinsically safe lighting should be used. If a gasoline-driven generator is used to power the lights, care must be taken to avoid contaminating the atmosphere in the rescue area with exhaust from the generator.

Communications

If the extrication area is remote from the incident command post (ICP)— that is, far enough away that the patient cannot be seen from the ICP or there is too much ambient noise to allow unaided verbal communication between the rescuers and the IC, some effective means of communication must be established. Depending upon conditions, everything from portable radios, hard-wired telephones, and cell phones can be used. However, each form of communication has its limitations, such as concrete walls making radios and cell phones unreliable, and stretching a communications cable from the ICP to the rescue area may be difficult and time consuming. Also, the means selected needs to be intrinsically safe.

Phase III: Machinery Extrication Operations

The process of actually extricating the patient can begin only after zero mechanical state has been achieved. Determining the method of extrication can be a very difficult decision. The following four critical factors must be addressed when making this decision.

1. Time necessary to complete the extrication

2. Effects the extrication will have on the patient

3. Effects the extrication will have on rescuers

4. Effects (damage) the extrication will have on the equipment involved

Naturally, the rescuers' goal is to minimize each of the four factors. A solution that takes little or no time, does not further injure the patient, avoids risks to the rescuers, and causes no damage to the equipment is unlikely. Generally, a compromise will have to be made. Two things that should never be compromised are the effect the extrication will have on the patient and the rescuers. At no time should rescuers take steps that will cause further injury to the patient or will place rescuers in an excessive amount of danger.

The other two variables-time and possible damage to equipment-will help determine a final course of action. The time necessary to complete a certain procedure must be weighed against the patient's condition and ability to withstand that amount of waiting. A patient who has not sustained a lift-threatening injury will probably be able to withstand a longer extrication procedure, such as a disassembling operation. Patients whose lives are in danger will require quicker actions, such as those where the machine is forcibly compromised. In rare cases, either disassembly or forcing will be required regardless of the patient's condition, because the design of the machine will not permit any other option.

Once the atmosphere in the immediate extrication area is safe for rescue personnel to enter and do their work, they can begin stabilizing the machine, isolating energy sources, stabilizing and treating the patient, disentanglement, and extrication. Extrication can be accomplished in three basic ways: manipulative extrication, disassembling the machine, or forcing the machine. Whenever possible, the rescue operations in the sections that follow should be performed simultaneously, not sequentially.

Stabilizing the Machine

Because the structure and operation of the particular machine may not be obvious to rescue personnel, the machine operator or the plant maintenance mechanic may be able to provide vital information at this point. A technical expert can help the rescuers to free the patient in the shortest possible time and also help prevent mistakes that could injure the patient or extrication personnel.

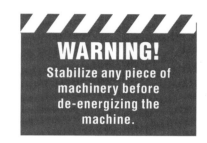

WARNING!
Stabilize any piece of machinery before de-energizing the machine.

The machine must be stabilized to prevent moving parts from either completing their cycle or returning to their original position when power is interrupted. Stabilizing the machine may have to be done with shoring, or it may involve strapping with chains, cables, webbing, ropes, or any combination of these.

Shoring. In situations with stamping or pressing machines that involve the vertical or horizontal movement of a piston or press, cribbing or shoring can be installed in the opening between the press plate and the receiver. The potential force involved dictates the cribbing pattern used. In some cases, simple 2 by 2 box cribbing may be sufficient. If the potential force is greater, a 3 by 3 (or more) box crib may have to be installed. As in other extrication operations, if wooden shoring is used, the pieces should be cut a couple of inches (50 mm) short of the length needed to fill the opening and wedges driven in to tighten the shore.

If pneumatic or hydraulic shores are used to stabilize the machine or the rescue area, the length can be adjusted without the use of wedges. However, it is critically important to make sure that the shore will not slip because of metal-to-metal contact. Whenever possible, pneumatic or hydraulic struts should be installed at 90 degrees to the object to reduce the tendency to slip.

Strapping. Depending upon the type of machine component involved, it may be necessary to strap it in place using whatever means available. The strapping used must be sufficiently strong for the potential load. In some cases, chains looped through a component and around a stable anchor point can be tightened to prevent movement of the component. In other cases, it will be necessary to install two straps or chains in direct opposition on the same component.

Other means of strapping that may be used are cable/chain-tensioning devices such as come-alongs. Two-inch (50 mm) nylon webbing can also be used to strap machine components in place if an adequate means of tensioning the webbing is available. Even rope can be used in some cases.

Isolating Energy Sources

Once the machine has been stabilized, its energy source can be isolated. Isolating the source of energy may be as simple as flipping a switch or closing a valve. Electrical switches should be locked in the OFF position with a padlock and a tag attached that warns of the danger of turning the power back on before authorized. If lockout/tagout devices are not available, a rescuer with a portable radio should be assigned to stay at the switch to prevent anyone from turning the power back on before it is safe to do so. The same precautions should be used with pneumatic or hydraulic valves that supply energy to the involved machine.

Patient Treatment and Stabilization

Once the machine has been stabilized and its energy source isolated, the process of treating and stabilizing the patient can begin. EMS personnel usually carry out this part of the operation; however, if they are not immediately available, the rescuers themselves will have to care for the patient. Once freed from entrapment, the patient should be packaged for transport in the most appropriate means available.

Manipulative Extrication

Manipulative extrications are the simplest of the three basic methods. Generally, they are also the quickest. Manipulative extrications rely on common sense instead of rescue tools. Manipulative extrications can be divided into two types: those where the patient is manipulated and those where the machine is manipulated.

Procedures where the patient is manipulated should be limited to situations where the patient is not injured, but happens to be caught in something. Examples of this includes a worker who has gotten a hand or arm caught in the opening of a small pipe or conduit, or someone who has tried to squeeze through a small opening and has become stuck.

A patient can often be freed by getting the person to relax the body part and then sliding it out, perhaps with a slight twisting motion. A lubricant may be useful in helping free the appendage. Substances such as vegetable oil or petroleum jelly may be used to reduce the friction between the patient and the mechanism of entrapment. If at any point in such an operation the patient appears to be in severe pain and little or no progress is being made, rescuers should stop and try another procedure.

The second type of manipulative extrication is to manipulate the entrapping mechanism in order to release the patient. Manipulating the mechanism means to operate it in a manner in which it is designed to be operated, to the advantage of the patient and the rescuer. This is different from disassembly or forcing procedures, which require manipulation beyond the normal operating features of the machine.

A person caught in an auger or screw-type mechanism who can be released by reversing the direction of the auger or screw is one example of manipulative extrication. Another example is a person whose hand is caught in an adjustable opening of a machine. The hand could be freed by adjusting the machine to provide a larger opening.

When attempting these procedures, it is highly desirable to have plant maintenance or other civilian personnel present who are familiar with the proper operation of the machine. Civilian personnel are more likely to ensure the machine is operated smoothly during the extrication attempt. If performing the maneuvers requires special skills, a person trained in operating the equipment should be allowed to do so under the close supervision of rescue personnel. No part of the machine should be operated if rescuers cannot be assured that the part will react as predicted.

Disassembling the Machine

There are many reasons that most industrial extrications are accomplished by disassembling the entrapping machinery. Frequently, the machine is too heavily built to be affected by standard extrication equipment. In other cases, the minor injuries suffered by the patient do not necessitate quick removal or damage to expensive, high tech equipment. Whatever the reason, disassembly procedures generally require the help of civilian personnel who are highly knowledgeable about the machinery involved **(Figure 10.26)**. This type of expert assistance will help minimize the time it takes to loosen or remove the parts entrapping the patient. Even with their higher level of expertise, civilians should be closely supervised by rescue personnel and should not attempt any moves without prior approval of the rescue personnel.

Sometimes a duplicate piece of machinery is on the premises. If time allows, this machine may be examined before beginning any manipulation or disassembly of the machine entrapping the patient. If the patient's condition permits, it may be wise to attempt the planned maneuver on the duplicate machinery to pinpoint any hidden dangers as well as quicker ways to do the job.

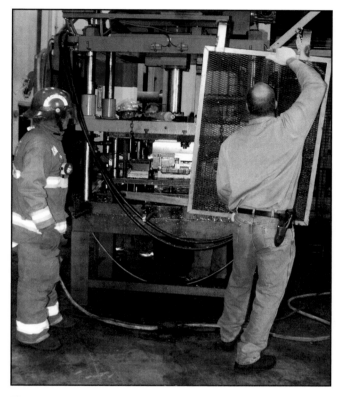

Figure 10.26 Machinery maintenance personnel can prove helpful in disassembling machinery components.

It may also be necessary to obtain special tools to accomplish disassembly operations. Most rescue companies do not carry the wide variety of mechanic's tools needed to take the machine apart. Examples of tools that may be needed are as follows:

- Large socket wrench sets
- Large box end wrenches
- Metric wrenches
- Allen wrenches

These tools are likely found on the premises as they are usually required in day-to-day activities. If tools from both the facility and the rescue company are being used, keep careful account so everything goes back to its proper place at the end of the incident. Representatives of the building occupants should be allowed to gather and keep track of any pieces that are removed from the machinery.

Protective guards and screens may have to be removed to access the bolts holding the main components in place. Rescuers should not become so fixated on the job of dismantling machinery that they waste time removing parts that don't require removal. The priority is to remove only those parts that are keeping the patient trapped.

In some cases, massive rollers or other similar components will have to be lifted off the patient. Because roller bearings and other parts have to be replaced on a regular basis, many industrial sites have overhead chain-hoists permanently installed to make these routine maintenance procedures faster and easier. Check the area above the machine for devices such as a chain-hoist track. If one is there, others can be assigned to move the hoist into place and get it ready for operation while the machine is being dismantled. If there is no overhead hoist, others can be assigned to erect a tripod and chain hoist over the component to be lifted. Still others can be assigned to clear the exit path that will be used when the patient is freed.

Rescuers must keenly observe every move made while the machine is being disassembled. Patients should be shielded from any further harm during this process. Before loosening or removing a part of the machine, rescuers must determine if the part could fall on or strike the patient. If a massive machine component were to fall back onto the patient, it could make a bad situation much worse. If this potential exists, take steps to support the part so this does not occur. As in any lifting operation — *lift an inch, crib an inch*. Causing further injury to the trapped patient is unacceptable — take every precaution to protect him or her during the rescue operation. Once the patient has been extricated from the machine, the patient can be packaged for transport to a medical facility.

Forcing the Machine

The least desirable alternative of the three basic industrial extrication strategies is to remove the patient by forcibly compromising the entrapping portions of the machinery. This method is least desirable because it is the least predictable and may cause extensive damage to the expensive machinery and may prove risky to the patient.

One of the main problems with this method is that rescue personnel are not accustomed to working on these types of machinery, thus they cannot be certain how a certain portion of a machine will act when pressure is applied to it. Another problem is that most rescue equipment is tailored to more common automobile accidents **(Figure 10.27)**. This equipment may be very difficult to use in an industrial setting and in many cases lacks the necessary power to be effective. Rescuers need to be well versed in operating their equipment and must be able to adapt the equipment, if possible, to the situation.

Rescuers should consult with equipment operators or maintenance personnel before attempting to force any piece or portion of a machine **(Figure 10.28)**. These people are more likely to know which parts of a machine are more vulnerable and how they will react when force is applied to them. They may also be able to estimate the amount of force needed to move the piece which will assist the rescuers in selecting the best tool for the job.

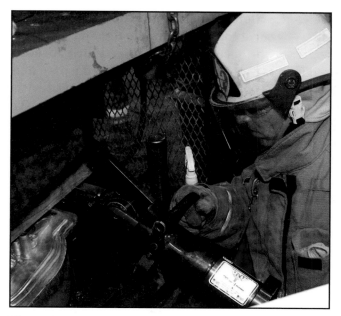

Figure 10.27 In some cases, automobile extrication tools and equipment may be used to force industrial machines in order to extricate an entrapped person.

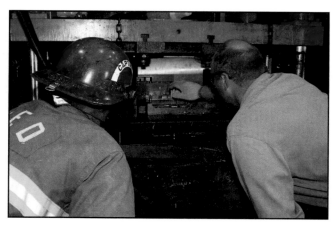

Figure 10.28 Machinery maintenance personnel can provide useful information about how a machine moves or can be moved.

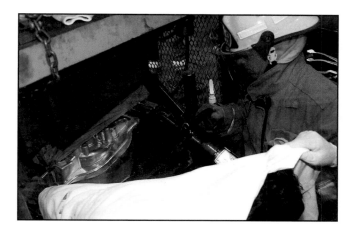

Figure 10.29 Rescuers should cover patients with a sheet, blanket, or tarp to protect the patient from sparks and small debris.

Protection of the patient and extrication personnel is critical during forcing operations. Patients should be shielded to protect them from any parts, pieces, or other flying hazards that may result from a forcing operation. Sheets, blankets, or tarps work very well for patient protection from sparks or very small pieces of debris **(Figure 10.29)**. If the patient is in danger of being hit by larger pieces of debris, then rescuers should place a sheet of plywood or metal between the work area and the patient. If cutting is being performed on metal parts that are in contact with the patient, then it may be necessary to apply water to the metal to keep it cool and prevent the patient from being burned. If there is a fire hazard associated with the extrication operation, charged and manned hoselines should be used to protect the patient and rescuers. Whenever forcing tactics are employed, extrication personnel should be wearing full personnel protective clothing and equipment, including eye protection.

When choosing tools to be used in a forcing operation, extrication personnel should choose those that will be the most controllable under the circumstances encountered. In some cases, it may be necessary to sacrifice a little speed to provide the control required for a safe operation. For example, if a patient is impaled by a long metal screw that is contained within a large mixing device; it may be necessary to cut the metal screw and transport the patient and the screw to a medical facility where it can be surgically removed. The type of cutting tool used must be consistent with the materials encountered and the level of safety required for the particular operation.

Phase IV: Termination

Once the extrication has been accomplished, rescue personnel can begin to terminate the incident. This phase should be conducted as described in Chapter 2, *Extrication Incident Management*.

Summary

Extrication incidents involving industrial or agricultural vehicles can be extremely challenging for rescue personnel. In order to function safely and efficiently at these incidents, personnel must be familiar with the anatomy and nomenclature of the types of vehicles and machinery that are common to their response areas. Regardless of the size or type of vehicle or piece of machinery involved in a particular incident, rescue personnel must keep in mind that their role is to protect themselves and others from harm, protect the trapped patients from further harm, and to free those patients as safely and as quickly as possible.

Review Questions

1. What are distinguishing features of each type of industrial and agricultural vehicle?

2. What are the hazards associated with industrial and agricultural vehicles?

3. What specific size-up concerns should an incident commander consider during industrial and agricultural vehicles extrication operations?

4. What methods can be used to stabilize industrial and agricultural vehicles during extrication operations?

5. What methods can be used to gain access to the interior of industrial and agricultural vehicles?

6. What tactics should an incident commander consider using during industrial and agricultural vehicle extrication operations?

7. What procedures can be used to perform extrication on industrial and agricultural machinery?

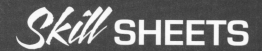
REMINDER: Not all agencies advocate the following procedures and practices. The following skill sheets present a snapshot of various procedures utilized during extrication operations. As always, local agency procedures and protocols must be followed.

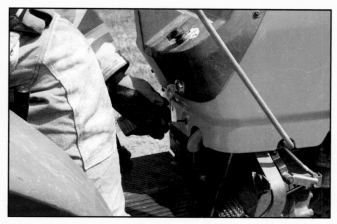

Step 1: Turn off the power to tractor or other piece of equipment powering the PTO shaft.

Step 2: Crib the implement to ensure firm support throughout the rescue.

Step 3: Attempt to telescope the two ends of the PTO shaft apart. It may be necessary to roll the tractor ahead to slide the stub shaft out of the front yoke, or to separate the shaft.

Step 4: Single-piece PTO shafts may have to be cut or disassembled at either end to free the patient.

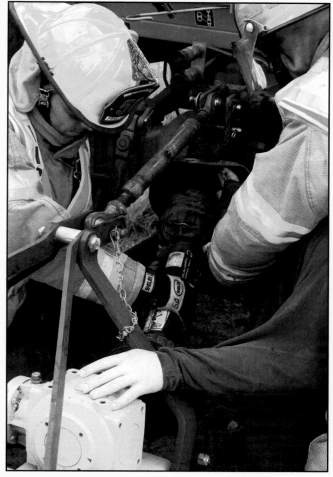

Step 5: It may be possible to free the patient by turning the shaft backward. Under no circumstances should tractor power be used to rotate the shaft!

Step 6: If the patient's clothes are caught in the section of the PTO, they must be cut loose to prevent further injury to the patient.

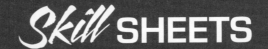

Step 7: Cervical spine and lower spine injuries are common with accidents involving PTO shafts if the patient's body is wrapped around the shaft. Sometimes, it is best to transport a stabilized patient still entangled with part of the PTO shaft. Extrication can be completed by a surgeon under hospital conditions.

Step 8: All amputated tissue should be transported to the hospital with the patient.

Step 9: If the accident involves complex or unfamiliar equipment, seek advice from a local implement dealer. This may prove to be faster and more efficient than the trial and error approach.

Step 10: Evaluate and maintain the integrity of the cribbing throughout the extrication.

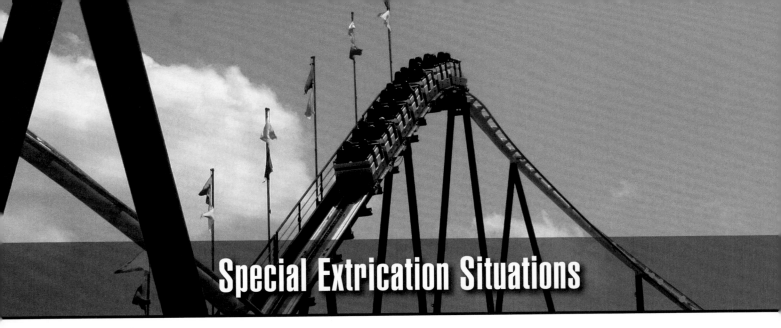

Special Extrication Situations

Chapter Contents

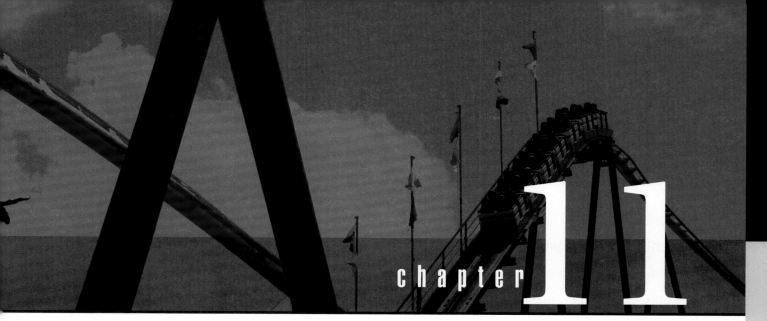

chapter 11

Key Terms

Job Performance Requirements

This chapter provides information that addresses the following job performance requirements (JPRs) of NFPA® 1001, *Standard for Fire Fighter Professional Qualifications* (2008), NFPA® 1006, *Standard for Technical Rescuer Professional Qualifications* (2008), and NFPA® 1670, *Standard on Operations and Training for Technical Search and Rescue Incidents* (2009).

NFPA® 1001 JPRs

6.4.1

6.4.2

NFPA® 1006 JPRs

5.2.2	10.1	10.1.3	10.1.7	10.1.10	10.2.2	10.2.5
5.2.3	10.1.1	10.1.4	10.1.8	10.2	10.2.3	
5.5.1	10.1.2	10.1.6	10.1.9	10.2.1	10.2.4	

NFPA® 1670 JPRs

8.2.2	8.3.4	12.2.2	12.3.3
8.2.3	8.4.2	12.2.3	12.3.4
8.3.2	12.1	12.3.1	12.4.1
8.3.3	12.2.1	12.3.2	12.4.2

Special Extrication Situations

Learning Objectives

1. Describe procedures for performing extrication on vehicles in structures.

2. Describe extrication procedures for vehicles in water.

3. Identify extrication procedures for multiple vehicle incidents.

4. Identify extrication procedures for recreational vehicle incidents.

5. Describe procedures for performing extrication on military vehicles.

6. Identify extrication procedures for armored vehicle incidents.

7. Describe extrication procedures for incidents involving emergency response vehicles.

8. Identify extrication procedures for incidents involving amusement park rides.

9. Describe extrication procedures for hanging vehicle incidents.

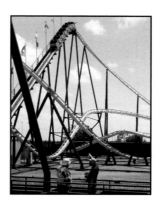

Chapter 11
Special Extrication Situations

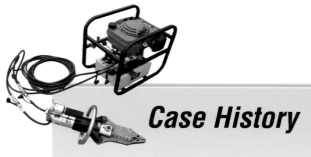

Case History

Rescuers in Florida were dispatched to an unusual vehicle into a structure response. The first responders to arrive on scene found an SUV had penetrated the wall of a single story garage almost six feet above ground level. The vehicle was balanced on the block wall with the rear of the vehicle outside the structure. The SUV held two patients.

The responders quickly sized up the structure, the vehicle, and the patients without disturbing anything. The patients' injuries were not severe, so an immediate extrication was not required. In addition to the hole punched in the side of the building by the vehicle, the building's structural integrity was heavily compromised. A technical rescue team was called to the scene to construct sufficient shoring to stabilize the structure prior to beginning patient extrication.

First, the team stabilized the vehicle with box cribs and rescue jacks. A 45 degree raker shore was constructed on the corner of the building to stabilize the front wall of the garage. Technical rescuers then built a T-shore inside the structure to stabilize the roof and walls. With the structure stabilized, rescuers turned their attention to the two patients. The rescuers were able to gain access into the vehicle, package, then remove the patients. The two patients were transported to local hospitals to be treated for minor injuries.

This chapter, unlike preceding chapters, focuses on the most unusual types of vehicle extrication situations. Some firefighters and other rescue personnel handle vehicle extrication incidents virtually every day, while others handle them less often but with some regularity. Those who deal with more or less routine incidents often become quite adept at handling them. However, there is a danger of these rescuers becoming complacent and overconfident. Regardless of how skilled and experienced rescuers are at handling routine incidents, when the situation is clearly unusual, they may find that they are less than fully prepared. It is imperative that adequate pre-incident planning be done and that the appropriate level of training and equipment be provided. Pre-incident planning should identify resources available within and outside of the agency that might be needed during special extrication situations and how these resources can be obtained when needed.

Regardless of how unusual the situation, the steps involved in handling an unusual incident safely and effectively are essentially the same as those in any other vehicle extrication incident: make an assessment of the situation, assume command of the incident, develop an incident action plan (IAP), and implement the plan. An IAP outlines the incident goals and objectives and specifies how the available resources are to be organized and deployed. The operational units within the incident organization then determine how to deal with hazards at the scene, stabilize the vehicles involved, stabilize and package the trapped patients, and extricate them from the vehicles. Finally, the plan specifies how the scene is to be restored and the incident terminated.

This chapter applies the steps involved in more commonly found incidents to incidents that are considered "special" or more rare. Any number of factors can cause a particular vehicle extrication incident to be considered a "special" situation. Common factors that can change an otherwise routine incident into one that is clearly special are as follows:

- Environment in which the incident occurred
- Number of vehicles involved
- Number of trapped patients
- Presence of fires or the potential for fires or explosions
- Presence of a large quantity of hazardous materials

The first-arriving responder at a special incident must be able to recognize that the situation is not routine, is beyond the capabilities of the responding rescue resources, and that a technical rescue or other specialized resources should be called. Answering the following questions will aid responders in recognize a situation that is not routine:

- How many vehicles are involved and what are their conditions?
- Did the vehicle crash into a structure? If so, what are the conditions of the structure and the vehicle? The condition of the structure must be the first concern followed by that of the vehicles. Vehicles hold a minimal amount of people compared to that of a structure. If the structure were to fail, many more people will be injured.
- Did the vehicle come to rest in a body of water? Is the vehicle under the water?
- Are there multiple vehicles involved? What types of vehicles and what are their conditions?
- Will heavy-duty tow trucks be needed? Will cranes, barges, or other specialized resources be needed to handle this incident?
- If the incident concerns an amusement ride, is the ride simply stalled or is it crushed? Are the people riding the attraction in an elevated position or located at ground level?

Ensuring Safety of On-Scene Personnel

It is vitally important that the first-arriving responder prevent on-scene personnel from endangering themselves and others in their zeal to rescue trapped vehicle occupants. Those in charge of these incidents must not allow their personnel to develop tunnel vision and rush into the scene before it is safe to do so — thereby adding more patients to the incident. It is essential that all rescuers remember that they did not cause the problem, they are not responsible for the patients being in that situation, and they are not obligated to sacrifice themselves in a heroic attempt to save a patient.

After answering questions about the scene and discovering that the incident qualifies as a special situation, rescuers must transform the information and plan they have created into action. This application of information to affect a rescue in special situations is the real challenge for responders. This chapter discusses several special situations with an emphasis on helping rescuers meet the challenges of the situation. For purposes of this discussion, special vehicle extrication situations are those that involve any of the following:

- Vehicle in a structure
- Vehicle in water
- Multiple vehicles
- Recreational vehicles (RVs)
- Military vehicles
- Armored vehicles
- Emergency response vehicles **(Figure 11.1, p. 456)**
- Amusement park rides **(Figure 11.2, p. 456)**
- Hanging vehicles

The sections that follow discuss each of these special situations in turn with an emphasis on the following aspects of the incident:

- Size-up
- Vehicle Stabilization
- Gaining Access
- Process

NOTE: Throughout this chapter, unless otherwise stated, stabilization, gaining access, and extrication can all be accomplished using the equipment and techniques found in Chapter 4, *Extrication Equipment*, and Chapter 5, *Extrication Techniques*.

Vehicle in Structure

In this context, the term structure refers to any stationary man-made object into which a vehicle has crashed **(Figure 11.3, p. 456)**. The object could be a building, bridge abutment, or tunnel.

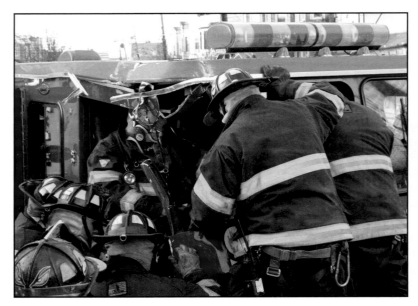

Figure 11.1 Rescuers must occasionally perform extrication on emergency response vehicles such as this fire apparatus. *Courtesy of Ron Jeffers.*

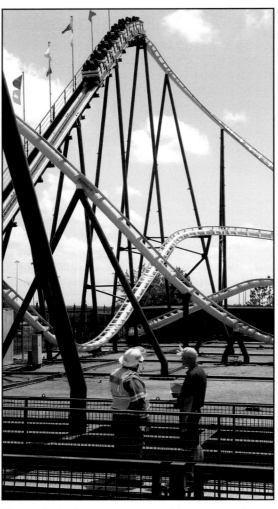

Figure 11.2 Amusement park rides can provide unique challenges for extrication personnel.

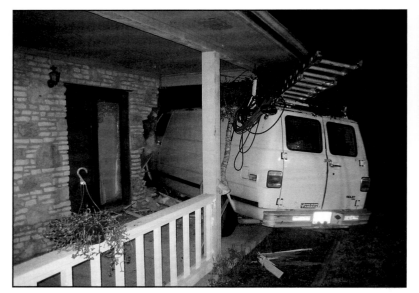

Figure 11.3 When vehicles collide with buildings, rescuers must take into account the stability of a structure as well as vehicle extrication procedures. *Courtesy of Buda (TX) Fire Department.*

Size-Up: Vehicle in Structure

First, the integrity of the structure must be assessed along with the other items normally associated with the assessment of a vehicle extrication scene. The first question to be asked is: Has the structure been damaged to the point that a collapse is likely? If the answer is yes, then the structure should be stabilized by a structural collapse rescue team or other qualified personnel. While waiting for the structural collapse team to arrive, on-scene personnel should be used to establish and maintain control of the scene, and perform any other duties that would not require them to enter the collapse danger zone. Request the response of the local building department if there is any question as to the instability of the structure.

NOTE: Storefront glass windows are typically non-load bearing and normally do not require structural stabilization to effect rescue.

Once the structure has been stabilized, the process of assessing the condition of the vehicle may be relatively quick and easy. Before the vehicle is stabilized, the assessment of the trapped patients must be somewhat rapid. At this point, all that is necessary is to confirm that there are patients in the vehicles, and what their general conditions are. Depending upon the type of vehicle and the type of structure, patient assessment may be very difficult and time consuming. If the vehicle cannot adequately be assessed in place, the cost/benefit of pulling the vehicle out of the structure may have to be considered. Since removal could be very risky for any trapped patients, it should be considered only in the most extreme situations.

The point here is to assess how the patients are entrapped and what will be needed to extricate them. Questions that should be considered are as follows:

- Are patients trapped because the structure into which the vehicle crashed will not allow the vehicle's doors to be opened?
- Are patients trapped by some part of the vehicle having collapsed around them?
- Are special tools, equipment, and other resources needed to free the patients?

Vehicle Stabilization: Vehicle in Structure
Once structural collapse is no longer a consideration, rescue personnel can begin to stabilize the vehicle. Given adequate space in which to operate, stabilizing a vehicle in a building, regardless of its position, is the same as described in the earlier chapter that focused on that type of vehicle.

If the shoring needed to stabilize the building so restricts the operating space around the vehicle that rescuers cannot maneuver as necessary to stabilize the vehicle, then the cost/benefit of pulling the vehicle from the building must be considered. As mentioned earlier, moving the vehicle before the occupant is stabilized can be very risky. Therefore, this option should be considered only in the most extreme situations.

Gaining Access: Vehicle in Structure
Once the structure and the vehicle have been stabilized, the tools and techniques used to gain access into the vehicle are the same as those described in Chapter 5, *Extrication Techniques*. However, if the vehicle is inside the building, operating space may be limited and extrication personnel must be careful not to disturb or dislodge any of the shoring that is supporting the structure.

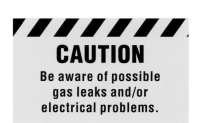

CAUTION
Be aware of possible gas leaks and/or electrical problems.

Extrication Process: Vehicle in Structure

The same space limitations and other environmental challenges that affected the vehicle stabilization and access processes may also affect the disentanglement and extrication processes. It may be necessary to package patients so that the litters in which they are placed can be manipulated in a variety of ways (even vertically) to avoid the shoring used to stabilize the building. As in the other phases of the operation, rescuers must be careful not to disturb or dislodge the structural shoring.

Vehicle in Water

Even in areas with very arid climates, vehicles sometimes leave the roadway and come to rest in a body of water. The water may be in a swimming pool, canal, bayou, swamp, river, estuary, lake, or even the ocean.

A submerged vehicle would have its passenger compartment totally under the water, while a partially submerged vehicle would have a portion of the passenger compartment above the water. Both determinations should be made with the vehicle resting on the bottom of the waterway. Partially submerged vehicles may be floating, only to become submerged. Rescuing patients from a floating vehicle is one of the most hazardous scenarios a team will face.

Size-Up: Vehicle in Water

If a vehicle has crashed into a body of water, the first question that must be answered is: Can rescue personnel do what must be done to extricate any trapped patients without having to enter the water? If the answer is no, then appropriately trained personnel should be utilized. On-scene personnel should be used to establish and maintain control of the scene, and perform any other tasks that would not require them to enter the water, especially if the vehicle fell from a great height into the water, or if the vehicle and its occupants have been submerged for more than an hour. Under these circumstances, the operation is almost certainly a body recovery and not a rescue. If the agency has one or more rescue boats, personnel trained in boat-based rescue operations can perform those tasks that can be done from the boat.

The overall situation — the type of vehicle, the nature of the body of water, how much of the vehicle is above the surface of the water, and in what position the vehicle came to rest — can make the process of assessing the vehicle's condition relatively easy or quite difficult. Much of the vehicle damage may be hidden below the waterline **(Figure 11.4)**. The vehicle may be entirely submerged making damage assessment virtually impossible without entering the water.

Depending upon how much of the vehicle is visible above the water, it may be possible to see into the vehicle and determine the number of patients and their conditions. In other cases, it may only be possible to determine that there are patients inside the vehicle and a more thorough assessment of their conditions will have to be delayed until the vehicle is pulled from the water and stabilized.

Assessing the extrication problems involved in this situation may have to wait until the vehicle is pulled from the water. A properly trained and equipped dive rescue team should be called at the first indication that a vehicle is in a body of water.

Vehicle Stabilization: Vehicle in Water

In most cases, there is little that anyone can do to stabilize a vehicle that is immersed in water except secure the vehicle to the shore with rope, chain, cable, or webbing attached to a secure anchor point. The major challenge may be to prevent the vehicle from sinking to the bottom or being swept downstream. Depending upon the vehicle's position and the amount of the vehicle above the water's surface, it may be necessary to pull the vehicle from the water before attempting any other extrication activities.

Gaining Access: Vehicle in Water

If the vehicle is still in the water, there is a remote possibility that the occupants could be surviving by taking advantage of a pocket of air trapped inside the vehicle passenger compartment. A dive rescue team may be best able to provide vehicle occupants with spare SCUBA devices in the event the vehicle becomes submerged. If rescuers attempt to cut through the roof or to remove the rear window, any trapped air will escape and allow the vehicle to sink and possibly drown the occupants.

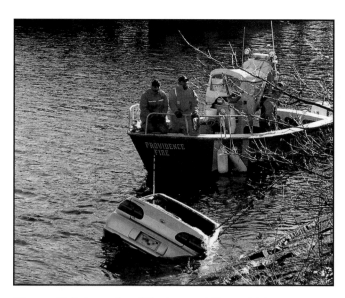

Figure 11.4 It can be difficult to stabilize vehicles that enter deep water. *Photo by Michael Porowski.*

Once the vehicle has been pulled from the water, there are two important considerations as follows:

1. Electrically powered extrication tools and equipment must be used only where contact with water is unlikely.

2. Rescue personnel in this situation should make sure that their actions do not cause the vehicle to roll back into the water.

> **CAUTION**
> Creating openings in a submerged vehicle may allow air trapped in the vehicle to escape.

Extrication Process: Vehicle in Water

If the vehicle is still submerged in the water, only rescuers trained in water rescue should attempt the disentanglement and extrication of trapped patients. Once the vehicle has been pulled from the water, the extrication process is the same as in any other vehicle extrication incident with that type of vehicle, with the exception of the cautions mentioned in the previous section.

Multiple Vehicle Incident

A multiple vehicle incident that qualifies as a special situation is one that involves more vehicles than the responsible agency can handle. If the responsible agency has to call for mutual aid or other outside assistance because of the number of vehicles involved, the incident meets the criteria for a special situation.

Size-Up: Multiple Vehicles

In sizing-up this type of incident the first question should be: Is there anything in the situation that would put rescue personnel or others at greater risk than any other vehicle extrication incident? If so, the needed resources should be called immediately. While waiting for the additional resources to arrive, on-scene personnel should be used to establish and maintain control of the scene, and perform any other duties that would not require them to enter the hot zone before the hazard has been mitigated.

The problems associated with assessing the condition of multiple vehicles involved in a single incident have less to do with the environment and more to do with the sheer number of vehicles involved. Vehicular triage — a sorting of the vehicles into categories of damage, is the beginning of this type rescue. Some may have superficial damage to the front and rear; others may have suffered significant structural damage and deformation that will require major manipulation to provide access to their occupants. In these types of collisions, there is a greater than normal threat of fires being initiated by the uncontrolled release of flammable liquids in close proximity to a variety of ignition sources. Fire crews with portable fire extinguishers and charged hoselines (1½-inch [38 mm] minimum) with foam capability should be standing by.

A multiple-vehicle incident is likely to also involve multiple casualties. This may indicate a need for several medical triage teams working at once. Depending upon the number of vehicles involved, weather conditions, darkness, and other factors, simply identifying the exact number of trapped patients may be a challenge. Especially at night, it is critical that this phase of the operation be well organized to reduce the chances of any patient being overlooked.

Vehicle Stabilization: Multiple Vehicles

The prospect of having to stabilize a large number of damaged vehicles at the same time can be very daunting. Based on the results of the vehicular triage performed earlier, the process can be organized and efficient. Each team should be responsible for stabilizing one vehicle at a time.

Gaining Access: Multiple Vehicles

Because these incidents often involve a series of rear-end collisions, access to the front and rear of the vehicles may be extremely limited. Otherwise, the tools and techniques involved in gaining access into many vehicles are the same as those used for gaining access into any passenger vehicle.

Extrication Process: Multiple Vehicles

Disentangling and extricating patients from vehicles involved in a multiple-vehicle incident can be very challenging because the vehicles may be in a variety of positions and environments. Some vehicles may be accordioned between other vehicles at their front and rear. Other vehicles may be wedged under or resting on top of other vehicles **(Figure 11.5)**. While even other vehicles may be in different positions — on their sides or upside down. Some vehicles may be in different locations – pushed into a ditch, off of a bridge or cliff, or into a body of water. Each extrication team must focus on one vehicle at a time. Based on the condition of the patients and the vehicle, the team must determine the best way to remove the vehicle from around the patients and to remove the patients from the wreckage.

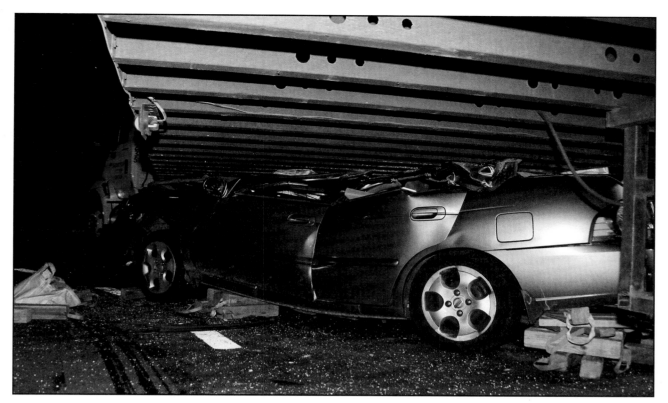

Figure 11.5 Multiple vehicle incidents may result in one vehicle overriding or underriding another. *Photo by Brian Wozniak/Newtown Fire Association.*

Recreational Vehicles (RVs)

Incidents involving recreational vehicles (RVs) are those in which motor homes, travel trailers, etc., have crashed. There may or may not be other types of vehicles involved.

Size-Up: RVs

These incidents may put rescue personnel and others at greater than normal risk if a liquefied petroleum gas (LPG) or other fuel tank or associated piping has been damaged and is leaking. Under these circumstances, on-scene personnel should be used to establish and maintain control of the scene, and perform any other duties that would not require them to enter the hot zone until the flammability hazard has been mitigated.

Assessing the damage to RVs involved in collisions may be less challenging than assessing other types of vehicles, unless the RV is in one of the hazardous environments already discussed. The structures of most RVs make them highly susceptible to damage but relatively easy to access. Most of these vehicles are constructed on a chassis with a rigid frame and are built more like mobile homes than highway vehicles.

Motor homes and travel trailers normally have a small number of occupants compared to some other vehicles, but this may or may not be true in any particular incident. If the RV was parked when struck by another vehicle, there could be several patients in the RV as well as in the other vehicle. In any case, the process of locating all of the patients and assessing their conditions must be as thorough and organized as in incidents involving other types of vehicles.

Because of the relatively lightweight construction of most RVs, basic extrication tools and equipment are all that are likely to be required. However because of ever changing vehicle construction technology, and the possibility of alterations made by the vehicle owner, this cannot be assumed. This phase of the operation must also be done thoroughly and conscientiously.

Vehicle Stabilization: RVs

Stabilizing an RV may be more like stabilizing a bus, as described in Chapter 7, *Bus Extrication*, than stabilizing any other type of vehicle. Whether or not rescuers use techniques for stabilizing a passenger vehicle or stabilizing a bus will largely depend upon the size of the RV involved in the accident.

Gaining Access: RVs

Because of the relatively light construction of most RVs, entry is likely to be quick and easy. However, the ease of entry should not be viewed as an excuse for rescuers to become complacent and ignore safety. As mentioned in this chapter and earlier chapters, RVs have hazards associated with them that rescuers will not encounter with other types of vehicles.

Extrication Process: RVs

Depending upon the type of RV involved and other variables in the particular incident, disentangling and extricating patients from these vehicles may be relatively simple or quite challenging. In a collision, the furnishings and other contents of the RV may turn its interior into a shambles. This mass of material can make disentangling and extricating the patients much more difficult. Even verifying that all the patients have been located may be difficult.

If a RV leaves the roadway and rolls over several times before coming to rest at the bottom of a steep slope, the vehicle may disintegrate as it tumbles leaving a trail of objects and occupants on the hillside. However, if the steepness of the slope would require more than low-angle rescue, a technical rescue team should be called in to extricate the patients. Otherwise, extricating patients from RVs requires the same techniques and equipment described in Chapter 7, *Bus Extrication*.

Military Vehicles

Incidents involving military vehicles are those that include but are not limited to light and heavy trucks, High Mobility Multipurpose Wheeled Vehicles (HMMWV), tanks, personnel carriers such as Mine Resistant Ambush Protected (MRAP) vehicles, aircraft tugs, and munitions loaders **(Figures 11.6a and b)**. Accidents involving these types of vehicles can pose significant hazards to the rescuer. Some vehicles involved in an accident may have munitions on board ranging from small arms ammunition to large munitions carried by aircraft.

Size-up: Military Vehicles

Incidents involving military vehicles or machinery pose a greater risk to the rescuer mainly due to the material the vehicle is manufactured with and the payload these vehicles can carry. It is essential that prior to arrival of emer-

High Mobility Multipurpose Wheeled Vehicles (HMMWV or Humvee) — A 4-wheel drive military vehicle that replaced earlier Jeep and MUTT vehicles.

Personnel Carriers — Armored fighting vehicles designed to transport infantry to a battlefield.

Mine Resistant Ambush Protected (MRAP) Vehicles — A series of armored fighting vehicles designed to survive ambushes and improvised explosive device (IED) attacks.

Aircraft Tugs — Special, low-profile vehicles designed to tow aircraft on the airport ramp or push aircraft backwards away from an airport gate. Also called *pushback tractors* or *tugs.*

Munitions Loaders — A military vehicle used to transport and load/off-load bombs and other munitions from military aircraft.

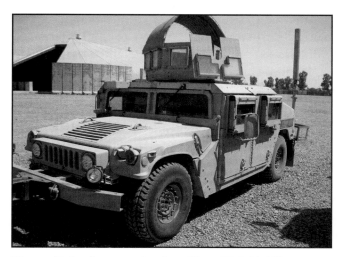

Figure 11.6a An example of a military High Mobility Multipurpose Wheeled Vehicles (HMMWV) or Humvee. *Courtesy of Kevin Ferrara.*

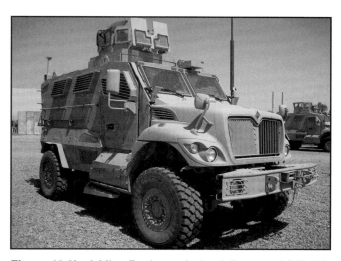

Figure 11.6b A Mine Resistant Ambush Protected (MRAP) vehicle. *Courtesy of Kevin Ferrara.*

gency response personnel, the telecommunicators relay information pertaining to the contents of the vehicles involved if able to do so. This type of information may not be able to be transmitted via radio due to security protocols. Meanwhile, the first-arriving rescuer should establish the appropriate control zones until the contents of the vehicle can be verified. Verification may be obtained from military personnel on scene or through telephone or individual messenger. This communication should be directed to a contact at the military installation the vehicle departed from. Military vehicles involved in an accident may need to be secured by military security forces prior to arrival. The nonmilitary rescuer may or may not be permitted to enter the accident scene until military personnel have secured the vehicle.

Assessing military vehicles involved in an accident is somewhat similar to any other vehicle assessment. The difference lies in the construction of the vehicle. If armored vehicles are involved, these vehicles may not have visible damage to the exterior. However individuals inside the vehicle may have some type of injury. Rescuers should note the type of material with which the vehicle is constructed. Armored vehicles such as tanks and personnel carriers may have a thick layer of material that cannot be penetrated by normal cutting devices **(Figure 11.7)**. While non-armored vehicles may be accessible by circular type saws and other cutting devices, a thorough inspection of the vehicle construction material should be conducted prior to attempting access.

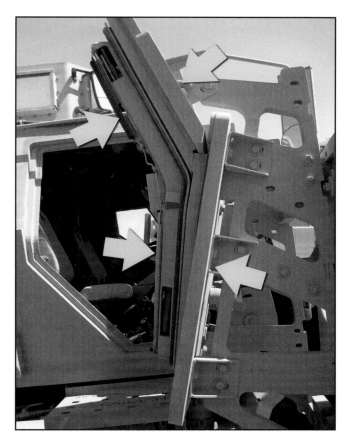

Figure 11.7 The thickness of military vehicle armor can make it difficult for rescue personnel to breach the armored areas into a vehicle's passenger compartment. *Courtesy of Kevin Ferrara.*

Military vehicles normally have a relatively small crew on board, but the number of personnel on board may vary. Military patients may be located either inside or outside the vehicle. Military patients may have helmets and other military equipment attached to themselves as well as weapons and ammunition. If possible, without causing further injury to the patient, the military equipment the patient is carrying may be removed. If the weapon and ammunitions is removed, it must be relocated and secured preferably by law enforcement personnel.

Because of the medium to heavy construction of military vehicles and machinery, basic extrication tools and equipment may not be feasible for accessing the injured patients. It is essential that any extrication efforts regarding military vehicles and machinery be performed thoroughly.

Vehicle Stabilization: Military Vehicles

While the techniques for stabilizing passenger vehicles may be appropriate for most military vehicles, the excessive weight of some military vehicles, especially armored vehicles, can pose significant challenges for rescue personnel. Rescuers must carefully assess whether or not they have sufficient stabilization equipment to handle this excess weight. If not, rescuers should seek outside sources who have the necessary equipment to stabilize the vehicle.

Gaining Access: Military Vehicles

Unless the military vehicle or machinery is positioned in a unique position, the tools and equipment as described in earlier chapters may be able to be utilized in gaining access. Rescuers should be aware that some military vehicles may not be able to be accessed using basic extrication tools commonly found on a rescue apparatus. Additional resources may need to be acquired after the initial assessment has been conducted. In addition, military vehicles found in unusual positions increase the difficulty of gaining access because the available path of entry may not allow the use of common tools and equipment.

Extrication Process: Military Vehicles

Military vehicles are unique due to the composition of the materials the vehicle or machinery is constructed from as well as the unique payloads they may be carrying. These vehicles may contain equipment that during a collision may become loose and strike occupants.

Armored Vehicles

Incidents involving armored vehicles those that include, but are not limited to the following:

- Armored military vehicles
- Armored trucks commonly found in transport of currency **(Figures 11.8)**
- Armored vehicles such as those used for dignitary and Presidential motorcades.

Size-up: Armored Vehicle

Incidents involving armored vehicles or machinery pose a greater risk to the rescuer mainly due to the material with which the vehicle is manufactured. The materials used in constructing armored vehicles are greater in weight and more resistant to basic extrication tool usage. The glass found on most armored vehicles is sometimes called bullet proof due to its thickness. It may require additional time to access the interior of the vehicle.

Assessing armored vehicles involved in an accident is somewhat similar to any other vehicle assessment. The difference lies in the construction of the vehicle. Armored vehicles may not have visible damage to the exterior. However individuals inside the vehicle may have some type of injury. Rescuers should note the type of material with which the vehicle is constructed. Armored vehicles such as currency transport type vehicles may have a thick layer of material that normal cutting devices cannot penetrate. If the normal route of access is unfeasible, an alternate route should be considered. Most armored vehicles do not allow the rescuer to easily access the hinges on the doors, so a special cutting device such as a plasma cutter may need to be requested.

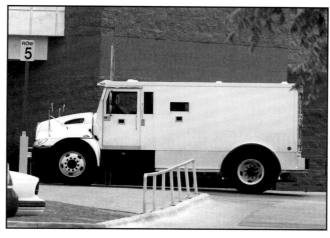
Figure 11.8 An armored currency transport vehicle.

The number of passengers inside an armored vehicle may vary. Currency and valuable cargo transports usually carry a small crew armed with weapons while dignitary transport vehicles may have a greater number of security personnel and weapons on board. Careful consideration should be made to secure any loose weapons found. No matter what type of armored vehicle is involved in an accident, it is essential that an accurate accountability is established as to who the original occupants of the vehicle were. Depending on the situation, rescuers may or may not be authorized access to the occupants until verification or security measures have been established.

Because of the medium to heavy construction of armored vehicles, basic extrication tools and equipment may not be feasible for accessing the injured patients. It is essential that any extrication efforts regarding armored vehicles and machinery be performed thoroughly with extreme caution.

Vehicle Stabilization: Armored Vehicle

While the techniques for stabilizing passenger vehicles may be appropriate for most armored vehicles, the excessive weight of some of these vehicles can pose significant challenges for rescue personnel. Rescuers must carefully assess whether or not they have sufficient stabilization equipment to handle this excess weight. If not, rescuers should seek outside sources who have the necessary equipment to stabilize the vehicle.

Gaining Access: Armored Vehicle

Rescuers should be aware that some armored vehicles may not be accessed using basic extrication tools commonly found on a rescue apparatus due to the construction materials found on the armored vehicle. Additional resources may need to be acquired upon initial assessment being conducted. In addition, armored vehicles found in unusual positions increase the difficulty of gaining access because the available path of entry may not allow the use of common tools and equipment.

NOTE: The transport company may need to be contacted to dispatch a key to gain access to the vehicle and to send personnel to secure the cargo.

Extrication Process: Armored Vehicle

Armored vehicles are unique due to the composition of the materials the vehicle or machinery is constructed from as well as the unique payloads they may be carrying. Because of the composition of the armored materials, rescuers need to understand the limitations of their extrication tools and equipment. While the extrication techniques are similar to other such operations, the tools may be insufficient to complete the extrication process.

Emergency Response Vehicles

Incidents involving emergency response vehicles (such as ambulances, fire apparatus, and law enforcement vehicles) are very unique due to the fact that the rescuers must be rescued. Emergency response vehicles carry a wide variety of unique equipment that would not commonly be found in passenger and light duty transport vehicles. Should an emergency response vehicle become involved in an accident, additional care must be considered regarding patient assessment and packaging based on the equipment the personnel maybe wearing, such as weapons, bullet-proof vest, and SCBAs.

Size-up: Emergency Response Vehicles

Incidents involving emergency response vehicles pose a significant risk to the rescuer due to the amount of loose equipment these vehicles carry. For example, a patient transport apparatus may have onboard oxygen cylinders as well as various biohazard items such as loose needles, drugs/medication, and blood that could contaminate or injure the rescuer as well as the patient. The presence of these hazards are potential dangers for rescuers but may already have had an effect on patients. The first-arriving rescuer should ascertain the types of hazards present, how many patients are involved, and the degree of entrapment.

Assessing emergency response vehicles is similar to assessing military or heavy duty vehicles. Because of the weight and dimensions of emergency response vehicles, care should be taken to ensure that all vehicles involved are stabilized prior to performing extrication activities. Rescuers should use caution when performing extrication activities on patient transport apparatus due to the possibility of oxygen cylinders being present.

Emergency response vehicles are normally operated with a relatively small crew, however based on the activities the crew was performing prior to the accident, the number of personnel on board could vary. As in the case of patient transport apparatus personnel, individuals located in the rear of the vehicle may not be secured with seat restraints. If this is the case, rescuers may expect some type of trauma upon assessment.

Due to their construction, emergency response vehicles could pose a challenge for basic extrication tools and equipment. It is crucial that caution be utilized when performing any extrication activities regarding emergency response vehicles due to the contents they may have on board. Rescuers should be aware of the type of equipment the emergency response vehicle may be carrying because that equipment may be beneficial in assisting extricating patients.

Vehicle Stabilization: Emergency Response Vehicle

While the techniques for stabilizing passenger vehicles may be appropriate for many emergency response vehicles, the excessive weight of some of these vehicles can pose significant challenges for rescue personnel. Rescuers must carefully assess whether or not they have sufficient stabilization equipment to handle this excess weight. If not, rescuers should seek outside sources who have the necessary equipment to stabilize the vehicle.

Gaining Access: Emergency Response Vehicle

Gaining access into emergency response vehicles will vary depending on the severity of the accident, degree of patient entrapment, hazards present, as well as construction type of the vehicle involved. Rescuers must familiarize themselves with these type of vehicles found in their local jurisdictions. Significant training on these vehicles will allow the rescuer to access the patient more quickly ultimately increasing the chance of survival for the patient.

Extrication Process: Emergency Response Vehicle

Emergency response vehicles vary in construction and occupancy load. Depending on the severity of damage, extrication may range from easily performed to in-depth and time consuming **(Figure 11.9)**. It is essential that rescue personnel receive training on these type of vehicles so that they are familiar with how to successfully gain access and extricate trapped occupants.

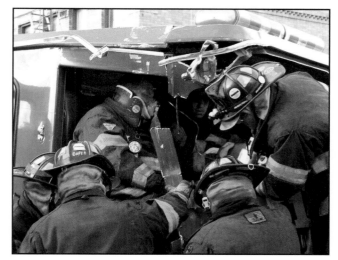

Figure 11.9 Rescuers working to extricate the officer of this fire apparatus. *Courtesy of Ron Jeffers.*

Special Considerations: Emergency Response Vehicles

Some emergency vehicles such as law enforcement cars may contain vehicle cages, police dogs, or weapons. The sections that follow identify what actions should be taken when these items are encountered.

Law Enforcement Vehicle Cages

Law enforcement vehicle cages may pose a significant obstacle to rescuers due the construction type and method of installation. Some cages may have a sliding window constructed from Plexiglas® that would allow rescuer access to the rear passenger compartment. Other cages are constructed with either a wire or steel mesh surrounded by heavy gauge roll bars that totally separates the front passenger compartment from the rear **(Figure 11.10)**. In this case, rescuers must gain access to the rear passenger compartment through the rear doors or rear window. Rescuers should know that most law enforcement vehicles have reinforced doors and windows that may not be breached easily. It is the responsibility of the rescuers to become familiar with what types of law enforcement vehicles are found in their local jurisdiction.

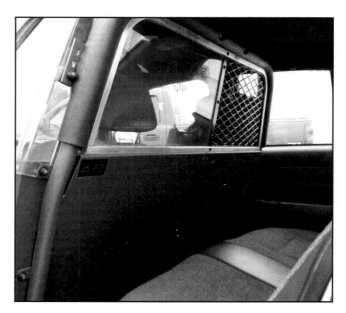

Figure 11.10 A Plexiglas® and steel mesh barrier between the front and back seats of a law enforcement vehicle. *Courtesy of Alan Braun, University of Missouri Fire and Rescue Training Institute.*

Police Dogs

Some police departments may have a K9 (canine) or police dog assigned to their department. If a police dog vehicle is involved in an accident, rescuers should take care when attempting to gain access into such a vehicle. Rescuers should be cautious if the police dog is injured as it may become aggressive when confronted by rescuers. If the vehicle is not involved in fire, is stabilized, and the dog appears uninjured, the dog may be left in place until resources with appropriate retrieval equipment arrive on scene to assist in removing the dog.

Weapons

Weapons may range from knives to ammunition to high caliber rifles. In any case, a vehicle involved in an accident transporting any type of weapon, the weapon(s) should be secured as quickly as possible prior to removing patients. Depending on the type of vehicle weapons may be carried in a variety of locations, for example in the trunk, passenger compartment stowage points, or on the officers' persons. These weapons may need to be secured by a specific individual or agency; typically law enforcement personnel, prior to rescuers gaining access to the vehicle **(Figure 11.11)**. If rescuers themselves secure any type of weapon, it must immediately be turned over to law enforcement personnel who can then secure it.

Amusement Park Rides

Amusement park ride incidents may include several different potential dangers for rescuers and others. Many of these vehicles are powered by high-voltage electricity in an electro-magnetic drive system, and others are attached to a gear-driven chain similar to a conveyor. In addition, many of these vehicles travel on or are suspended from elevated tracks that add the element of height to the other potential dangers.

Size-Up: Amusement Park Rides

In amusement park ride incidents, the scene assessment questions that need to be answered are as follows:

- Has the means of locomotion been turned off, and if not, does the vehicle need to be stabilized before that is done?

- Is the vehicle on an elevated track that is beyond the reach of standard fire service ground ladders or aerial devices **(Figure 11.12)**?

- Is the vehicle located in a confined area such as a tunnel? If so, a technical rescue team should be called. In that case, on-scene personnel should be used to establish and maintain control of the scene, and support the technical rescue team when it arrives.

The uniqueness of these vehicles can make damage assessment difficult. Therefore, pre-incident planning is essential to familiarizing local rescue personnel with the construction of these vehicles. Larger amusement parks and theme parks have maintenance and engineering staff solely dedicated to the upkeep of their attraction rides. These types of rides undergo a rigorous and thorough maintenance schedule. Rescuers should seek the advice of these professionals if an incident occurs on this type of a vehicle **(Figure 11.13)**.

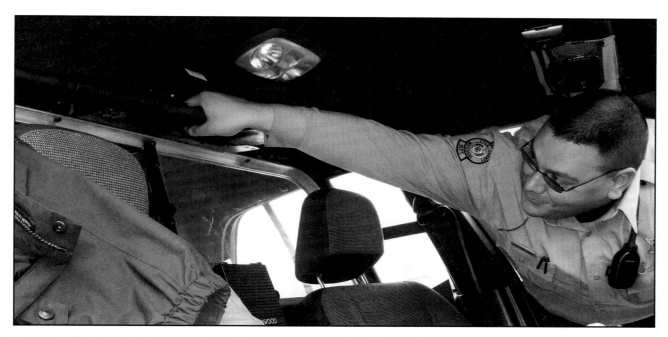

Figure 11.11 Designated personnel need to secure weapons found in wrecked law enforcement vehicles. *Courtesy of Alan Braun, University of Missouri Fire and Rescue Training Institute.*

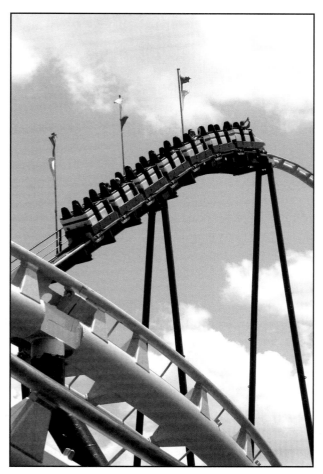

Figure 11.12 Some amusement park rides are taller than fire service ground ladders and aerial devices can reach.

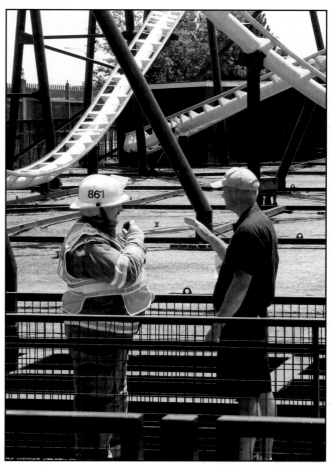

Figure 11.13 Amusement park engineers and maintenance personnel can provide valuable technical assistance during extrication operations on amusement park rides.

Assessing the condition of the patients of an amusement park ride incident may in some ways be easier than assessing patients in other types of vehicles. The difference lies in the fact that the design of the vehicles used in amusement park rides are usually more open than most highway vehicles, so the patients are often more visible from outside of the vehicle.

Since the tools and techniques of freeing patients from entrapment in an amusement park ride are the same as those used in other types of vehicles, the differences in the extrication assessment may relate more to the environment than the vehicle. If the vehicle is at ground level or close to it, the extrication needs will be the same as those of any other vehicle with a similar passenger load. However, if the vehicle is on an elevated track or in a confined area, the problems are likely to be quite different. If the vehicle is beyond the reach of standard fire service ground ladders or aerial devices, a technical rescue team should be called in to rig the necessary rope rescue systems.

Also, the attitude of the vehicle and the manner in which the car is attached to its tracks has a major bearing on the extrication. The passenger carrying cars typically ride on top of a track or are suspended underneath a track and the ride may turn up to 360 degrees on a front to back axis and/or a side to side axis. This presents rescuers with an infinite number of positions that a ride may be found. For example in each of the following scenarios careful planning is required in order to safely mitigate the emergency:

- Patients seated upside down with the track on top of their seats
- Patients seated upside down with the track at their heads
- Patients seated upright with the track underneath the seats
- Patients seated upright with the track above their heads

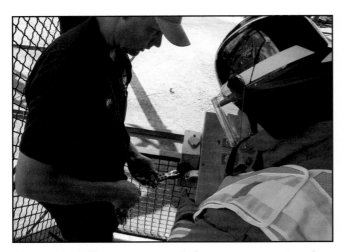

Figure 11.14 The power controls for an amusement park ride should be shut off and locked out/tagged out.

Vehicle Stabilization: Amusement Park Rides

The tools and techniques used to stabilize an amusement park ride may be more like stabilizing a piece of industrial machinery, as discussed in Chapter 10, *Industrial/Agricultural Vehicle and Machinery Extrication*, than stabilizing a highway vehicle. The parks engineering staff may perform lockout/tagout and vehicle stabilization before the arrival of rescue personnel **(Figure 11.14)**. Rescuers should refer to the expertise of the parks engineering staff for information regarding individual ride systems. These staff members work on the rides daily and should be considered subject matter experts. However, if the vehicle has derailed and is on the ground, the stabilization tools, techniques, and equipment will be the same as those for any other vehicle of similar size.

Gaining Access: Amusement Park Rides

Because of the open design of most of these vehicles, gaining access into them should not be a major challenge unless the crash caused serious deformation of the vehicle or if the vehicle has come to rest upside down. Many rides have different types of safety restraint device actuators. Some operate by the turn of a common wrench or a custom designed tool specific to that ride. Other actuators operate with the use of a hand-held magnet. The best way to prepare for this type of emergency is through joint training with park personnel. Maintaining a good working relationship with park management and personnel is essential.

Extrication Process: Amusement Park Rides

Considering the open design of most of these vehicles, disentangling and extricating patients may be easier than in other types of vehicles — unless the vehicle is upside down. If the vehicle is upside down, the process of packaging and extricating these patients may be protracted. The previously mentioned safety restraint device actuators usually open an entire row of devises simultaneously. If the rescue team responded to an incident involving a passenger compartment which was upside down with the track located on top of the seats, the entire row of patients may have to be removed at the same time. Consider securing the safety devices at each seat in place to avoid accidental discharge from the ride. In this scenario, remove each patient individually according to patient triage criteria.

Hanging Vehicles

In this context, a hanging vehicle incident is one in which a vehicle has crashed through a guardrail on a bridge, highway overpass, cliff, or an embankment and has come to rest with the cab or passenger compartment hanging above an abyss. The goal in this type of incident is to prevent rescue personnel, patients, or the occupied portion of the vehicle, from falling to whatever lies beneath it.

Size-Up: Hanging Vehicle

The first question that must be answered in these incidents is: Can the trapped patients be reached from below with standard fire service ground ladders or aerial devices? If the answer is no, then a technical rescue team should be called in to rig the necessary rope rescue systems. While waiting for the technical rescue team, on-scene personnel should be used to establish and maintain control of the scene.

An important safety consideration during scene assessment, and until the vehicle can be stabilized, is to keep everyone — rescue personnel and all others — out of the area directly below the hanging vehicle. Should all or part of the vehicle come loose before it has been stabilized, anyone below it may be in serious jeopardy.

Another obvious safety consideration is controlling vehicular traffic near the scene. Traffic should be stopped in both directions and detoured around the scene at a sufficient distance to ensure that traffic-generated vibration will not affect the stability of the hanging vehicle.

Getting close enough to assess the damage to a vehicle that is hanging from a high point may be extremely dangerous. The vehicle may be ready to come loose and plunge downward or the location the vehicle is hanging from may be in danger of collapsing. Assessing the damage to the vehicle may have to be done from some distance away using binoculars.

Getting close enough to the vehicle occupants to determine their number and assess their conditions — without putting rescue personnel at serious risk — may be extremely difficult. This, too, may have to be done from a distance.

Determining how the trapped patients will have to be removed from their precarious situation may influence the decisions about what tools and techniques can be used to accomplish that. If rescue personnel will have to work from scaffolding or some other platform — perhaps one suspended from a crane boom — only the types of tools and equipment that are appropriate for use under those conditions should be selected. In most cases, only those tools and equipment that are fully portable and self-contained will be used. Those that require cords and hoses connected to power units mounted on rescue vehicles may not be safe and effective to use in these situations.

Vehicle Stabilization: Hanging Vehicle

Stabilizing a vehicle that is hanging from some precipice may be the most challenging of any vehicle stabilization situation. The height of the vehicle above the ground (or water) can make this potentially one of the most dangerous situations for rescuers and trapped patients alike. When devising a plan to stabilize the vehicle the following must be considered:

- Type of vehicle involved
- Height above the surface below
- Likelihood of the vehicle falling

While there may be variables in the specific situation that would dictate otherwise, initial stabilization may have to be provided by securing the vehicle to bombproof anchor points with as many ropes, chains, or pieces of webbing as can be applied quickly and safely **(Figure 11.15)**. Again, depending upon the specific circumstances, it may be desirable or necessary to stabilize the hanging portion of the vehicle with a sling suspended from the boom of a crane or heavy recovery vehicle.

Figure 11.15 A hanging vehicle must be anchored to prevent further movement

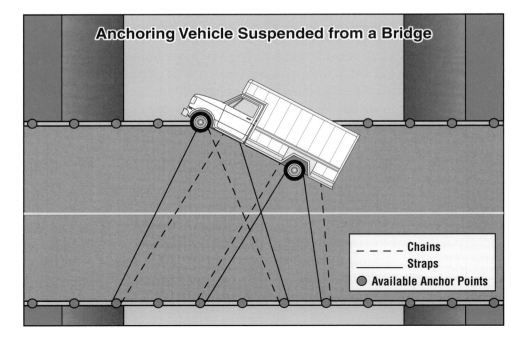

Anchoring Vehicle Suspended from a Bridge

_ _ _ _ Chains
_____ Straps
● Available Anchor Points

Gaining Access: Hanging Vehicle

In these situations, being able to reach the part of the vehicle that is hanging may be as difficult as gaining access into it. Once the hanging part has been reached, a stable platform must be created so that rescue personnel have a safe place from which to work. Under ideal circumstances, such as a vehicle hanging from a highway overpass, rescuers may be able to work from an aerial device positioned on the highway below. In other situations, it may be necessary to suspend a platform from the boom of a crane positioned below the point from which the vehicle is hanging. If the vehicle is hanging from a bridge over a river, estuary, or other body of water, it may be necessary to put the crane on a barge in order to reach the hanging vehicle **(Figure 11.16)**. As mentioned earlier, if the hanging part of the vehicle cannot be reached with standard fire service ground ladders or aerial devices, a technical rescue team should be called to handle this phase of the operation.

Extrication Process: Hanging Vehicle

Once a safe working platform has been created, disentangling and extricating patients from a hanging vehicle may be relatively routine. Depending upon the circumstances, it may be necessary to provide each patient with fall protection in addition to the normal packaging for extrication.

Summary

Special vehicle extrication situations are those that are unusual in some significant way. They may be special because of the environment in which they occurred, the number of vehicles and/or patients involved, or because of the presence of hazardous materials or some other threat that could put rescuers or others at greater than normal risk.

As in any other vehicle extrication incident, the key word in special situations is safety. Part of maintaining safety in special extrication situations is recognizing that the situation is unusual and that it may be beyond the operational capabilities of those responding to it. Another aspect of conducting these special operations safely is avoiding the tunnel vision that can induce some to exceed their operational limits and put themselves and others in jeopardy, perhaps adding more patients to the incident. If these operations are to be done safely, they must be conducted calmly, methodically, and according to agency protocols and standard operating procedures.

Review Questions

1. What is the first size-up consideration in a situation involving a vehicle in a structure?

2. What tools and equipment can be used to stabilize a vehicle that is in water?

3. What are some of the challenges rescuers face when performing extrication at a multiple vehicle incident?

4. What hazards do rescuers face at an extrication operation involving a recreational vehicle?

5. What challenges do military vehicles pose to rescuers during vehicle extrication operations?

6. Who should rescuers contact during an extrication operation on an armored vehicle?

7. What challenges and hazards can rescuers expect to encounter when performing extrication on a law enforcement vehicle?

8. Who can provide valuable technical assistance to rescuers at an amusement park ride extrication incident?

9. What equipment can be used to reach hanging vehicles?

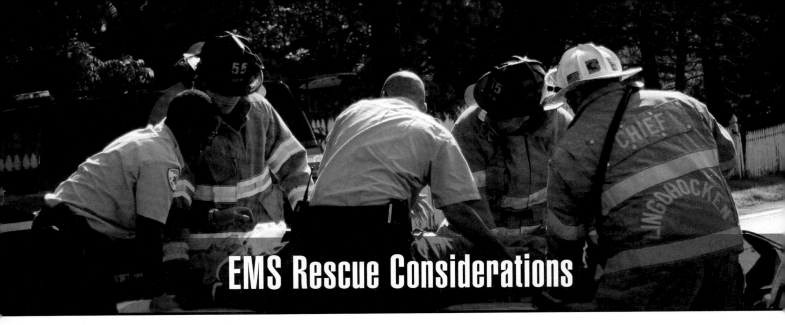

EMS Rescue Considerations

Chapter Contents

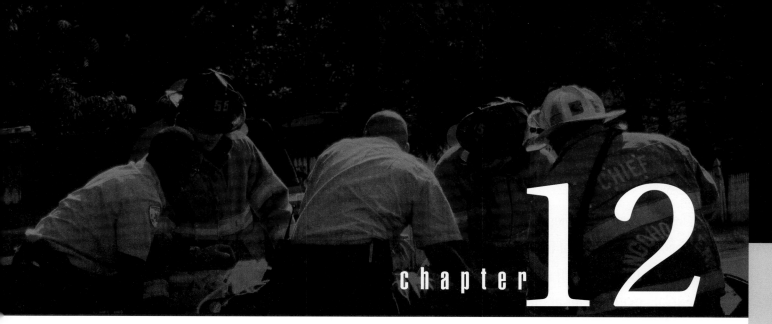

chapter 12

Key Terms

Job Performance Requirements

This chapter provides information that addresses the following job performance requirements (JPRs) NFPA® 1006, *Standard for Technical Rescuer Professional Qualifications* (2008), and NFPA® 1670, *Standard on Operations and Training for Technical Search and Rescue Incidents* (2009).

NFPA® 1006 JPRs

5.3.1	10.1.8
5.3.2	10.1.9
5.3.3	10.2.5

NFPA® 1670 JPRs

8.3.4	12.3.4
8.4.2	12.4.2

Learning Objectives

1. Describe key principles of trauma care.

2. Describe the types of injuries associated with each mechanism of injury.

3. Identify types of farm equipment injuries.

4. Explain methods for administering care in the field for various injuries, exposures, and conditions.

5. Describe procedures for coordinating with medical personnel.

6. Identify patient packaging and removal procedures.

7. Describe post incident follow up and education procedures.

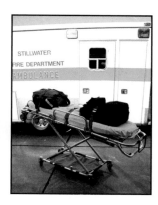

Chapter 12
EMS Rescue Considerations

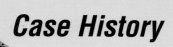

Case History

Fire and rescue crews were dispatched to a motor vehicle accident in a rural area involving a collision between a pontoon boat and trailer and a mini-van. The boat trailer had separated from the towing truck and, decelerating rapidly, was struck by the mini-van that was following close behind. Rescuers found that one pontoon of the boat had penetrated the mini-van windshield and struck the driver of the mini-van in the head.

The boat and trailer as well as the mini-van were quickly stabilized and the patient was immobilized and extricated from the mini-van. Firefighter/paramedics intubated the patient and provided oxygen therapy. They also began two IV lines. Because of a heavy fog in the area, a helicopter flight was not possible, so the patient had to be transported by ground ambulance to a trauma center approximately 50 miles away. Prior to arriving at the trauma center, the patient went into cardiac arrest. Attempts by the paramedics and trauma center personnel failed to resuscitate the patient.

This chapter discusses the care of the extended entrapped patient and the kinetic energy's associated with vehicle collisions. As outlined in previous chapters safety of rescue personnel is the main priority and full personal protective equipment (PPE) must be worn at all times during the extrication of patients. It is highly desirable for all rescuers to have at least some formal basic first aid or emergency medical technician (EMT) training.

NOTE: The information in this chapter is general in nature. Each jurisdiction should have its own emergency medical service (EMS) protocols that must be followed as closely as possible.

Principles of Trauma Care

The primary focus of an extrication operation is to remove the patient or patients safely from the entrapping mechanism. To care for the patient or patients, rescuers should understand the role of triage in mass casualty incidents (MCI) and how to coordinate the roles of the various medical groups that are part of the Incident Command System (ICS).

Mass Casualty Incident — An incident that results in a large number of casualties within a short time frame as a result of an attack, natural disaster, aircraft crash, or other cause that is beyond the capabilities of local logistical support.

Many jurisdictions have varying definitions of what constitutes a MCI and when field triage protocols can be employed. Simply defined, a MCI is any incident where the need for patient care overwhelms the resources available. Incidents where the resources are not overtaxed by the incident are usually termed Multiple Patient Incidents (MPI). At an MPI, normal treatment and transportation protocols of routine daily operations should be followed. While many responders tend to think of MCI events as large scale acts of terrorism, natural disasters, and crashed passenger jets, it is more likely that responders will be utilized at MCI events of a smaller scale such as a multiple vehicle collision, bus accidents, and train derailments. Responders should be familiar with MCI and triage protocols so that can be rapidly be employed when a MCI event happens in their jurisdiction. Rescuers at MCI events need to have a basic understanding of the Golden Hour, triage, and patient disentanglement as addressed in the following sections.

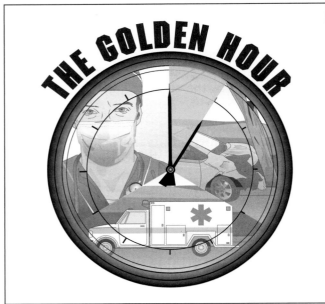

Figure 12.1 To increase their chances of survival, trauma patients should receive medical treatment at hospital facilities within the Golden Hour.

Golden Hour

The Golden Hour refers to the concept that trauma patient suffering from internal bleeding should be treated, packaged, transported, and delivered to a surgeon in under an hour. The Golden Hour begins at the moment of crisis or impact if in an accident **(Figure 12.1)**.

NOTE: In addition to the Golden Hour maxim, there is the Platinum Ten Minutes. The Platinum Ten Minutes is the maximum on scene time goal that EMS units strive for when caring for trauma patients.

At incidents of severe trauma, especially internal bleeding, no external treatment can replace the needed surgery. If the internal bleeding is not corrected early enough, the patient could suffer from, and potentially succumb to, shock. As part of the appropriate care for a patient that has injuries causing internal bleeding, transportation decisions should be made, according to local protocol, to transport the patient to a trauma center capable of handling the injuries.

Triage

Triage, a French word that means sorting, is a process of identifying the most critically injured patients that have the highest chance of survival with the appropriate medical care at a MCI. Triage needs to be done in coordination of the principle of the greatest good for the greatest number of people. The person assigned the role of triage should be one of the most knowledgeable EMS responders on the scene. At times triage may be done by experienced EMT Basics and EMT Intermediates, thus freeing up EMT Paramedics to work in the treatment area providing advanced life support skills to multiple patients.

The first unit at a MCI event should begin triage immediately, and this should be reported to the next arriving unit so that they can set up command. While command needs to be established and triage implemented quickly, efforts should be taken to control the walking wounded also. These patients can wander off and often self transport to the closest hospital. These patients can easily overwhelm that facility taking staff away from arriving patients with more critical injuries. Triage tags are commonly used to identify the level of injuries sustained by a patient **(Figure 12.2)**.

When performing triage, patients are classified into the following four categories listed in decreasing priority:

- **Red - Treatable Life Threatening Injuries** – These patients may present rescuers with some or all of the following:
  - airway and breathing difficulties
  - severe bleeding
  - reduced level of consciousness
  - large surface area burns
  - airway burns
  - shock

- **Yellow - Serious But Not Immediate Life Threatening Injuries** - These patients may or may not be able to walk on their own. These patients may present rescuers with some or all of the following:
  - burns (without airway involvement)
  - major fractures or joint injuries
  - potential spinal injuries

- **Green – Walking Wounded** – These patients may present with some or all of the following:
  - minor fractures
  - minor joint injuries
  - minor soft tissue injuries

- **Black – Deceased or Mortally Wounded** - These patients may present rescuers with some or all of the following:
  - exposed brain tissue or decapitation
  - cardiac arrest
  - severed trunks
  - incineration

NOTE: Patients in cardiac arrest must be triaged black when resources are limited. If resources become available, these patients can be retriaged to a red level priority.

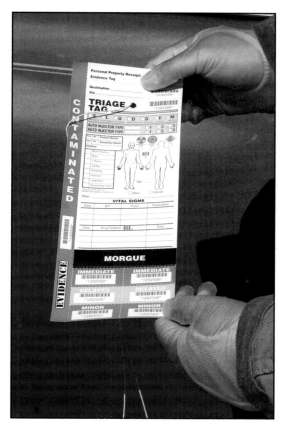

Figure 12.2 An example of a triage tag.

Patient Disentanglement

Trauma in the setting of vehicle collisions and other emergencies where patients become entrapped in machinery is challenging. Not only does the patient need highly skilled and competent medical care, the patient also needs responders proficient in modern extrication techniques. These extrication techniques are used to disentangle the patient from whatever is entrapping them. Using this method the patients are not removed from the vehicle, rather the vehicle is removed from around them so that proper packing and stabilization can be accomplished **(Figure 12.3, p. 482)**.

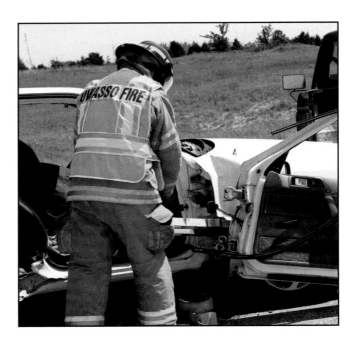

Figure 12.3 A rescuer performing extrication techniques to reach a patient.

Mechanisms of Injury

Discussed below are common causes and injury patterns found in a variety of accidents. These are intended to be a guide and injuries are not limited to those listed, responders should always maintain a high index of suspicion when evaluating patients.

Fatality in the Same Vehicle

When assessing the mechanism of injury of patients, factors such as fatality in the same vehicle must be considered. The forces that where applied to the body of the deceased were similarly applied to that of the surviving patient(s). In some cases it may also be necessary to remove a deceased victim in order to best access a viable patient. A deceased victim should be treated with care and dignity when being moved. Trauma center staff should be informed that patient they are receiving was in the same vehicle as a deceased victim so that they too can understand the violent forces that may have been placed upon the patient during the collision.

There are five basic types of collisions: head-on impact, side impact, rear impact, rotational impact, and rollover. Each one has its own predictable pattern of injury. Being aware of the mechanism of collision will allow rescuers to help diagnosis and treat your patient.

Head-on Impact Collision

A head-on impact occurs when a car hits another vehicle or an immovable object, such as a tree. The greater the car's speed, the greater the energy, the greater the damage. When the car stops, its occupants continue to travel forward. Patients take one of two possible pathways of motion and energy, either up and over or down and under. Each pathway has a distinctive pattern of injury, which can be affected by the use of a seat belt.

Injury Patterns: Blunt and Penetrating Trauma

Blunt trauma is an injury caused by a blow or force that does not penetrate through the skin or other tissues in the body. The majority (50-75%) of blunt force trauma occurs in the abdomen.

Penetrating trauma is the result of an object passing through body tissue. There are times when the object may pass completely through the body, such as bullet and other times when an object may become impaled in the tissue.

Vehicle manufactures have worked over the years to engineer out objects that may penetrate a vehicle occupant during a collision. There are many items along the roadside that an cause penetrating trauma such as guardrails, sign posts, and fence posts. There are also items in a vehicle or its load that cause penetrating trauma such as rebar, pipe, or smaller dimension wood. If an object becomes impaled, it shall not be removed from the patient's body, this needs to be done in surgery. In some cases the impaled object may need to trimmed in size in order to transport the patient. Care should be taking to not vibrate or move the object in the patient. Impaled objects should be stabilized to prevent further internal injury.

Face, Head, and Neck Injuries

Obvious clues of face, head, and neck injuries are hair, tissue, or blood on the windshield. Also the windshield may be cracked in a classic bull's-eye or spiderweb pattern. A damaged windshield on the passenger side can be either from a passenger or from an air bag. The patient's face can sustain extensive soft tissue damage, however the bleeding may not be serious as it looks. Airway problems may also be present if there is bleeding from the mouth, nose, or face. Skull fractures may occur as well and almost all head injuries have the potential to cause damage to the brain. Brain tissue can compress and rebound against the opposite sides of the skull, which is very rough or jagged.

Energy can travel down the neck, causing the potential for cervical-spine injury. The neck may be flexed or extended too far, resulting in whiplash injuries or fractures. An impact to the top of the head can cause compression fractures of the cervical spine. Hitting the steering wheel or dashboard can also injury the anterior neck. Cartilage rings in the trachea (windpipe) may be separated or crushed, which would impair breathing.

Chest Injuries

When the chest strikes the steering wheel, the ribs and sternum may break. The heart may be compressed and bruised, making it unable to pump blood effectively. The aorta may be torn, resulting in life threatening bleeding. As the lungs are compressed, they can be bruised or ruptured. Broken ribs can also injure the lungs and heart.

Abdominal Injuries

When the abdomen strikes the steering wheel, the liver, spleen and other organs are compressed-or lacerated. These injuries can cause internal bleeding that can be identified by abdominal pain and/or firmness.

Other Injuries from Head-on Collisions

In the down and under pathway of motion, a body slides under the steering wheel. The knees strike the dashboard and energy travels up the legs. The abdomen and then the chest strike the steering wheel. Common injuries include a dislocated hip and a broken patella (kneecap), femur (thigh bone), or pelvis. When an airbag is deployed a passenger can tend to go under the bag, sustaining serious lower extremity injuries.

Side Impact Collision

The side impact is often called a T-bone collision. The occupant closest to impact absorbs more energy than the occupant on the opposite side. As the energy of the impact is absorbed, the patient's body is pushed sideways and the head moves in the opposite direction. The following injuries commonly occur:

Face, Head, and Neck Injuries

The patient's head often impacts the door post. This impact can result in skull injury, brain injury, injuries to the neck and even cervical fractures.

Chest Injuries

If the vehicle door slams against the occupant's shoulder, the clavicle may fracture. If the arm is caught between the door and the chest, or if the door impacts against the chest directly, suspect broken ribs and possible breathing problems. Fractures low in rib cage can also injure liver and spleen.

Abdominal/Pelvic Injuries

Lateral impact to the pelvis often causes fractures of the pelvis and femur. Damage to the iliac arteries and internal organs, such as the bladder, can also occur.

Other Injuries from Side Impact Collisions

The person on the opposite side of the car is subject to similar head and neck injuries. In addition, if there is more than one person sitting on a seat, heads can often collide.

Rear Impact Collision

Rear impact occurs when a car is struck from behind by another vehicle traveling at greater speed. The car that is hit accelerates suddenly, and the occupant's body is slammed suddenly backwards into the seat, and then forward. Rescue personnel should suspect the same kind of injuries as discussed for head-on collisions. If positioned properly, a headrest will prevent the head from whipping back. If the headrest is not in place or not properly fitted to occupant, suspect injury to the neck.

Rotational Impact

A rotational impact is one that occurs off center. The car strikes an object and rotates around it until the car either loses speed or strikes another object. The sturdiest structures in the car, such as steering wheel, dashboard, door posts, and windows, are the ones that cause the most serious injuries. A variety of injury patterns may occur, therefore responders should look for the same kind of injuries found in head-on and side impact collisions.

Rollover

During a rollover, car occupants change direction every time the car does. Every fixture inside the car becomes potentially lethal. A specific pattern of injury is impossible to predict. An aggressive head to toe exam may find severe soft tissue injuries, multiple broken bones, and crushing injuries resulting from the car rolling over parts of the occupant. Patients are often ejected in this type of accident ejected patients also have much higher chance of spine injury or death.

Soft Tissue Injury – Damage to human tissue that encloses bones or joints, such as muscles, tendons, or ligaments.

Ejections from Vehicles

Data from NHTSA's Fatality Analysis Reporting System (FARS) show that the ejection rate among fatally injured passenger vehicle occupants has remained at over 20 percent since the early 1980s. The risk of fatality in a crash is over three times as great for an ejected occupant compared with a non-ejected occupant (i.e., person retained in the vehicle). Patients that are ejected are subjected to unprotected collision with the vehicle they were in as they exit it, the ground, trees, buildings or even other vehicles. Because of the many possibilities for blunt trauma to a patient during the collision event, ejected patients are high priority patients. Emergency responders should use caution when approaching a scene to ensure they do not further injure an ejected patient. Searches of the area around a vehicle collision scene should be conducted to account for patients that may have been ejected.

Farm Equipment Injuries

Farm equipment injuries can occur in variety of ways. As with road automobiles, mechanisms that cause the injuries should be understand what internal injuries may be present in the patient. The major categories of injures from equipment include penetrating, crushing, twisting, and tearing. These mechanisms can occur independently or in combination with each other. Another consideration is wound contamination from grease, oil, rust or other items on the equipment.

Power Take Off (PTO) Injuries

PTO shaft accidents often cause massive traumatic injuries due to the amount of force involved with the rotating shaft. If the patient's clothes are caught in the section of the PTO attached to the tractor, they must be cut loose to prevent further injury to the patient such as airway and respiratory compromise, or compartment syndrome in an extremity (see section later in this chapter for more information on compartment syndrome) **(Figure 12.4, p. 486)**. Cervical spine and lower spine injuries are common with accidents involving PTO shafts if the patient's body is wrapped around the shaft. Proper stabilization of the victim is necessary to prevent further injury.

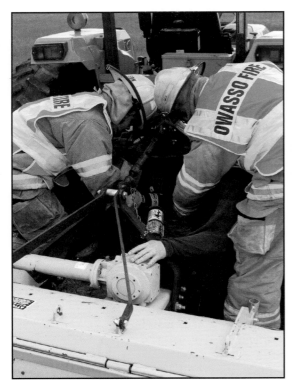

Figure 12.4 Rescuers disentangling a patient from a PTO shaft.

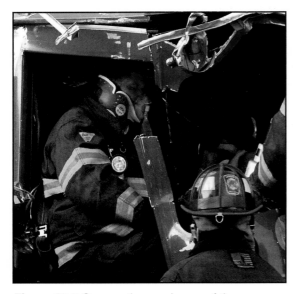

Figure 12.5 Oxygen therapy is one of the common emergency medical care procedures rescuers administer in the field. *Courtesy of Ron Jeffers.*

Oxygen Therapy – The administration of oxygen through a mask or tube in the nose to increase the amount of oxygen in the patient's blood.

Hydraulic Fluid Injections

Injuries from hydraulic fluid injection are rare, however the Fluid Power Safety Institute has conducted a study that indicates that over 99% of the people who service, repair, and troubleshoot hydraulic systems have been subjected to the exact dynamics that trigger a high-pressure injection injury. Many hydraulic systems are not de-energized even after lockout/tagout. A pin-hole leak in a hydraulic hose that is under pressure can release hydraulic fluid at a speed of about 600 (183 m) feet per second. Hydraulic fluid released at such a high pressure can puncture protective clothing such as gloves and coveralls and penetrate skin from a distance of as much as 4 inches (101.6 mm). When the fluid enters the body of an exposed victim, it begins to kill tissue. Definitive medical treatment usually involves surgery to remove the fluid.

Administering Care in the Field

The types and severity of injuries that a victim of a vehicle accident may incur are almost limitless. Rescuers and medical personnel must be prepared to provide a full array of patient care procedures to include:

● Protecting patients from hazards, including hazardous extrication activities

● Immobilizing the cervical spine

● Supporting the airway, breathing, and circulation (the ABCs)

● Providing psychological support through extrication

● Providing oxygen therapy (usually high-flow oxygen by mask) **(Figure 12.5)**

● Maintaining body temperature

● Monitoring cardiac activity

● Administering certain life support medications

● Immobilizing and packaging the patient for removal

Rescuers should also keep in mind that monitoring a patient during rescue is just as important as conducting the initial evaluation. Patients' conditions can change dramatically during the rescue attempt and their care should be managed accordingly.

There are a number of common injuries frequently seen in vehicle accidents and those patients that have been entrapped for extended amount of time. These include but are not limited to the following:

● Fractures and lacerations

● Hypovolemia

● Hypothermia

- Respiratory difficulties
- Crush/compartment injuries
- Partial/full amputation

NOTE: The information that follows on these types of injuries and their treatment should be considered general in nature. It is expected that rescuers and emergency medical personnel will be familiar with and follow local treatment protocols established by the medical control within the authority having jurisdiction.

Fractures and Lacerations

Orthopedic and soft-tissue injuries are associated with the force of a vehicle accident. Also the potential is high for cervical injury. Precautions such as cervical immobilization, use of cervical collars, and appropriate removal devices can have a very positive effect on patient survival **(Figure 12.6)**.

Orthopedic Injury – An injury to the bones, mainly the extremities.

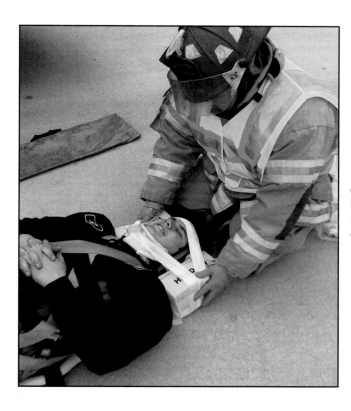

Figure 12.6 Vehicle accidents commonly cause cervical spine injuries. *Courtesy of Alan Braun, University of Missouri Fire and Rescue Training Institute.*

Hypovolemia – Shock

Hypovelemia, or loss of blood volume, can occur as a result of impact and injuries to the body. Shock as a result of hypovolemia is a life-threatening complication. Rescuers must stop the bleeding and provide oxygen and intravenous fluid replacement if possible. Bleeding or other complications may recur when objects that are compressing bleeding sites are removed during extrication known as crush injury.

Hypothermia

In addition to injuries from a vehicle accident the patient may also develop hypothermia (decreased body temperature) due to exposure to cold temperatures. Wet clothing, lack of normal heating, weather, and duration of exposure during extrication increases the possibility of hypothermia. To lessen the effects of this problem, rescuers must protect the patient from the environment during rescue operations.

A victim who is suffering from hypothermia needs aggressive basic techniques designed to rewarm his or her core body temperature. Rewarming a patient can be accomplished by administering:

- Warm IV fluids
- Warm oxygen and warmed blankets (at least keep the oxygen tank warm)
- Warm air, through the use of a heater/blower that resembles ventilation equipment but blows warm air into the vehicle during extrication efforts

Hazardous Materials Exposure

Many transportation related hazardous materials leaks are due to vehicle collisions. Exposure to hazardous materials is a concern for both rescuers and victims. Ideally, the patient should be removed from the source of any hazardous material, but this is not possible with an entrapped patient. In this situation, the material should be removed from the patient if possible by cleansing the skin gently and, depending on the substance, flushing with large amounts of water. Cleansing should remove most of the contaminant. Respiratory protection should also be provided for the victim if the material poses an inhalation danger and extrication will be delayed.

Crush Injury and Compartment Syndrome

The body's muscle tissues are extremely vulnerable to sustained pressure. In a vehicle entrapment, compression may be caused by structural components of the vehicle such as posts, steering wheel, and dash or by the patient's own body weight. The time frame until a crush injury occurs depends upon the amount of pressure exerted and on patient factors.

Crush Injury

Crush injuries occur as a result of crushing pressure on certain parts of the body, typically the lower extremities that restrict blood flow to the injured area. As with compartment syndrome, the injured tissue dies and gives off toxins. Then a sudden release of pressure, which occurs when the victim is released from the entrapment, allows the toxins to flow into the bloodstream. Toxins can have an effect on other organs in the body and possibly cause death.

To minimize the effects of crush syndrome, rescuers can recognize it as a possibility and provide treatment before patient extrication. If available, advanced life support personnel familiar with crush syndrome should provide treatment for the patient. The following are appropriate for prerelease treatment:

- High-flow oxygen by nonrebreather mask
- Large volumes of intravenous fluids
- Cardiac monitoring
- Certain medications

Compartment Syndrome

Usually found in heavy machinery or very prolonged vehicle extrications in rural areas or severe accidents, compartment syndrome can occur when a patient's limb has been trapped for over 60 minutes. Beyond this time frame the crushed tissue in the involved limb begins to give off toxins, which decreases the potential for saving the limb. If allowed to continue, the limb swells until the skin is stretched to its maximum. These patients will need advanced life support care and aggressive surgery to save the limb.

Field Amputations

Victims of vehicle accidents may suffer partial or total amputation of one or more limbs. Rescuers and EMS personnel should treat the victim and handle the limb according to local protocols. On rare occasions, field surgical amputations of arms or legs may be necessary to remove a trapped person before they expire. Such a drastic measure should be performed *only* after it has been determined that it is the *only* way a patient can be extricated and/or saved. Amputations create not only a psychological impact but also a biohazard. In these situations the rescuers' roles will be one of support for medical personnel (surgeons) who perform the procedure in the field. Jurisdictions should have protocols in place for this type of event.

Coordinating with Medical Personnel

Extrications often present problems for rescuers, some of these are difficulty in reaching trapped victims, instability of the vehicle, and the necessity to coordinate the care of many patients. Some of the chief problems include the following:

- Inherent delay in reaching trapped patients, so there is progression of trauma/medical problems beyond that normally seen in prehospital trauma management.

- Unusual medical problems, such as crush syndrome, haz mat injuries, and others that rescuers and emergency medical personnel do not face on a regular basis.

- The inability to "scoop and run" with seriously injured victims. Victims may be trapped and require a prolonged extrication process or egress from the vehicle.

- Medical system chaos secondary to loss of communications, overwhelmed/compromised EMS providers and hospitals, loss of medical personnel in the incident, and medical workers occupied with personal/family calamity related to the event.

While trauma systems vary in jurisdictions, it is good practice to notify the receiving hospital of severely injured trauma patient as early as possible when an accurate assessment of injuries has been made. This allows medical facility emergency department staff to prepare for the patient and have specialty services ready upon arrival of the patient. In cases where hospitals are only recognized as a Level 2 Trauma Centers, surgeons and other members of the surgical team may have to be called back to the hospital.

Patient Packaging and Removal

Any responder that performs vehicle extrication should have a good working knowledge of how a patient is immobilized and removed from the vehicle after the disentanglement process is done. It is understood that not all extrication responders have EMT or First Responder Training. Assistance of these responders may still be needed to secure the patient on the device and carry to the waiting ambulance cot. The guiding principle should be that the spinal column be treated as one bone that needs to be immobilized from the base of the skull to tailbone. The sections that follow describe techniques and equipment used to package patients and protect them from further aggravating spinal injuries.

NOTE: Trauma patients (especially those complaining of head, neck, or back pain) should be removed from the vehicle in a manner that does not compromise spinal integrity. Ideally, this should be in a straight line with the direction of the patient's orientation.

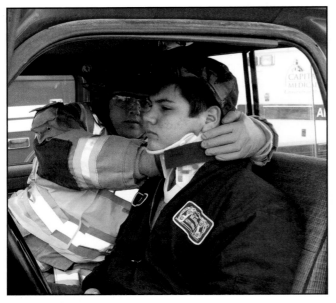

Figure 12.7 A rescuer continuing to maintain manual stabilization of a patient's cervical spine until immobilization is complete. *Courtesy of Alan Braun, University of Missouri Fire and Rescue Training Institute.*

Cervical Spine (C-Spine) Immobilization

Once the area has been made safe, cervical spinal immobilization of the victim is a primary concern for rescuers. Immobilization should occur as soon as the head and neck are free, with a minimum of a rigid cervical collar. Once the collar is placed, a rescuer should continue manual stabilization until total immobilization is complete **(Figure 12.7)**. Even though a patient has been trapped for an extended period without c-spine immobilization, the mechanism of injury potential is great because the patient may not have had the ability to move his head to aggravate the injury until rescue personnel can finish extrication. It could be considered poor medical care to bend or twist an injured patient in order to remove them from the side of the vehicle unless no other option exists.

Almost every person that has to be extricated from a vehicle after collision will need to have some form of spinal immobilization. Manual stabilization may be applied and then replaced by a cervical immobilization device that is rigid. C-spine immobilization devices are not adequate alone; they should be used in conjunction with a long spine board and possibly a seated spinal immobilization device. The cervical immobilization device will need to be measured for appropriate sizing. Newer devices are on the market that allow for adjustment from different sizes in all in one unit.

Long Boards

Long boards are also known as long spine boards or full body immobilization devices. Extrication responders should almost think of this as a full body splint. When properly applied, it immobilizes the head, neck, torso, pelvis, and extremities of the patient **(Figure 12.8)**.

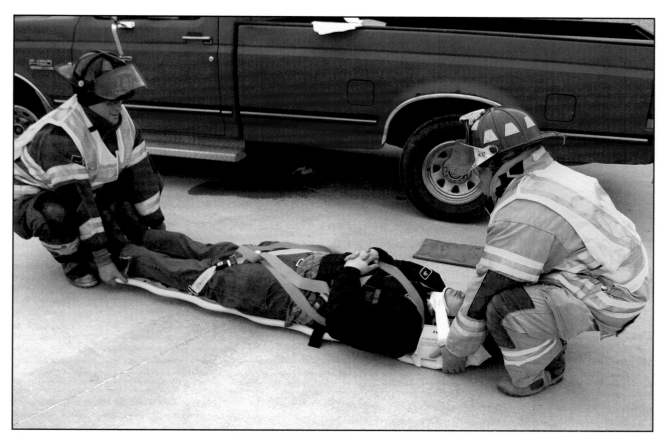

Figure 12.8 A patient immobilized on a long backboard and ready to be transferred to an ambulance. *Courtesy of Alan Braun, University of Missouri Fire and Rescue Training Institute*

Seated Spinal Immobilization Device

Seated spinal immobilization devices, such as the Kendrick Extrication Device (KED®) or wooden short board, are designed to immobilize a suspected spinal injured patient that is found seated. While they can be used in other applications they are most often used when treating patients or vehicle collision. These devices allow immobilization of the head, neck and torso **(Figure 12.9)**. Then the patient can be moved to a long board. This device should only be used on a stable or non-critical patient.

Life Support Products (LSP) Half Back Splint

A device similar to the KED® is the Life Support Products (LSP) Half Back Splint. This device provides the same advantages as the KED® but is unique in that it can be attached to a rigging system and used to raise or lower the patient while maintaining spinal immobilization. This device may also be used as a harness for rescuers after the spinal immobilization is removed. It allows patient removal from a confined space with very limited access.

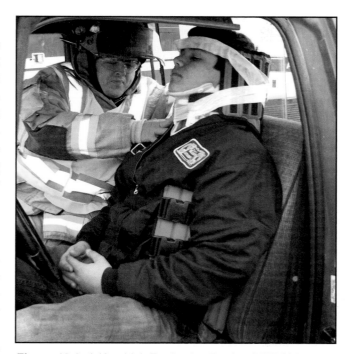

Figure 12.9 A Kendrick Extrication Device (KED®) is used to immobilize a patient found in a seated position. *Courtesy of Alan Braun, University of Missouri Fire and Rescue Training Institute.*

Children in Car Seats

If a child in child passenger safety seat needs to be immobilized for transport to a hospital, and the integrity of the seat is intact, the child can be immobilized in the seat **(Figure 12.10)**. Taking the seat as a single unit and securing it in the ambulance is considered the safest method for immobilization of children and infants.

Basket Type Litter

The basket type litter has been the standard for patient removal over rough terrain for many years. It is designed for lifting and lowering the patient with a rigging system or for being hand carried **(Figure 12.11)**. This device is not used by itself for spinal immobilization. Due to its size, it is not easily used in a confined space or limited access area. This device is bulky and will require two rescuers to carry it to the patient unless it is moved by a rigging system.

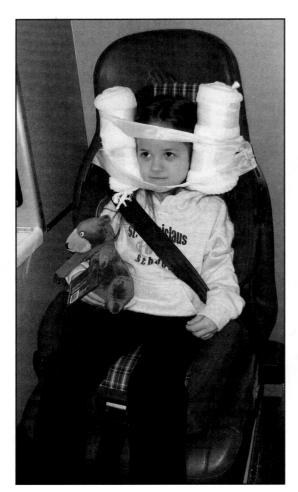

Figure 12.10 If a child's passenger safety seat is intact, the child can be immobilized and transported in the seat. *Courtesy of Alan Braun, University of Missouri Fire and Rescue Training Institute.*

Psychological Concerns of the Patients

Patient evaluation begins as soon as there is voice contact with the patient. When rescuers establish contact with the patient they need to remember that the person has been entrapped in vehicle and unable to get out. It is vital that rescuers remember to communicate with the patient in order to provide additional support.

Once contact has been established, a patient that is trapped in a vehicle or piece of equipment will be terrified at being alone. Rescuers must communicate as completely as possible if it is necessary to leave the patient to get additional equipment, reposition equipment, and so on. At times during an extrication, a patient may need to be covered to protect the patient from glass of debris. A rescuer should be assigned to stay with the patient and explain what is happening.

Follow Up on Patient Information

Following up on patients provides responders with valuable feedback to improve future patient care and extrication practices. The run review, also known as the After Action Review (AAR), provides a process to gather information on the call.

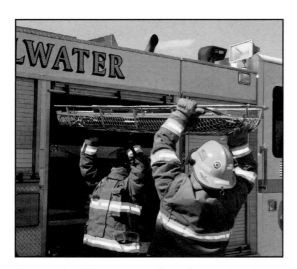

Figure 12.11 Rescuers pulling a basket litter from an apparatus.

Health Insurance Portability and Accountability Act (HIPAA)

The Health Insurance Portability and Accountability Act (HIPAA) was enacted by Congress in 1996 to set a national standard for electronic transfers of health data. U.S. Department of Health and Human Services (DHHS) is charged with establishing administrative rules. Because of well publicized changes, some emergency response units have questioned whether or not they could conduct Quality Assurance/Improvement AARs of incidents as previously done.

It is allowable under HIPAA to conduct reviews for educational purposes, but all identifiable information (name, social security number, age, date, address) must be removed from the presentation before open discussion in a Quality Assurance/Improvement AAR occurs. The responders directly involved in patient care can discuss specifics of the call with other medical professionals who cared for that patient during the incident but all others are to be censored from the Protected Health Information.

After Action Review (AAR) – A formal review or debrief process conducted by the participants and those responsible for the project or event to analyze *what* happened, *why* it happened, and *how* it can be done better.

Summary

Patient care is the essence and primary purpose of any rescue operation. Extrication scenes pose a significant number of challenges to rescuers not necessarily found in other types of incidents. These include the potential for a large number of patients, patients who are inaccessible by simple means, and patients who are trapped by forces that are beyond the use of standard fire service tools. All agencies that participate in extrication incidents should ensure that they have sound operating procedures for handling the medical needs of their patient(s) and a good interagency working relationship between responders who perform the extrication and those who provide medical treatment.

Review Questions

1. What is the "Golden Hour?"

2. What types of injuries are caused by head-on impact collisions?

3. What are two common injuries associated with farm equipment?

4. What patient care procedures must rescuers and medical personnel be prepared to provide in the field?

5. What devices can be used to provide spinal immobilization during patient packaging and removal?

6. What tactics should an incident commander consider using during industrial and agricultural vehicles extrication operations?

7. What is the purpose of post incident patient follow up and education?

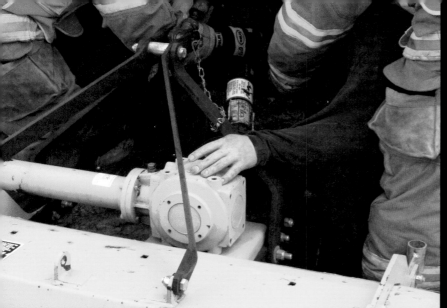

Appendices

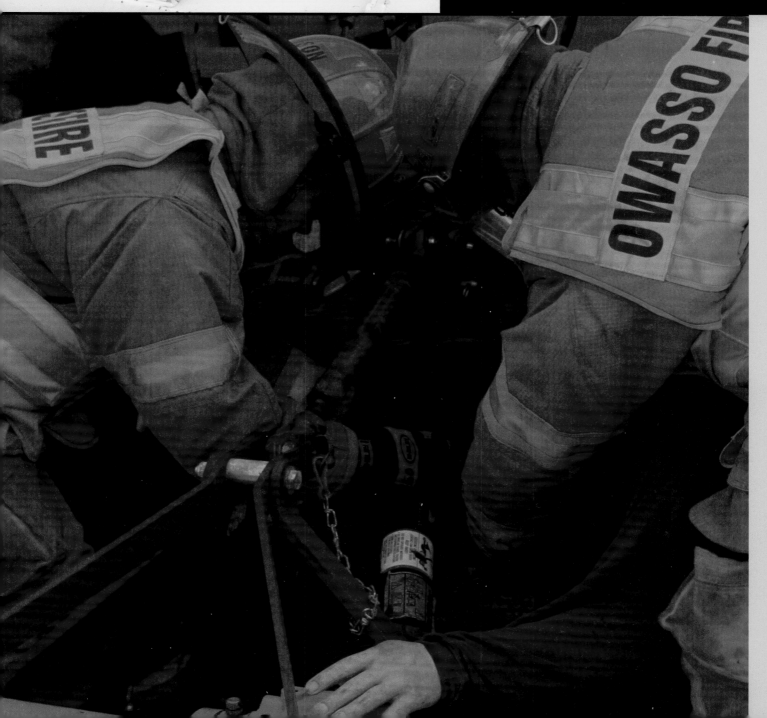

Appendix A
NFPA® Job Performance Requirements (JPRs) With Page References

NFPA® 1001 (2008) JPR Numbers	Chapter References	Page References
6.4.1	1, 3, 4, 5, 6, 7, 8, 9, 10, 11	15-21, 84-88, 98-99, 137-139, 142-171, 177-264, 270-296, 302-354, 362-381, 383-412, 419-448, 455-474
6.4.2	1, 2, 3, 4, 5, 6, 7, 8, 9, 10, 11	25-26, 32, 33, 34, 40, 89-109, 142-171, 177-264, 270-296, 302-354, 362-381, 388-412, 419-448, 455-474

NFPA® 1006 (2008) JPR Numbers	Chapter References	Page References
4.1.1	1, 2	12-15, 31-32
4.1.2	1, 2	12-15, 31-32
4.2	1	17
4.3	1, 4	18-20
4.3.1	1, 3, 4	19, 69, 142-171
4.3.2	1, 2, 3, 4	20, 32, 34-35, 38, 39, 40, 60-61, 63, 69, 142-171
5.1	1	20-21
5.2.1	1, 2, 4, 5	20, 31, 32, 38, 39, 43-45, 47, 48, 49, 51-52, 54, 141-142, 178-179
5.2.2	1, 2, 5, 6, 7, 8. 9, 10, 11	19, 38-44, 177-179, 285, 325, 369-371, 397-399, 427-429, 456-457, 458, 459-460, 461-462, 462-464, 464-465, 466, 468, 471
5.2.3	1, 2, 3, 4, 5, 6, 7, 8, 9, 10, 11	19, 23, 25, 26, 32-60, 69, 85-86, 89, 104, 121-171, 178-179, 188-189, 192, 194, 217-218, 275-285, 311, 317, 321, 323-325, 329-331, 362-371, 388-399, 418-427, 456-473
5.2.4	1, 2	18, 31-64
5.2.5	1, 2	19, 26, 42
5.2.6	2	51
5.2.7	1, 2, 3, 10	24, 64-65, 418, 446

NFPA® 1006 (2008) JPR Numbers	Chapter References	Page References
5.3.1	2, 7, 9, 12	34, 43, 48, 49, 50, 331, 339, 398-399, 406, 480-481
5.3.2	7, 8, 9, 12	311, 320, 325, 333, 334, 338, 339, 340, 341, 376, 401, 402, 486-489, 490-492
5.3.3	1, 2, 12	26, 49, 63, 480-481, 489-493
5.4.1	2, 4	63, 64, 121-129
5.4.2	2, 4	63, 64, 121-171
5.5.1	4, 5, 8, 9, 10, 11	147-149, 192-199, 373, 400, 441, 471, 472
10.1	1, 2, 3, 5, 7, 10, 11	19, 22, 31-65, 177-264, 325-354, 418-448, 453-473
10.1.1	1, 2, 3, 5, 6, 7, 10, 11	19-24, 31-65, 69-111, 178-187, 217, 270-294, 325-354, 418-446, 453-473
10.1.2	1, 2, 5, 6, 10, 11	19, 23, 25, 52-60, 178-179, 188-189, 192, 194, 217-218, 275-285, 418-427, 455, 457, 458, 459-460, 461, 463, 471
10.1.3	1, 2, 3, 5, 6, 7, 10, 11	23, 26, 37, 43-44, 61, 91, 92-95, 99-100, 104-105, 108, 183, 185, 217, 275, 282, 283, 284-285, 287, 293, 328, 331, 428, 454
10.1.4	1, 3, 4, 5, 6, 7, 10, 11	19, 23, 25-26, 78, 85, 87-88, 111-112, 143-149, 179-199, 220-232, 269, 286-288, 292, 325-329, 429-433, 441, 454, 457, 459, 460, 462, 464, 465, 467, 470, 472
10.1.5	1, 3, 4, 6, 7, 10	19-21, 23, 25, 89-97, 100-104, 107-111, 121-129, 151-153, 156-157, 281-282, 285, 311, 317, 321, 322, 324-325, 327-331, 436, 442
10.1.6	1, 2, 3, 5, 6, 7, 10, 11	18, 19, 22-24, 43-44, 60, 62, 78, 84, 98-99, 199-212, 217-219, 233-264, 270-285, 302-323, 331-354, 432-433, 442-446, 457, 458, 460, 461-462, 463, 464-465, 466, 470, 472
10.1.7	1, 2, 3, 4, 5, 6, 7, 10, 11	18, 19, 22-24, 43-44, 60, 62, 78, 84, 98-99, 149-171, 199-212, 217-219, 233-264, 270-285, 289-294, 302-323, 331-354, 432-433, 442-448, 457, 459, 460, 462, 464, 465, 467, 470-471, 473
10.1.8	2, 4, 5, 6, 7, 10, 11, 12	49, 62, 149-171, 177-264, 291-294, 340-342, 433-434, 442-446, 447-448, 458, 459, 460, 462, 464, 466, 467, 471, 473, 481-486, 489-492
10.1.9	2, 7, 10, 11, 12	44, 49, 63, 443, 444, 471
10.1.10	1, 2, 4, 10, 11	24, 63-65, 142-171, 446, 454
10.2	1, 2, 5, 7, 8, 9, 10, 11	19, 22-24, 31-65, 177-264, 359-381, 386-412, 434-446, 462-468
10.2.1	1, 2, 3, 5, 7, 8, 9, 10, 11	19, 22-24, 31-65, 70, 73-78, 79-83, 178-199, 325-354, 360-375, 386-404, 434-440, 462-468
10.2.2	1, 2, 4, 5, 7, 8, 9, 10, 11	19, 23, 26, 38, 41, 42, 44, 48, 49, 62, 143-149, 180-199, 325-329, 371-373, 399-400, 441, 464, 465, 467

NFPA® 1006 (2008) JPR Numbers	Chapter References	Page References
10.2.3	1, 2, 5, 7, 8, 9, 10, 11	18, 19, 22, 62, 199-213, 217-219, 329-354, 362-364, 374-381, 390-399, 401-412, 437, 464, 465, 467
10.2.4	1, 2, 4, 5, 7, 8, 9, 10, 11	18, 19, 22-23, 62, 149-171, 199-212, 217-219, 233-264, 331-354, 374-381, 401-412, 442-448, 464, 466, 467
10.2.5	4, 5, 7, 8, 9, 10, 11, 12	149-179, 177-264, 331-354, 375-381, 405-412, 442-448, 464, 466, 467, 481-485

NFPA® 1670 (2008) JPR Numbers	Chapter References	Page References
4.1.1	1, 2	18, 31, 33
4.1.2	1	18
4.1.3	1	18
4.1.3.1	1, 2	16, 32-33
4.1.3.2	1	18
4.1.4	1, 3, 4	15, 18-20, 140-171
4.1.5	1	18-20
4.1.6	1, 2	15, 17-18, 21, 33-34
4.1.7	1	17
4.1.8	1	18
4.1.9	1, 2	17, 34
4.1.10.1	1	18
4.1.10.1.1	1	18
4.1.10.1.2	1	18
4.1.10.2	1	18
4.1.10.3	1	20
4.1.10.4	1	20
4.1.10.5.1	1	20
4.1.10.5.2	1	20
4.1.11	1	15
4.1.12.1	1	18
4.1.12.2	1	18
4.1.12.3	1	12, 15
4.1.12.4	1	15

NFPA® 1670 (2008) JPR Numbers (cont.)	Chapter References	Page References
4.2.1	1	15-16
4.2.2	1	15-16
4.2.3	1	20
4.2.4	1	16, 20
4.2.5	1	20
4.2.6	1	15
4.2.7	1	15
4.2.8	1	15
4.3.1	1	16
4.3.1.1	1	16
4.3.1.2	1	16-17
4.3.2	1	16
4.3.3	1	16
4.3.4	1	16
4.4.1.1	1, 4	15, 20-21, 121-171
4.4.1.2	1, 4	20-21, 121-171
4.4.1.3	1	20
4.4.2.1	1, 4	15, 20-21, 121-129
4.4.2.2	1, 4	20-21, 122
4.4.2.3	1, 4	21, 121
4.4.2.4	1, 4	21, 125-129
4.4.2.4.1	1, 4	21, 125-129
4.4.2.4.2	1	21
4.4.2.4.3	1	21

NFPA® 1670 (2008) JPR Numbers (cont.)	Chapter References	Page References
4.4.2.4.4	1, 4	21, 127
4.5.1.1	1, 3	15-20
4.5.1.2	1, 4	15-29, 121-129
4.5.1.3	1, 4	17, 121-129
4.5.1.4	1, 2	17, 34
4.5.1.5	1	17
4.5.2.1	1, 2	17, 32, 35
4.5.2.2	1	17
4.5.3.1	1, 2	18, 32, 45
4.5.3.2	1	18
4.5.3.3	1, 2	18, 32, 34, 48, 51-52
4.5.3.4	1	17-18, 21
4.5.3.5	1	18
4.5.4	1	17
4.5.5.1	1	16
4.5.5.2	1	16
8.1	1	15-24
8.2.1	1	18-19
8.2.2	1, 8, 9, 10, 11	19-20, 359, 361, 369-370, 387-388, 406, 428, 454
8.2.3	1, 2, 3, 5, 6, 7, 8, 9, 10, 11	19, 36, 37, 38, 39-40, 44, 45-47, 52-60, 178-179, 188-189, 192, 194, 217-218, 275-285, 311, 317, 321, 322, 323-325, 361-371, 386-399, 423-429, 434-439, 456-457, 458, 459-460, 461-462, 462-464, 464-465, 466, 468-470, 471-472
8.3.1	1	18-19
8.3.2	1, 8, 9, 10, 11	19-20, 359, 361, 369-370, 387-388, 406, 428, 454

NFPA® 1670 (2008) JPR Numbers (cont.)	Chapter References	Page References
8.3.3	1, 2, 5, 6, 7, 8, 9, 10, 11	19, 34-35, 39-40, 60-61, 178-264, 270-294, 296, 311, 317, 321, 323-325, 362-371, 386-397, 423-428, 434-439, 453-473
8.3.4	1, 2, 5, 6, 7, 8, 9, 10, 11, 12	19, 31-34, 37-45, 47-48, 52-63, 178-264, 270-294, 296, 302-354, 362-381, 386-412, 418-448, 453-473, 481-492
8.4.1	1	18-20
8.4.2	1, 2, 3, 5, 6, 7, 8, 9, 10, 11, 12	19-20, 31-34, 37-45, 47-48, 52-63, 178-264, 270-294, 296, 302-354, 360-381, 386-412, 418-448, 453-473, 481-492
12.1	1, 10, 11	18-20, 434-448, 468-471
12.2.1	1, 10, 11	18-20, 434-448, 468-471
12.2.2	1, 10, 11	19-20, 428, 454
12.2.3	1, 2, 10, 11	19, 34-38, 44, 46-47, 49, 52-60, 431, 433-440, 468-471
12.3.1	1, 10, 11	18-20, 434-448, 468-471
12.3.2	1, 10, 11	19-20, 428, 454
12.3.3	1, 2, 10	19-20, 34-35, 39-40, 60-61, 431, 433-440, 468-471
12.3.4	1, 2, 10, 11, 12	19-20, 31-34, 37-45, 47-48, 52-63, 434-448, 468-471, 481-492
12.4.1	1, 10, 11	18-20, 434-448, 468-471
12.4.2	1, 10, 11, 12	19-20, 434-448, 468-471, 481-485

Appendix B
Hybrid Vehicle Emergency Response Guide Websites

The following websites contain links to online and downloadable emergency response guides for hybrid vehicles. Many of these sites were created by the vehicle manufacturers themselves as a service to the Fire and Emergency Services. Others have been created by Fire and Emergency Services personnel to spread reliable knowledge regarding safety and procedures at incidents involving hybrid vehicles. These websites were current at the time this manual went to print.

NOTE: Some manufacturers of hybrid vehicles provide hard copy versions of the emergency response guides for their hybrid products through their dealerships.

Hybrid Manufacturer's Emergency Responder Links:
http://www.extrication.com/ERG.htm

Scene of the Accident:
http://www.sceneoftheaccident.org/ERGs.aspx

This site has links to ERGs for a wide variety of hybrid automobiles. This site is also one of the few sites that has any information about the Mazda Tribute.

General Motors Service Technical College:
http://www.gmstc.com/FirstResponder.aspx

Toyota Scion Lexus Technical Information System:
https://techinfo.toyota.com

Follow the link on the front page titled, "Emergency Response & Hybrid Information."

Ford Motorcraft:
http://www.motorcraftservice.com/vdirs/retail/default.asp

Use the menu on the left to enter "Quick Guides" then "Escape/Mariner Hybrid Emergency Response Guide."

Nissan Altima:

http://www.nissanusa.com/pdf/techpubs/altima_hybrid/2007/2007_Altima_Hybrid_FRG.pdf

http://www.nissanusa.com/pdf/techpubs/altima_hybrid/2008/2008_Altima_Hybrid_FRG.pdf

http://www.nissanusa.com/pdf/techpubs/altima_hybrid/2009/2009_Altima_Hybrid_FRG.pdf

Honda Hybrid Emergency Response Guides:

https://techinfo.honda.com/rjanisis/logon.asp

Follow the link on the left for "Hybrid and other Emergency Response Guides."

U.S. Department of Energy Updates on Hybrid and Fuel Cell Vehicles:

http://www.fueleconomy.gov/feg/fuelcell.shtml

http://www1.eere.energy.gov/vehiclesandfuels/technologies/systems/index.html

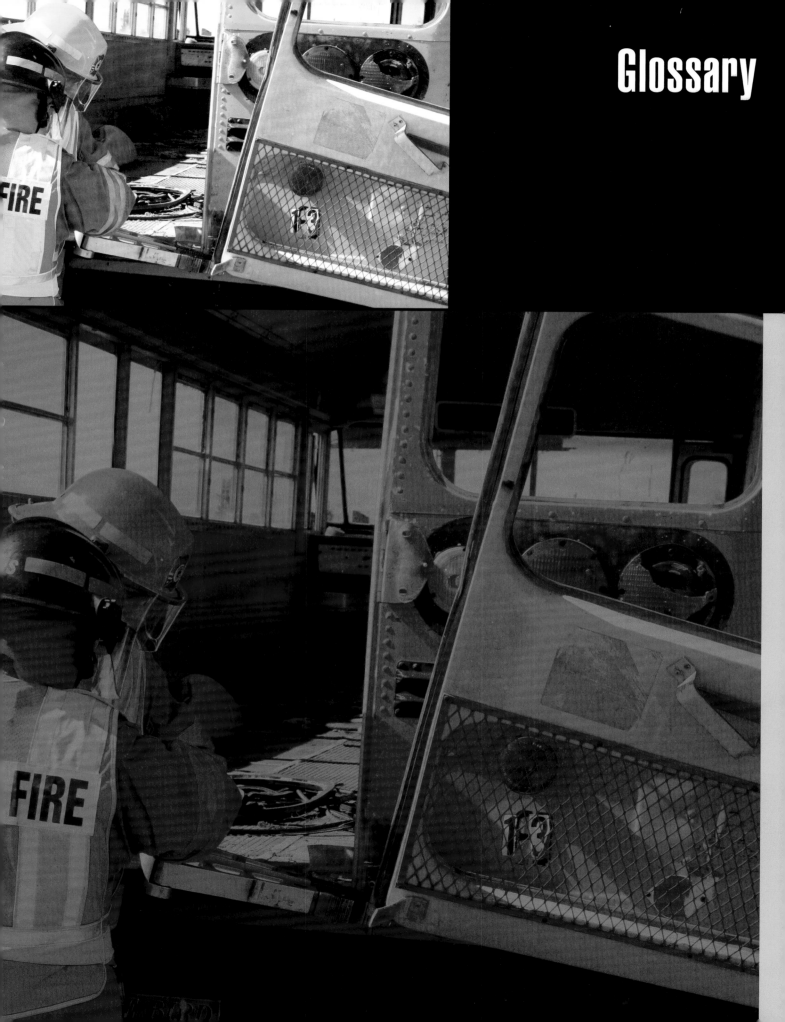

Glossary

Glossary

A

Access Hole — 1) Starter hole into which a cutting tool may be inserted to continue cutting a piece of sheet metal. (2) Space made in a door crack with a manual prying tool to facilitate the placement of a spreading tool.

Accessibility — Ability of fire apparatus to get close enough to a structure or emergency scene to conduct emergency operations.

Accident — Sequence of unplanned or uncontrolled events that produces unintended injury, death, or property damage; the result of unsafe acts by persons who are unaware or uninformed of potential hazards and ignorant of safety policies or who fail to follow safety procedures.

Acetylene [c_2h_2] — Colorless gas that has an explosive range from 2.5 percent to 100 percent; used as a fuel gas for cutting and welding operations.

Action Plan — Written plan of how objectives are to be achieved. *See* Incident Action Plan.

Actual Mechanical Advantage — Something less than the theoretical mechanical advantage, due to the friction in a system.

Advanced Life Support — Advanced medical skills performed by trained medical personnel, such as the administration of medications, or airway management procedures to save a victim's life.

A-Frame — Vertical lifting device that can be attached to the front or rear of the apparatus. It consists of two poles attached several feet (meters) apart on the apparatus and whose working ends are connected to form the letter A. A pulley or block and tackle through which a rope or cable is passed is attached to the end of the frame.

After Action Reviews — Learning tools used to evaluate a project or incident to identify and encourage organizational and operational strengths and to identify and correct weaknesses.

AHJ — Abbreviation for authority having jurisdiction.

Air Bag — (1) Inflatable bag designed into the steering wheel, dashboard, or doors of an automobile that inflates immediately when the vehicle is impacted. (2) Large inflatable bag onto which persons can leap to escape danger. (3) *Also see* Air Lifting Bag.

Air Chisel — *See* Pneumatic Chisel/Hammer.

Aircraft Tugs — Special, low-profile vehicles designed to tow aircraft on the airport ramp or push aircraft backwards away from an airport gate. Also called *pushback tractors* or *tugs*.

Air Lifting Bag — Inflatable, envelope-type device that can be placed between the ground and an object and then inflated to lift the object. It can also be used to separate objects. Depending on the size of the bag, it may have lifting capabilities in excess of 75 tons (68 040 kg).

Air Line Connection — *See* Chuck.

Air-Purifying Respirator (APR) — Respirator with an air-purifying filter, cartridge, or canister that removes specific air contaminates by passing ambient air through the air-purifying element; may have a full or partial facepiece.

Aisle — A passageway between sections of seats in rows.

All Clear — Signal given to the incident commander that a specific area has been checked for victims and none have been found or all found victims have been extricated from an entrapment.

ALS — *See* Advanced Life Support.

American National Standards Institute (ANSI) — Voluntary standards-setting organization that examines and certifies existing standards and creates new standards.

Anchor Point — Solid base or point from which pulling or pushing operations can be initiated.

Anchor System — The total combination or anchor points, slings, and carabiners used to create attachment points for a rope rescue system.

Antisubmarine Device — Any device designed to prevent a driver from sliding forward and become wedged or trapped beneath the dashboard of a vehicle.

A-Post — Front post area of a vehicle where the door is connected to the body.

Armormax® — A combination of numerous synthetic fibers used to form an opaque composite ballistic armor.

Articulated Transit Bus — A passenger carrying bus constructed with two sections (a tractor and a trailer) which are connected by a pivoting joint.

Assessment Stop — Distant location that is safe for the first responders to stop and evaluate the situation, to complete donning their protective clothing and SCBA, and to report conditions to the communications center.

Attack Hose — Hose between the attack pumper and the nozzle(s); also, any hose used in a handline to control and extinguish fire. Minimum size is 1½ inch (38 mm).

Attack Line(s) — (1) Hoseline(s) connected to a pump discharge of a fire apparatus ready for use in attacking a fire (may or may not be preconnected); contrasted to supply lines connecting a water supply with a pump. (2) Fire streams used to attack, contain, or prevent the spread of a fire.

Auger — (1) Screwlike shaft that is turned to move grain or other commodities through a farm implement. (2) Tool for boring holes in floors.

Authority Having Jurisdiction — Term used in codes and standards to identify the legal entity, such as a building or fire official, that has the statutory authority to enforce a code and to approve or require equipment. In the insurance industry it may refer to an insurance rating bureau or an insurance company inspection department.

Automatic Aid — Written agreement between two or more agencies to automatically dispatch predetermined resources to any fire or other emergency reported in the geographic area covered by the agreement. These areas are generally where the boundaries between jurisdictions meet or where jurisdictional "islands" exist.

B

Basic Life Support — Maintenance of airway, breathing, and circulation, as well as basic bandaging and splinting, without the use of adjunctive equipment.

Bird Cage Construction — See Integral Construction.

Blank — A thin piece of metal inserted between flanges in a pipe system to isolate part of the system.

Blank Flange — A device that attaches to the end of a pipe in order to cap the end.

Block and Tackle — Series of pulleys (sheaves) contained within a wood or metal frame. They are used with rope to provide a mechanical advantage for pulling operations.

Blood Borne Pathogens — Pathogenic microorganisms that are present in the human blood and can cause disease in humans. These pathogens include (but are not limited to) hepatitis B virus (HBV) and human immunodeficiency virus (HIV).

BLS — *See* Basic Life Support.

Body-on-Chassis Construction — Method of school bus or recreational vehicle construction where the school bus body manufacturer installs the body unit onto a commercially available chassis constructed by another manufacturer.

"Bombproof" Anchor Point — Slang reference to an anchor that is absolutely immovable, such as a huge boulder, a large tree, or a fire engine; also synonymous for an anchor point capable of withstanding forces in excess of those that might be generated by the rescue operation or even catastrophic failure (and resultant shock load) of a raising or lowering system.

Box Crib — Stabilization platform constructed by creating opposing layers of pieces of cribbing.

B-Post — Post between the front and rear doors on a four-door vehicle, or the door-handle-end post on a two-door car.

Branch — Organizational level of an incident management system having functional/geographic responsibility for major segments of incident operations. The branch level is organizationally between section and division/sector/group.

Bumper — Structure designed to provide front or rear end protection of a vehicle.

Bumper Struts — Bumpers that incorporate energy absorbing struts to make them less vulnerable to damage in low-speed collisions.

C

Caisson — Protective hardened steel sleeves located inside automobile B- and C- posts that are designed to protect seatbelt pretensioners from being cut.

Carline Supports — Structural members used in the construction of buses. They are designed to strengthen the sidewall of the bus where it might come into contact with a car during a collision.

Cascade System — Three or more large air cylinders, each usually with a capacity of 300 cubic feet (8 490 L), that are interconnected and from which smaller SCBA cylinders are recharged.

Caternary Wire System — A series of overhead wires used to transmit electrical power to buses, locomotives, and trams at a distance from the energy supply point.

Center of Gravity — Point through which all the weight of a vehicle and its contents may be considered as concentrated so that if supported at this point, the vehicle would remain in equilibrium in any position.

Cervical Collar — Device used to immobilize and support the neck.

Cervical Spine — First seven bones of the vertebral column, located in the neck.

Chain of Command — (1) Order of rank and authority in the fire and emergency services. (2) The proper sequence of information and command flow as described in the National Incident Management System - Incident Command System (NIMS-ICS).

Channeling Devices — Items such as signs, road flares, and cones intended to guide traffic away from the active zones at an incident or accident.

Charged Line — Hose loaded with water under pressure and prepared for use.

Chassis — Basic operating system of a motor vehicle consisting of the frame, suspension system, wheels, and steering mechanism but not the body.

Cheater Bar — Piece of pipe added to a prying tool to lengthen the handle and provide additional leverage.

Chock — Wooden, plastic, or metal block constructed to fit the curvature of a tire; placed against the tire to prevent apparatus rolling. Also called a Wheel Block.

Circular Saw (Rotary Rescue Saw) — Gas- or electric-powered saw whose circular blade rotates at a high speed to produce a cutting action. A variety of blades may be used, depending on the material being cut. Also called Rotary Rescue Saw.

CISD — Abbreviation for Critical Incident Stress Debriefing.

Clevis Hook — A type of hook attached at the end of a rope, web sling, or chain engineered for rapid connection; commonly used during vehicle extrication and rescue incidents.

Coil Spring Suspension — A type of suspension system consisting of numerous elastic steel bodies wound spirally that recover their shape after being compressed, bent, or stretched.

Collision Beams — 1) Structural member within a vehicle door designed to prevent the door from collapsing inward if struck. 2) Heavy-gauge steel member strategically located in the sidewall of a bus. Its purpose is to limit penetration of an object into the passenger compartment.

Combine — Large, self-propelled machine that cuts, threshes, and cleans crops as it drives across a field.

Come-Along — Manually operated pulling tool that uses a ratchet/pulley arrangement to provide a mechanical advantage.

Command — (1) Act of directing, ordering, and/or controlling resources by virtue of explicit legal, agency, or delegated authority. (2) Term used on the radio to designate the incident commander. (3) Function of NIMS-ICS that determines the overall strategy of the incident, with input from throughout the ICS structure.

Command Post (CP) — The designated physical location of the command and control point where the incident commander and command staff function during an incident and where those in charge of emergency units report to be briefed on their respective assignments. CP may be co-located with Base. *See* Incident Command Post.

Commercial Chassis — Truck chassis produced by a commercial truck manufacturer. These chassis are in turn outfitted with a rescue or fire fighting body.

Commercial Motor Coach — Custom-built buses designed to carry groups of people to a specific destination, usually a long distance away. These buses may run regularly scheduled routes, or they may be specially chartered. Also called Charter Bus and Touring Bus.

Compartment Syndrome — Occurs when a patient's limb has been entrapped for four to six hours. At this point, the crushed tissue in the involved limb begins to give off toxins, which decreases the potential for saving the limb.

Composite Materials — Plastics, metals, ceramics, or carbon-fiber materials with built-in strengthening agents. These materials are much lighter and stronger than the metals formerly used for such aircraft components as panels, skin, and flight controls.

Compressed Air — Air under greater than atmospheric pressure; used as a portable supply of breathing air for SCBA or to operate pneumatic tools.

Contamination — Condition of impurity resulting from mixture or contact with foreign substance.

Control Zones — System of barriers surrounding designated areas at emergency scenes intended to limit the number of persons exposed to the hazard, and to facilitate its mitigation. At a major incident there will be three zones — hot (restricted), warm (limited access), and cold (support).

CP — Abbreviation for Command Post.

C-Post — Post nearest the rear door handle on a four-door vehicle. On a two-door vehicle, the rear roof post is considered to be the C-post.

Critical Incident Stress Debriefing (CISD) — Counseling designed to minimize the effects of psychological/emotional post-incident trauma on those at fire and rescue incidents who were directly involved with victims suffering from particularly gruesome or horrific injuries. *See* Post-Traumatic Incident Debriefing.

Crow Bar — Prying tool with a blade at either end. One end is significantly curved to provide additional mechanical advantage.

Crowd Control — Limiting access to an emergency scene by curious spectators and other non-emergency personnel.

Crush Points — Places within the frame of a vehicle that are designed to collapse, crush, deform, and otherwise absorb (not transmit) forces so as to minimize the impact on the passengers.

Crushable Bumpers — Polystyrene foam or fluoroelastomer devices designed to absorb energy by flexing when struck.

Curbside — Side of a trailer nearest the curb when trailer is traveling in a normal forward direction (right-hand side); opposite to roadside.

Custom Chassis — Truck chassis designed solely for use as a fire or rescue apparatus.

Cutting Tool — Any one of a number of hand or power tools used to cut a specific kind of material.

D

dB — Abbreviation for decibel.

Decibel — Unit for expressing the relative intensity of sounds on a scale from 0 for the least perceptible sound to about 130 for the average pain level; degree of loudness.

Decontaminate — To remove a foreign substance that could cause harm; frequently used to describe removal of a hazardous material from the person, clothing, or area.

Delayed Treatment — Classification for patients with serious but not life threatening injuries; these patients may need additional care but may not need that care immediately.

Disentanglement — That part of vehicle extrication that relates to the removal and/or manipulation of vehicle components to allow a properly packaged patient to be removed from the vehicle. Sometimes referred to as removing the vehicle from the patient.

Division — IMS organizational level having responsibility for operations within a defined geographic area. It is composed of a number of individual units that are assigned to operate within a defined geographical area.

Door/roof Posts — Also called pillars, these are the structural members that surround the doors and support the roofs of vehicles.

Drill — Exercise conducted to practice and/or evaluate training already received; the process of skill maintenance.

Driver's Side — The side of a vehicle that is on the same side as the vehicle's steering wheel.

Drive Train — *See* Power Train.

E

Egress — A means of exiting a vehicle.

Emergency Medical Services (EMS) — Initial medical evaluation/treatment provided to those who become ill or are injured.

Emergency Operations — Activities involved in responding to the scene of an incident and performing assigned duties in order to mitigate the emergency.

Emergency Response Guidebook (ERG) — A manual that aids emergency response and inspection personnel in identifying hazardous materials placards. It also gives guidelines for initial actions to be taken at hazardous materials incidents. Formerly the North American Emergency Response Guidebook (NAERG).

Emergency Responder — Qualified member of a fire and emergency services organization that provides search and rescue, fire suppression, medial, hazardous materials, or specialized protection services. The organization may be publicly or privately managed and funded.

Emergency Traffic — Urgent radio traffic; a request for other unit to clear the radio waves for an urgent message. Also called Priority Traffic.

EMS — Abbreviation for Emergency Medical Services.

Engine Company — Group of firefighters assigned to a fire department pumper who are primarily responsible for providing water supply and attack lines for fire extinguishment.

Enhanced 9-1-1 — Emergency telephone service that provides selective routing, automatic number identification (ANI), and automatic location identification (ALI).

Enhanced Performance Glass (EPG) — EPG type of laminated glass that provides higher levels of security as well as additional impact protection and sound proofing.

ERG — Abbreviation for Emergency Response Guidebook.

Explosion-Proof Equipment — Encased in a rigidly built container so it withstands an internal explosion and also prevents ignition of a surrounding flammable atmosphere; designed to not provide an ignition source in an explosive atmosphere.

Explosive Atmosphere — Any atmosphere that contains a mixture of fuel to air that falls within the explosive limits for that particular material.

Extension Ram — Powered, hydraulic tool designed especially for straight pushing operations that may extend as far as 63 inches (1 600 mm). Also called Ram.

Exterior (Vehicle) — All of the features of the outside of a vehicle. The exterior is composed of the vehicle's body panels, glass, bumpers, and other components.

Extrication — The removal and treatment of victims who are trapped by some type of man-made machinery or equipment.

Extrication Collar — Device used for spinal immobilization.

Extrication Group — The group within the Incident Management System that is responsible for extricating the victim(s).

F

Fairing — An auxiliary structure or the external surface attached to or part of the roof of a large truck that serves to reduce drag.

Farm Implement — General term used to describe farm machinery.

Fatality — Someone who has died as the result of the incident.

Fenders — The body material that surrounds the front tires. The fender starts at the front of the vehicle, proceeds around the front tire and ends at the fire wall.

Fiberglass — Composite material consisting of glass fibers embedded in resin.

Fifth Wheel — Device used to connect a truck tractor or converter dolly to a semi-trailer in order to permit articulation between the units. It is generally composed of a lower part consisting of a trunnion, plate, and latching mechanism mounted on the truck tractor (or dolly) and a kingpin assembly mounted on the semi-trailer.

Fifth-Wheel Pickup Ramp — Steel plate designed to lift the front end of a semi-trailer to facilitate the engagement of the kingpin into the fifth wheel.

Fire Apparatus — Any fire department emergency vehicle used in fire suppression or other emergency situation.

Firewall (Vehicle) — The partition between the engine compartment and the passenger compartment of a vehicle. It is designed to protect vehicle occupants from the engine and its associated hazards.

First Aid — Immediate medical care given to a victim until he or she can be transported to a medical facility.

First Responder (EMS) — (1) First person arriving at the scene of an accident or medical emergency who is trained to administer first aid and basic life support. (2) Level of emergency medical training, between first aider and emergency medical technician levels, that is recognized by the authority having jurisdiction.

Flagger — An individual assigned to direct the flow of traffic using a flag, flashlight, paddle, wand, sign, or other device.

Fluid — Any substance that can flow, has a definite mass and volume at constant temperature and pressure but no definite shape, and that is unable to sustain shear stresses. Fluids include both gases and liquids. Common fluids encountered during extrication operations include gasoline, diesel fuel, coolant fluid, hydraulic fluid, brake fluid, and human body fluids such as blood.

Folding Jack — Common type of lifting jack. The frame of the folding jack is made of metal bars of equal lengths fastened in the center to form Xs. This jack has limited use and is considered safe only for light loads.

Force — (1) To break open, into, or through. (2) Simple measure of weight, usually expressed in pounds or kilograms.

Forcible Entry — (1) Techniques used by fire personnel to gain entry into buildings, vehicles, aircraft, or other areas of confinement when normal means of entry are locked or blocked. (2) Entering a structure or vehicle by means of physical force, characterized by prying open doors and breaking windows, leaving visible indicators of illegal entry if pry marks and certain window breakage are present upon the first firefighters' arrival.

Frame — (1) The chassis of some automobiles. (2) Part of an opening that is constructed to support the component that closes and secures the opening such as a door or window.

Front (Vehicle) — The front of the vehicle is generally defined by the direction the driver faces during normal travel or operation. Generally indicated by the headlights.

Front-impact Air Bags — A supplemental restraint system designed to deploy air bags to absorb passenger impacts during a frontal collision. These air bags are activated through a system of inertia switches located forward of the passenger compartment and by microelectronic controls that may be located under the front seats or in the console between the front seats.

Front-impact Collision — Occurs when a vehicle collides head on with another vehicle or object.

Frostbite — Local freezing and tissue damage due to prolonged exposure to extreme cold.

Fulcrum — Support or point of support on which a lever turns in raising or moving something.

Full or Rigid Frames — Automobile construction (also known as body-on-frame construction) consisting of a steel ladder frame that is constructed using two parallel beams that run along the long axis of the vehicle to form a chassis. Cross members are bolted and welded between these beams to provide rigidity and support. This chassis then supports the powertrain and the vehicle body is bolted to the frame.

Full Structural Protective Clothing — Protective clothing including helmets, self-contained breathing apparatus, coats and pants customarily worn by firefighters (turnout or bunker coats and pants), rubber boots, and gloves. It also includes covering for the neck, ears, and other parts of the head not protected by the helmet or breathing apparatus. When working with hazardous materials, bands or tape are added around the legs, arms, and waist. *See also* Personal Protective Equipment (PPE).

Full Trailer — Truck trailer constructed so that all of its own weight and that of its load rests upon its own wheels; that is, it does not depend upon a truck tractor to support it. A semitrailer equipped with a dolly is considered a full trailer.

G

Generator — Auxiliary electrical power generating device. Portable generators are powered by small gasoline or diesel engines and generally have 110- and/or 220-volt capacities.

Gin Pole — A vertical lifting device that may be attached to the front or the rear of the apparatus. It consists of a single pole that is attached to the apparatus at one end and has a working pulley at the other. Guy wires also may be used to stabilize the pole.

Gloves — Part of the firefighter's or rescuer's protective clothing ensemble necessary to protect the hands.

Gross Vehicle Weight Rating (GVWR) — the maximum allowable total weight of a road vehicle or trailer when loaded to include the weight of the vehicle itself plus fuel, passengers, cargo, and trailer tongue weight.

Group — ICS organizational subunit responsible for a number of individual units that are assigned to perform a particular a specified function at an incident (extrication, transportation, EMS, etc.).

Group Commander/Supervisor — Person in charge of a group within the Incident Command System.

H

Hailing — Technique used during physical search; involves calling out to victims and listening for responses.

Halfboard — Device used for spinal immobilization and patient removal; can be used as a lifting harness.

Halligan Tool — Prying tool with a claw at one end and a spike or point at a right angle to a wedge at the other end. Also called Hooligan Tool.

Handline — Small hoseline (2 inch [65 mm] or less) that can be handled and maneuvered without mechanical assistance.

Handline Nozzle — Any nozzle that can be safely handled by one to three firefighters and flows less than 350 gpm (1 400 L/min).

Handsaw — A saw that is operated by hand rather than a power source. Especially useful for cutting objects that require a controlled cut but are too big to fit in the jaws of a scissors-type cutter or unsuitable for cutting with a power saw.

Hand Tool — Tool that is manipulated and powered by human force.

Hardware — (1) A general term used for small equipment made of metal such as hand tools. (2) Ancillary equipment used in rope systems, for example, carabiners, pulleys, and figure-eight plates.

Hauling System — Mechanical advantage system that is constructed of rope and appropriate hardware and is designed for lifting a load.

Hazard Area — Established area from which bystanders and unneeded rescue workers are prohibited.

Hazard and Risk Assessment — Formal review of the hazards and risk that may be encountered while performing the functions of a firefighter or emergency responder; used to determine the appropriate level and type of personal and respiratory protection that must be worn.

Hazardous Atmosphere — Atmosphere that may or may not be immediately dangerous to life and health but that is oxygen deficient, that contains a toxic or disease-producing contaminant, or that contains a flammable or explosive vapor or gas.

Hazardous Chemical — Defined by the Occupational Safety and Health Administration (OSHA) as any chemical that is a physical hazard or a health hazard to employees.

Hazardous Material — (1) Any material that possesses an unreasonable risk to the health and safety of persons and/or the environment if it is not properly controlled during handling, storage, manufacture, processing, packaging, use, disposal, or transportation. (2) Substances or materials in quantities or forms that may pose an unreasonable risk to health, safety, or property when stored, transported, or used in commerce (DOT).

Hazardous Materials Incident — Emergency, with or without fire, that involves the release or potential release of a hazardous material.

Hazardous Substance(s) — Any substance designated under the Clean Water Act and the Comprehensive Environmental Response, Compensation and Liability Act (CERCLA) as posing a threat to waterways and the environment when released.

Head Protection Systems (HPS) — Air bags that deploy from a narrow opening between the headliner and the top of the door frame to protect passengers' heads.

Heat Stress — Combination of environmental and physical work factors that make up the heat load imposed on the body. The environmental factors that contribute to heat stress include air, temperature, radiant heat exchange, air movement, and water vapor pressure. Physical work contributes to heat stress by the metabolic heat in the body. Clothing also has an effect on heat stress.

Heat Stroke — Heat illness caused by heat exposure, resulting in failure of the body's heat regulating mechanism; symptoms include high fever of 105° to 106° F (40.5° C to 41.1° C); dry, red, hot skin; rapid, strong pulse; and deep breaths, convulsions. May result in coma or possibly death. Also called Sunstroke.

Heavy Rescue Vehicle — Large rescue vehicle that may be constructed on a custom or commercial chassis. Additional equipment carried by the heavy rescue unit includes A-frames or gin poles, cascade systems, larger power plants, trench and storing equipment, small pumps and foam equipment, large winches, hydraulic booms, large quantities of rope and rigging equipment, air compressors, and ladders.

Helmet — Protective headgear worn by firefighters and rescue personnel that provides protection from falling objects, side blows, the fire environment elements, and eye injuries.

High Mobility Multipurpose Wheeled Vehicles (HMMWV or Humvee) — A 4-wheel drive military vehicle that replaced earlier Jeep and MUTT vehicles.

High-Strength Low-Alloy (HSLA) Steel — An alloy steel developed to provide better mechanical properties or greater resistance to corrosion than carbon steel. HSLA steels are different from other steels in that they are made to meet specific mechanical properties.

HPS — *See* Head Protection Systems.

Hydration — (1) Act or process of combining with water. (2) Condition of having adequate fluid in body tissues through adequate fluid intake. (3) Chemical process in which concrete changes to a solid state and gains strength.

Hydraulic Jack — Lifting jack that uses hydraulic fluid power supplied from a manually operated hand lever.

Hydroplaning — Condition in which moving tires on a vehicle are separated from pavement surfaces by steam and/or water or liquid rubber film, resulting in loss of mechanical braking effectiveness.

Hypothermia — Abnormally low or decreased body temperature. Also called Systemic Hypothermia.

I

IC — Abbreviation for Incident Commander.

ICS — Abbreviation for Incident Command System.

IDLH — Abbreviation for Immediately Dangerous to Life and Health. *See* Immediately Dangerous to Life and Health.

Illumination Unit — A portable light generating unit capable of providing 3 to 6 lights of 500 watts each with extension cords from 500 to 1000 feet for the purpose of providing specified level of illumination capacity.

Immediate Treatment — Classification for patients with the most serious injuries at an incident and will require packaging and movement to a health care facility as soon as possible.

Immediately Dangerous to Life and Health (IDLH) — Any atmosphere that poses an immediate hazard to life or produces immediate irreversible, debilitating effects on health. A companion measurement to the PEL, IDLH concentrations represent concentrations above which respiratory protection should be required. IDLH is expressed in ppm or mg/m3.

Impaled — (1) Condition resulting when a victim's head or other appendage pierces a stationary object such as a windshield. (2) Condition resulting from a foreign object becoming lodged in some portion of a victim's body.

Impaled Object — Object that has caused a puncture wound and remains embedded in the wound.

Incident — An emergency or non-emergency situation or occurrence (either human-caused or natural phenomenon) that requires action by emergency services personnel to prevent or minimize loss of life or damage to property and/or natural resources.

Incident Action Plan (IAP) — Written or unwritten plan for the disposition of an incident. The IAP contains the overall strategic goals, tactical objectives, and support requirements for a given operational period during an incident. All incidents require an action plan. On relatively small incidents, the IAP is usually not in writing. On larger, more complex incidents, a written IAP is created for each operational period, and is disseminated to units assigned to the incident. When written, the plan may have a number of forms as attachments.

Incident Command Post — Location at which the incident commander and command staff direct, order, and control resources at an incident; may be co-located with the incident base.

Incident Command System (ICS) — (1) System by which facilities, equipment, personnel, procedures, and communications are organized to operate within a common organizational structure designed to aid in the management of resources at emergency incidents. (2) Management system of procedures for controlling personnel, facilities, equipment, and communications so that different agencies can work together toward a common goal in an effective and efficient manner. (3) Recommended method of establishing and maintaining command and control of an incident. It is an organized approach to incident management, adaptable to any size of type of incident.

Incident Commander (IC) — Person in charge of the incident management system and responsible for the management of all incident operations during an emergency.

Incident Safety Officer (ISO) — Member of the Command Staff responsible for monitoring and assessing safety hazards and unsafe conditions during an incident and developing measures for ensuring personnel safety. The ISO is responsible for the enforcement of all mandated safety laws and regulations and departmental safety-related SOPs. On very small incidents, the IC may act as the ISO.

Insurance Institute for Highway Safety (IIHS) — An independent research organization funded by a host of well-known insurance companies. The IIHS focuses on both crash avoidance and the crashworthiness of vehicles.

Integral Construction — Method of construction used on all types of buses. The manufacturer assembles the vehicle starting with the frame and chassis assembly and proceeds item by item to the finished vehicle. Also called Bird Cage Construction.

Integral Frame — See Unitized Body.

Interior (Vehicle) — The interior of a vehicle is composed of the passenger compartment and may contain, depending on the vehicle, the storage compartment.

Inverter — Auxiliary electrical power generating device. The inverter is a step-up transformer that converts the vehicle's 12- or 24-volt DC current into 110- or 220-volt AC current.

J

Jack — Portable device used to lift heavy objects with force applied by a lever, screw, or hydraulic press.

Jackknife — Condition of truck tractor/semitrailer combination when their relative positions to each other form an angle of 90 degrees or less about the trailer kingpin.

Jaws — *See* Powered Hydraulic Spreader.

K

Kendrick Extrication Device (KED)® — Device used to assist with spinal immobilization and patient packaging for removal.

Kevlar® — The trademarked name of a lightweight, very strong para-aramid synthetic fiber. It is used in many products to include bicycle tires, sails, body armor, and armor components for vehicles.

Kick Panels — The vertical panel walls of a vehicle that are enclosed by several structural members.

Kilopascal (kPa) — Metric unit of measure for pressure; 1 psi = 6.895 kPa, 1 kPa = 0.1450 psi.

Kilowatt (KW) — Measurement of rate of heat release measured in the number of Btu per second (equivalent to ten 100-watt light bulbs).

Kinematics — One branch of the study of dynamics that defines the motion of objects without addressing mass and force or the factors that lead to the motion. In terms of accidents, kinematics describe the effects of collisions on vehicles.

Kinematics of Injury — The types of injuries suffered by vehicle occupants that vary depending upon the type of collision incurred.

Kinetic Energy — The energy possessed by a moving object.

Kingpin — Attaching pin on a semitrailer that connects with pivots within the lower coupler of a truck tractor or converter dolly while coupling the two units together.

Knee Bolsters — A protective systems designed help prevent the driver of a vehicle from sliding forward and becoming wedged under the dashboard in an accident. Also called "antisubmarine" devices.

Kneeling — The ability of some buses to lower the front end of the bus to curb level for ease of passenger boarding.

kPa — Abbreviation for *Kilopascal*.

KW — Abbreviation for kilowatt.

L

Label — A four-inch-square diamond-shaped marker required by federal regulations on individual shipping containers containing hazardous materials and which are smaller than 640 cubic feet (18 m3).

Latch — Spring-loaded part of a locking mechanism that extends into a strike within the door frame.

Leading Block — A pulley or snatch block used to change the direction of the fall line in a block and tackle system. This does not affect the mechanical advantage of the system.

Leaf Spring Suspension — A type of suspension system consisting of several long, narrow, layers of elastic metal bracketed together.

Light Rescue Vehicle — Small rescue vehicle usually built on a 1-ton or ½-ton chassis. It is designed to handle only basic extrication and life-support functions and carries only basic hand tools and small equipment.

Lightweight Transparent Armor® (LTA) — Polycarbonate bulletproof glass sheets bonded together to form windows and windshields for armored vehicles and structures.

Limited Access (Warm) Zone — Large geographical area between the support zone and the restricted zone. The area for personnel who are directly aiding rescuers in the restricted zone. This would include personnel who are handling hydraulic tool power plants, fire personnel handling standby hoselines, and so on. This zone should contain the decontamination area and the safe haven. Personnel in this zone should not get in the way of rescuers working in the restricted zone.

Litter — *See* Stretcher.

Livestock — Cattle, horses, sheep, and other useful animals raised or kept on a ranch or farm.

Lock Mechanism — Moving parts of a lock, which include the latch or bolt, lock cylinder, and articulating components.

Lockout/Tagout Device — A device used to secure any power switches on a machine to prevent accidental or otherwise undesirable re-energization of the machine.

Logistics — Function of the ICS responsible for seeing that the details necessary to sustain the incident are handled. This includes such areas as food, shelter, supply, and communications.

Logroll — Method for placing a patient onto a backboard by turning the patient as a unit, first onto the side, then onto the back.

Long Backboard — Board used to package patient with suspected spinal injury.

M

Maintenance — Keeping equipment or apparatus in a state of usefulness or readiness.

Manual on Uniform Traffic Control Devices (MUTCD) — U.S. DOT Federal Highway Administration publication that identifies the types of traffic control devices that should be used to establish work areas and identify incident scenes as well the methods for deploying these devices.

Marrying Vehicles — Attaching two vehicles to one another in such a fashion that the two vehicles move as one, stable object.

Mass Casualty Incident — An emergency incident involving the injury or death of a number of victims that is beyond what the jurisdiction is routinely capable of handling. *See* Multi-Casualty Incident.

Mass Transportation — Any mode of transportation designed to carry large numbers of people at the same time.

Mechanical Advantage — (1) Gain in force, when levering, by moving the fulcrum closer to the object. (2) Used in rope rescue and to lift heavy objects, this refers to the advantage created when levers, pulleys, and tools are used to make work easier. (3) The ratio of the force applied by a simple machine, such as a lever or block and tackle, to the force applied to the machine by the user.

Mechanical Trauma — Injury, such as an abrasion, puncture, or laceration, resulting from direct contact with a fragment or a whole container.

Mechanism of Injury — The forces placed on the victim's body by the collision.

Medium Rescue Vehicle — Rescue vehicle somewhat larger and better equipped than a light rescue vehicle. This vehicle may carry powered hydraulic spreading tools and cutters, air bag lifting systems, power saws, oxyacetylene cutting equipment, ropes and rigging equipment, as well as basic hand equipment.

Miller Board — Board used to package a patient with suspected spinal injury; may also be used with a harness for lifting the patient.

Mine Resistant Ambush Protected (MRAP) Vehicles — A series of armored fighting vehicles designed to survive ambushes and improvised explosive device (IED) attacks.

Minor Treatment — Classification for patients with minor injuries; they may simply require first aid and may even be able to be transported to medical facilities in private vehicles without the care of EMS staff.

Mitigate — (1) To cause to become less harsh or hostile; to make less severe, intense or painful; to alleviate. (2) Third of three steps (locate, isolate, mitigate) in one method of sizing up an emergency situation.

Mock (Staged) Incident — A simulated emergency that allows responders to test their skills under realistic conditions. Also called staged incident.

Monocque — Construction technique in which an object's external skin supports the structural load of the object.

Motor Vehicle Accident (MVA) — Term used when one vehicle hits a stationary object or another vehicle.

Mouse — To tightly wrap or cover the open end of a hook with a material to prevent an object from slipping off the hook.

Multi-Casualty Incident — Emergency incident involving the injury or death of a number of victims beyond what the jurisdiction is routinely capable of handling. Also called mass casualty incident.

Multiple Patient Incident (MPI) — An incident where the emergency response resources are not overtaxed by the number of patients involved.

Munitions Loaders — A military vehicle used to transport and load/off-load bombs and other munitions from military aircraft.

Muscle Cars — High performance, American cars made from 1964 to 1974 or modeled from cars built during that time; usually 2-door, rear wheel drive, mid-sized vehicles with oversized, V8 engines.

MUTCD — Abbreviation for Manual on Uniform Traffic Control Devices.

Mutual Aid — Reciprocal assistance from one fire and emergency services agency to another during an emergency based upon a prearrangement between agencies involved and generally made upon the request of the receiving agency.

MVA — Abbreviation for motor vehicle accident.

N

Nader Pin — The bolt on a vehicle's door frame that the door latches on to in order to close the door.

Nader Safety Lock — Vehicle door safety lock; required by law on all passenger vehicles built since 1973.

National Fire Protection Association (NFPA) — Nonprofit educational and technical association located in Quincy, Massachusetts devoted to protecting life and property from fire by developing fire protection standards and educating the public.

National Highway Traffic Safety Administration (NHTSA) — Agency within the U.S. Department of Transportation (DOT) that publishes annual summary reports of fatal highway accidents.

National Incident Management System - Incident Command System — The U.S. mandated system that defines the roles, responsibilities, and standard operating procedures used to manage emergency operations. Also be referred to as NIMS- ICS.

National Transportation Safety Board (NTSB) — Agency within the U.S. Department of Transportation (DOT) that maintains a fire-related data base on aircraft and railway accidents, as well as highway accidents involving hazardous materials injuries.

NFPA® — Abbreviation for National Fire Protection Association. A national organization that sets standards for fire service equipment.

NHTSA — Abbreviation for the U.S. National Highway Traffic Safety Administration.

NTSB — Abbreviation for the U.S. National Transportation Safety Board.

O

Occupational Safety and Health Administration (OSHA) — U.S. federal agency that develops and enforces standards and regulations for occupational safety in the workplace.

Orthopedic Injury — An injury to the bones, mainly the extremities.

OSHA — See Occupational Safety and Health Administration.

Outside Aid — Assistance from agencies, industries, or fire departments that are not part of the agency having jurisdiction over the incident.

Override Collision — Occurs when a striking vehicle collides with another vehicle and comes to rest on top of the vehicle being struck.

Oxygen Therapy — The administration of oxygen through a mask or tube in the nose to increase the amount of oxygen in the patient's blood.

P

Packaging — Readying a patient for transport.

Pantograph — A mechanical linkage device which maintains electrical contact with a contact wire and transfers power from the wire to the traction unit of electric buses, locomotives, and trams.

Passenger Side — The passenger side of a vehicle is found opposite of the steering wheel.

Patient — A person who is receiving medical care.

Patient Assessment — The process of examining a patient to determine injuries or illness.

Perimeter Control — Establishing and maintaining control of the outer edge or boundary of an incident scene.

Personal Protective Equipment (PPE) — General term for the equipment worn by firefighters and rescuers; includes helmets, coats, pants, boots, eye protection, gloves, protective hoods, self-contained breathing apparatus, and personal alert safety systems (PASS devices). Also called Bunker Clothes, Protective Clothing, Turnout Clothing, or Turnout Gear.

Personnel Accountability System — A method for identifying which emergency responders are working on an incident scene.

Personnel Carriers — Armored fighting vehicles designed to transport infantry to a battlefield.

Placard — A sign that is affixed to each side of a structure or a vehicle transporting hazardous materials to inform responders of fire hazards, life hazards, special hazards, and reactivity potential. The placard indicates the primary class of the material and, in some cases, the exact material being transported; required on containers that are 640 cubic feet (18 m³) or larger.

Plan of Operations — Clearly identified strategic goal and the tactical objectives necessary to achieve that goal. Included are assignments, authority, responsibility, and safety considerations.

Plug — Patch to seal a small leak in a container such as a vehicle's fuel tank or radiator.

Plymetal Panels — Railcar floor panels constructed of plywood sheets covered by sheets of metal, usually aluminum.

Pneumatic Chisel/Hammer — Pneumatic chisel is useful for extrication work; designed to operate at air pressures between 100 and 150 psi (700 kPa and 1 050 kPa). During periods of normal consumption, it will use about 4 to 5 cubic feet (113 L to 142 L) of air per minute. Also called Air Chisels, Pneumatic Hammers, or Impact Hammers.

Pneumatic Lifting Bag — Inflatable, envelope-type device that can be placed between the ground and an object and then inflated to lift the object. It can also be used to separate objects. Depending on the size of the bag, it may have lifting capabilities in excess of 75 tons (68 040 kg).

Pneumatic Power — Power derived by using the properties of compressed air at rest or in motion; generally used with a pressure regulator.

Pneumatic Shoring — Shores or jacks with movable parts that are operated by the action of a compressed gas.

Pneumatic Tools — Tools that receive their operating energy from compressed air.

Portable Equipment — Those items carried on the fire or rescue apparatus that are not permanently attached to or a part of the apparatus.

Portable Radio — Hand-held, self-contained transceiver radio used by personnel to communicate with each other when away from the vehicle radio. A portable radio draws upon power from its own battery and uses its case along with an antenna to make up the antenna place. Portable radios do not have much power. They generally transmit 1 to 5 watts and have limited coverage areas. Duration of battery and duty cycles depend upon their power source. *Also called Handi-Talki.*

Porta-Power — Manually operated hydraulic tool that has been adapted from the auto body business to the rescue service. This device has a variety of tool accessories that allows it to be used in numerous applications.

Position — (1) Specific assignment during a fire operation. (2) To spot an apparatus for maximum effective use.

Post-Incident Analysis — General overview and critique of the incident by members of all responding agencies (including dispatchers) that should take place within two weeks of the actual incident.

Post-Incident Stress — Psychological stress that affects emergency responders after returning from a stressful emergency incident.

Post-Traumatic Incident Debriefing — Counseling designed to minimize the effects of post-incident trauma. Also called Critical Incident Stress Debriefing.

Post-Traumatic Stress Disorder (PTSD) — A disorder caused when persons have been exposed to a traumatic event where they have experienced, witnessed, or been confronted with an event or events that involve actual death, threatened death, serious injury, or threat of physical injury to self or others. *Also called post-traumatic stress syndrome.*

Potential Energy — Stored energy possessed by an object that can be released in the future to perform work once released.

Pounds Per Square Inch (PSI) — U.S. unit for measuring pressure. Its metric equivalent is kilopascals.

Powered Hydraulic Shears — Large rescue tool whose two blades open and close by the use of hydraulic power supplied through hose from a power unit.

Powered Hydraulic Spreaders — Large rescue tool whose two arms open and close by the use of hydraulic power supplied through hose from a power unit. This device is capable of exerting in excess of 20,000 pounds (900 kg) of force at its tips. *Also called Jaws.*

Power Take-Off (PTO) — Rotating shaft that transfers power from the engine to auxiliary equipment. All farm tractors are designed to operate the PTO shaft at either 540 or 1,000 revolutions per minute.

Power Tool — Tool that acquires its power from a mechanical device such as a motor or pump.

Power Train — Includes all of the parts that create and transfer power to the surface being traversed. Sometimes called the drive train.

PPE — Abbreviation for Personal Protective Equipment.

Pre-Incident Plan — Document, developed during pre-incident planning, that contains the operational plan or set procedures for the safe and efficient handling of emergency situations at a given location (such as a specific building or occupancy). Also called Preplan.

Pre-Incident Planning — Act of preparing to handle an incident at a particular location or a particular type of incident before an incident occurs. Also called Prefire Planning, Preplanning, Prefire Inspection, or Pre-Incident Inspection.

Pressure — Force per unit area exerted by a liquid or gas measured in pounds per square inch (psi) or kilopascals (kPa).

Priority Traffic — *See* Emergency Traffic.

Proceed With Caution — Order for incoming units to discontinue responding at an emergency rate. Units should turn off warning devices and follow routine traffic regulations. Also called Reduce Speed.

Products of Combustion — Materials produced and released during burning.

Protective Clothing — Includes the helmet, protective coat, protective trousers, protective hood, boots, gloves, self-contained breathing apparatus, and eye protection where applicable. *See* Personal Protective Equipment.

Protective Coat — Coat worn during fire fighting, rescue, and extrication operations.

Protective Hood — Hood designed to protect the firefighter's ears, neck, and face from exposure to extreme heat. Hoods are typically made of Nomex®, Kevlar®, or PBI® and are available in long or short styles.

Protective Trousers — Pants worn during fire fighting operations. Also called turnout pants; bunker pants; night hitches.

Pry — To raise, move, or force with a prying tool.

Prying Tools — Hand tools that use the principle of leverage to allow the rescuer to exert more force than would be possible without the tool. These tools are characterized by their long, slender shape and are constructed of hardened steel.

PSI — Abbreviation for Pounds Per Square Inch, a measurement of pressure. In fire protection, pressure is most often dealt with in units of pounds per square inch (psi).

Public Way — Parcel of land, such as a street or sidewalk, that is essentially open to the outside and is used by the public for moving from one location to another.

Pulley — (1) Small, grooved wheel through which the halyard is drawn on an extension ladder. (2) Wheel used to transmit power by means of a band, belt, cord, rope, or chain passing over its rim. (3) Steel or aluminum rollers used to change direction and to reduce friction in rope rescue systems.

Pumping Apparatus — Fire department apparatus that has the primary responsibility to pump water.

Q

Quarter Panels — The rear sections of the vehicle's body shell which include the rear fender and the C-post.

R

Radio Channel — Band of frequencies of a width sufficient to permit its use for radio communication.

Rapid Intervention Team (RIT) — Two or more fully equipped and immediately available firefighters designated to stand by outside the hazard zone to enter and effect rescue of firefighters inside, if necessary. Also known as Rapid Intervention Crew (RIC).

Rear (Vehicle) — Opposite end of the vehicle from the front. Usually indicated by the taillights.

Rear-impact Collision — Occurs when one vehicle is struck in the rear by another vehicle or if a vehicle backs into an object.

RECEO Model — One of many models for prioritizing activities at an emergency incident: Rescue, Exposures, Confine, Extinguish, and Overhaul.

Reciprocating Saw — Electric saw that uses a short, straight blade that moves back and forth.

Regenerative Braking — A mechanical system that reduces the speed of a vehicle by converting part of the vehicle's kinetic energy into another type of energy that can be fed back into a power system or stored for future use.

Rehab — Incident Command System (ICS) term for a rehabilitation station at a fire or other incident where personnel can rest, rehydrate, and recover from the stresses of the incident.

Rehabilitation —Allowing firefighters or rescuers to rest, rehydrate, and recover during an incident.

Relief Cut — Cut made to reduce resistance and to facilitate the bending of a portion of a car or other object.

Remote Power Outlet (RPO) — An AC power receptacle mounted on or in a vehicle and powered by an inverter from the vehicle's DC electrical system

Rescue — Removing a patient from an untenable or unhealthy atmosphere.

Rescue Company — Specialized unit of people and equipment dedicated to performing rescue and extrication operations at the scene of an emergency. Also called Rescue Squad or Rescue Truck.

Rescue Officer — Officer in charge of the rescue company.

Rescue Pumper — Specially designed apparatus that combines the functions of both a rescue vehicle and a fire department pumper.

Resources — All of the immediate or supportive assistance available, or potentially available, for assignment to help control an incident including personnel, equipment, control agents, agencies, and printed emergency guides.

Response — Call to respond.

Response District — Geographical area to which a particular apparatus is assigned to be first due on a fire or other emergency incident. Also called District.

Response Time — Time between when a fire and emergency services company is dispatched and when it arrives at the scene of an emergency.

Restricted (Hot) Zone — In a rescue or extrication operation, the area where the extrication is taking place. Only personnel who are performing the extrication procedures or attending directly to the victims should be in this zone. This avoids crowding and confusion among rescuers.

RIT — *See* Rapid Intervention Team.

Risk Assessment (Evaluation) — Determining the risk level or seriousness of a risk.

Risk Management Plan — Written plan that identifies and analyses the exposure to hazards, selection of appropriate risk management techniques to handle exposures, implementation of chosen techniques, and monitoring of the results of those risk management techniques.

Roadside — Side of the trailer farthest from the curb when trailer is traveling in a normal forward direction (left-hand side); opposite to "curbside."

Rocker Panels — The usually rounded narrow body panels on each side of an automobile below the doors and between the kick panel and the quarter panel.

Rollover — Involves a vehicle rolling sideways onto its side and possibly continuing onto its top, then the opposite side.

Rollover Protection — The use of roll bars and roll cages within automobiles to protect passengers in the event of a rollover.

Roof (Vehicle) — The vehicle body component above the passengers' heads that encloses the passenger compartment.

Rotary Rescue Saw — *See* Circular Saw.

Rotational Collisions — Caused by off center front or side impacts that forcefully turn the impacted vehicle horizontally inducing a spin to one or more of the accident vehicles.

S

Safety Glass (Laminated Glass) — Special glass composed of two sheets of glass that are laminated to a sheet of plastic sandwiched between them under high temperature and pressure. Primarily used for automobile windshields and some rear windows.

Safety Glasses — *See* Safety Goggles.

Safety Goggles — Enclosed, but adequately ventilated, goggles that have impact- and shatter-resistant lens to protect the eyes from dusts, chips, and other small particles; should be OSHA approved. Also called Safety Glasses.

Safety Guidelines/Safety Plan — Rules, regulations, or policies created and/or adopted by an organization that lists steps or procedures to follow that aid in reducing if not eliminating accident or injury.

Safety Officer — Member of the ICS Command Staff responsible to the incident commander for monitoring and assessing hazardous and unsafe conditions and developing measures for assessing personnel safety on an incident. Also referred to as the Incident Safety Officer.

Safety Shoes — Protective footwear meeting OSHA requirements.

Salvage Cover — Waterproof cover made of cotton duck, plastic, or other material used by fire departments to protect unaffected furniture and building areas from heat, smoke, and water damage; a tarpaulin. Also called Tarp.

SCBA — Abbreviation for Self-Contained Breathing Apparatus.

Scene Management — Those elements of incident command that include keeping those not involved in the incident from entering unsafe areas and protecting those in potentially unsafe areas through evacuation or sheltering in place.

School Bus — As defined by U.S. Federal Motor Vehicle Safety Standards, a passenger motor vehicle designed to carry more than 10 passengers, in addition to the driver, and which the Secretary of Transportation determines is to be used for the purpose of transporting preschool, primary, and secondary school students to or from such schools or school-related events.

Scoop Stretcher — Device used to package patient for removal from a confined environment; may be placed around the patient without lifting the patient.

Screw Jacks — Long, nonhydraulic jacks that can be extended or retracted by turning a collar on a threaded shaft.

Search Assessment — Search assessment and findings performed by search personnel.

Seat Belt Pretensioners — Protective devices designed to tighten the belts as the front-impact air bags deploy.

Secondary Device — Bomb placed at the scene of an ongoing emergency response that is intended to cause casualties among responders; secondary explosive devices are designed to explode after a primary explosion or other major emergency response event has attracted large numbers of responders to the scene.

Section — Organizational level of an incident command system having functional responsibility for primary segments of incident operations such as Operations, Planning, Logistics, and Finance/Administrative. The section level is organizationally between branch and incident commander.

Secure — (1) To make fast such as secure a line to a cleat or other stationary object. (2) Close in a manner to avoid accidental opening or operation.

Self-Contained Breathing Apparatus (SCBA) — Respirator worn by the user that supplies a breathable atmosphere that is either carried in or generated by the apparatus and is independent of the ambient atmosphere. Respiratory protection is worn in all atmospheres that are considered to be Immediately Dangerous to Life and Health (IDLH). Also called Air Mask or Air Pack.

Semitrailer — Freight trailer that when attached is supported at its forward end by the fifth wheel device of the truck tractor. Occasionally used to refer to a trucking rig made up of a tractor and a semitrailer.

Service Branch — Branch within the Logistics section of an Incident Command System; responsible for service activities at an incident. Components include the communications unit, medical unit, and foods unit.

Shackle — A U-shaped metal device that is secured with a pin or bolt across the device's opening. Another type of shackle is a hinged metal loop that is secured with a quick-release locking pin mechanism.

Shelter and Thermal Control — The process of protecting patients and rescuers from inclement weather and extreme temperatures.

Shims — Wedges used in pairs to tighten up a shoring system.

Shoring — General term used for lengths of timber, screw jacks, hydraulic and pneumatic jacks, and other devices that can be used as temporary support for formwork or structural components or used to hold sheeting against trench walls. Individual supports are called shores, cross braces, and struts.

Shoring Block — Shim for a jack.

Side-impact Collision — Occur when a vehicle is struck along its side by another vehicle (also called a T-bone collision) or if the vehicle slides sideways into another object.

Side-impact Protection Systems (SIPS) — Air bag systems designed to protect passengers during side-impact collisions. May be operated mechanically or powered by the vehicle's electrical system.

Simple Triage and Rapid Treatment (START) — Triage evaluation method for checking respiratory, circulatory and neurological function with the intention of categorizing patients in one of the four care categories: Immediate, Delayed, Minor, and Dead/Non-salvageable. The START method is recommended for use by first-arriving responders for initial and secondary field triage.

SIPS — *See* Side-impact Protection Systems.

Size-Up — Ongoing mental evaluation process performed by the operational officer in charge of an incident that enables him or her to determine and evaluate all existing influencing factors that are used to develop objectives, strategy, and tactics for extrication operations before committing personnel and equipment to a course of action. Size-up results in a plan of action that may be adjusted as the situation changes. It includes such factors as time, location, nature of incident, life hazard, exposures, property involved, nature and extent of vehicle or machinery incident, weather, and extrication facilities.

SKED® — Compact device for patient removal from a confined space with spinal immobilization; may be used as a lifting device with a harness.

Sleeper — A compartment built into or behind the cab of a large truck to be used by the driver for rest and relaxation.

Sliding Fifth Wheel — Fifth-wheel assembly capable of being moved forward or backward on the truck tractor to vary load distribution on the tractor and to adjust the overall length of combination.

Society of Automotive Engineers (SAE) — Organization of engineers in the automotive industry.

Soft Tissue Injury — Damage to human tissue that encloses bones or joints, such as muscles, tendons, or ligaments

SOG — *See* Standard Operating Procedure.

SOP — *See* Standard Operating Procedure.

Space Frames — Aluminum skeletons that are similar to aircraft frames upon which the aluminum, plastic, or composite skin of the vehicle's body is attached. The internal structure of these space frames provides the structural support for the vehicle while the skin provides aerodynamics, styling, and protection from the elements.

Spinal Immobilization — Stabilizing the victim's cervical spine (neck and back) to prevent severing of the spinal cord.

Spinal Precautions — Stabilizing the victim's cervical spine (neck and back) to prevent severing of the spinal cord under the assumption, based on mechanism of injury or actual findings, that the victim has an injury.

Squad — *See* Rescue Company.

Staging Area — Prearranged, temporary strategic location, away from the emergency scene, where units assemble and wait until they are assigned a position on the emergency scene and from which these resources (personnel, apparatus, tools, and equipment) must be able to respond within three minutes of being assigned. Staging area managers report to the incident commander or operations section chief if established.

Standard Operating Guidelines (SOGs) — *See* Standard Operating Procedures.

Standard Operating Procedures (SOPs) — Standard methods or rules in which an organization or a fire department operates to carry out a routine function. Usually these procedures are written in a policies and procedures handbook and all firefighters should be well versed in their content. A SOP may specify the functional limitations of fire brigade members in performing emergency operations. Sometimes called standard operating guidelines or SOGs.

Stand By — (1) To remain immediately available. (2) To clear the airwaves for a broadcast.

Standing Block — Block, in a block and tackle system, that is attached to a solid support and from which the fall line leads.

Step Block — Piece of cribbing with a tapered end specially designed for stabilization of automobiles. Also called a step chock.

Step Chock — *See* step block.

Strategic Goals — Overall plan that will be used to control the incident. Strategic goals are broad in nature and are achieved by the completion of tactical objectives.

Strategy — Overall plan for incident attack and control established by the incident commander.

Stretcher — Portable device that allows two or more persons to move the sick or injured by carrying or rolling while keeping the patient immobile.

Striking Tools — Tools characterized by large, weighted heads on handles. This category of tools includes axes, battering rams, ram bars, punches, mallets, hammers, sledgehammers or mauls, chisels, automatic center punches, and picks.

Super Bus — School bus with an extra-large carrying capacity. These buses may carry up to 84 people seated and over 100 people if standing is permissible.

Supervisor — (1) A person who is responsible for directing the performance of other people or employees. (2) ICS term for the individual responsible for command of a Division or Group.

Supplied Air Respirator — Atmosphere-supplying respirator for which the source of breathing air is not designed to be carried by the user; not certified for fire fighting operations. Also known as an Airline Respirator.

Support Branch — Branch within the logistics section of an incident command system; responsible for providing the personnel, equipment, and supplies to support incident operations. Components include the supply unit, facilities unit, and ground support units.

Support (Cold) Zone — Area encompassing the Limited Access (Warm) Zone and restricted to emergency response personnel who are not working in either the Restricted (Hot) Zone or the Limited Access (Warm) Zone. This zone may include the portable equipment and personnel staging areas and the command post. The outer boundary of this area should be cordoned off to the public.

T

Tactical Objectives — Specific operations that must be accomplished to achieve strategic goals. Objectives must be both specific and measurable.

Tactics — Methods of employing equipment and personnel on an incident to accomplish specific tactical objectives in order to achieve established strategic goals.

Tarp — *See* Salvage Cover.

Technical Rescue — Application of special knowledge, skills and equipment to safely resolve unique and/or complex rescue situations. This term has often been used interchangeably with rope rescue; however, it can refer to other disciplines, such as trench or confined space rescue, which require advanced knowledge to perform.

Telecommunicator — Person who works in the communications center and processes information from the public and emergency responders; also referred to as a *dispatcher*.

TERC — See Transportation Emergency Rescue Committee.

Terne Coated Steel — Cold rolled sheet steel that has hot-dip coated with a lead-tin alloy. This dull gray coating provides corrosion protection from contact with petroleum fuels.

Torque — (1) Force that tends to create a rotational or twisting motion. (2) Force that produces or tends to produce a twisting or rotational action.

Touring Bus — *See* Commercial Motor Coach.

Traction — (1) Act of exerting a pulling force. (2) The friction between a wheel and the surface on which it is rolling that permits the wheel to move forward and exert a pulling force.

Traffic Control — Important function of scene management that helps to control scene access and vehicular traffic in and out of the area. This function is generally handled by law enforcement personnel.

Trailer — Highway or industrial-plant vehicle designed to be hauled/pulled by a tractor.

Transit Bus — Vehicle designed to move a large number of people over relatively short distances. Most commonly found in urban or metropolitan areas that operate a mass transit system.

Transparent Armor — Ballistic protection materials used as windows for vehicles.

Transport Canada — Similar to the USDOT, it is the agency responsible for most of the transportation policies, programs, and goals set by the Government of Canada to make sure that the national transportation system is safe, efficient, and accessible to all its users.

Transportation Area — Location where accident casualties are held after receiving medical care or triage before being transported to medical facilities.

Transportation Emergency Rescue Committee (TERC) — Formed in 1986 to serve as a competent source of guidance and information on transportation emergencies for those involved in providing emergency services. The modern organization is composed of members who share their vehicle extrication expertise by conducting schools, seminars, and competitive exercises.

Transportation Group — Group within the Incident Command System responsible for seeing that all victims are transported to the appropriate medical facility.

Treatment Group — Group within the Incident Command System responsible for triage and the initial treatment of victims.

Triage — System used for sorting and classifying accident casualties to determine the priority for medical treatment and transportation.

Triage Tagging — Method used to identify accident casualties as to extent of injury.

Truck — Self-propelled vehicle carrying its load on its wheels; primarily designed for transportation of property rather than passengers.

Truck Tractor — Powered motor vehicle designed to pull a truck trailer.

Truck Trailer — Vehicle without motor power; primarily designed for transportation of property rather than passengers and is drawn by a truck or truck tractor.

Turnout Gear — Term used to describe personal protective clothing made of fire resistant materials that includes coats, pants, and boots. Also referred to as Turnout Clothing, Turnout Boots, Turnout Coat, Turnout Pants, Turnouts, or Bunker Gear. *See also* Personal Protective Equipment.

Type A School Bus — Van conversion-type school bus with a gross vehicle-weight rating of less than 10,000 pounds (4 536 kg).

Type B School Bus — Minibus-type vehicle with a gross vehicle-weight rating in excess of 10,000 pounds (4 536 kg).

Type C School Bus — Conventional school bus vehicle with a gross vehicle-weight rating well in excess of 10,000 pounds (4 536 kg). The engine is found ahead of the cab.

Type D School Bus — Cab-forward style school bus with a gross vehicle-weight rating well in excess of 10,000 pounds (4 536 kg). The engine is found in the front, rear, or midship of the vehicle.

U

Undercarriage — The part of a vehicle that contains the chassis or frame, drive train, and the floor pan.

Underride Collision — Occurs when a striking vehicle collides with another vehicle and comes to rest under the vehicle being struck.

Unibody — See Unitized Body.

Unified Command — In the Incident Command System, a shared command role that allows all agencies with responsibility for the incident, either geographical or functional, to manage the incident by establishing a common set of incident objectives and strategies. In unified command there is a single incident command post and a single operations chief at any given time.

United States Department of Transportation (USDOT) — Federal agency that regulates the transportation of hazardous materials. Formerly known as Interstate Commerce Commission.

Unitized Body — Automobile construction (also called unibody or integral frame) construction in which a vehicle's stress bearing elements and sheet metal body parts are built together as one unit instead of attaching the vehicle's body to a frame as in body-on-frame construction.

Utility Rope — Rope to be used in any situation that requires a rope — except life safety applications. Utility ropes can be used for hoisting equipment, securing unstable objects, and cordoning off an area.

V

Vehicle Rescue Technician (VRT) — Firefighter who is specially trained and certified to perform automobile extrications.

Vehicle Stabilization — Process of providing additional support to key places between an object of entrapment (in this case, a vehicle) and the ground or other solid anchor points to prevent unwanted movement.

Velocity — Speed; the rate of motion in a given direction. It is measured in units of length per unit time such as feet per second (meters per second) and miles per hour (kilometers per hour).

Victim — A person who suffers death, injury, or loss as a result of an act, circumstance, agency, or condition.

Vital Signs — Indicators of a patient's condition that reflect temperature, pulse, respirations, and blood pressure.

Voltage — The electrical force that causes a charge (electrons) to move through a conductor. Sometimes called the electromotive force (EMF). Measured in volts (V).

Volt(s) — Basic unit(s) of electrical potential and may be abbreviated either V or E. It is the difference in potential (electromotive force) needed to create a current of one ampere through the resistance of one ohm.

W X Y Z

Warning Devices — Any audible or visual devices, such as flashing lights, sirens, horns, or bells, added to an emergency vehicle to gain the attention of drivers of other vehicles.

Warning Lights — Lights on the apparatus designed to attract the attention of other motorists.

Weapons of Mass Destruction (WMD) — Any weapon or device that is intended or has the capability to cause death or serious bodily injury to a significant number of people through the release, dissemination, or impact of one of the following means: toxic or poisonous chemicals (or their precursors), a disease organism, or radiation or radioactivity.

Webbing — Synthetic nylon, spiral weave, tubular material used for creating anchors, lashings, and for packaging patients and rescuers.

Wedge — Angle-cut piece of timber used to snug up loads, fill in voids, or change the angle of thrust.

Weld — Joint created between two metal surfaces when they are heated and the two metals run together.

Wheelbase — The distance between a vehicle's front and rear axles.

Winch — Pulling tool that consists of a length of steel chain or cable wrapped around a motor-driven drum. These are most commonly attached to the front or rear of a vehicle.

Wire Cutters — Tool with approved, insulated handles to cut wire.

Wrecker — A vehicle that is usually equipped with a small crane, winch, or tilting bed assembly, and is used to transport damaged vehicles. The size and type of the wrecker depends on the type and size of the vehicle to be moved. Also referred to as a Tow Truck.

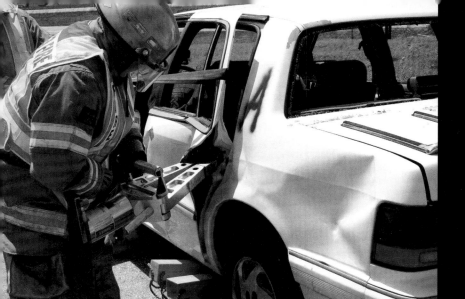

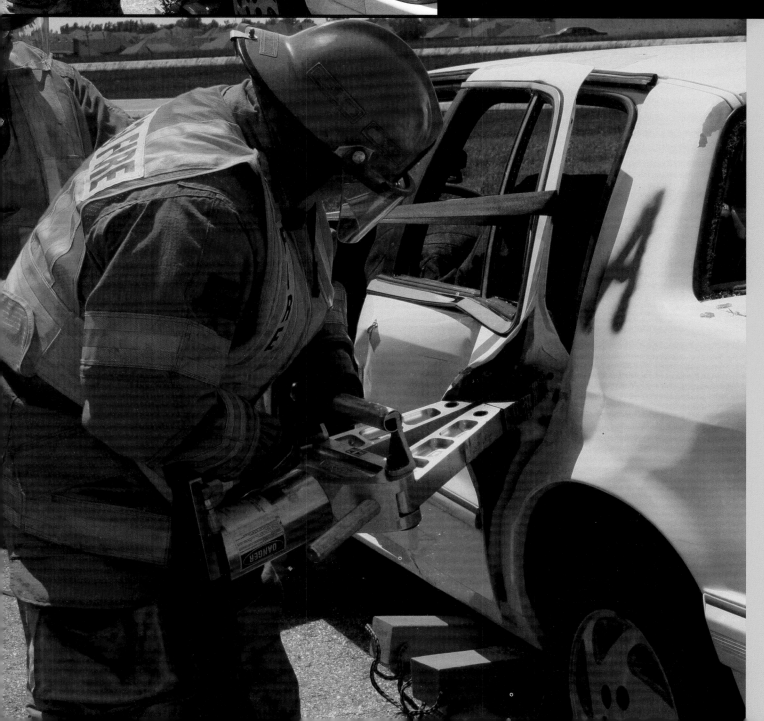

Index

Index by Nancy Kopper